D0215799

Women in Medicine

Women in Medicine
An Encyclopedia

Laura Lynn Windsor

A B C ● C L I O

Santa Barbara, California   Denver, Colorado   Oxford, England

Library of Congress Cataloging-in-Publication Data

Windsor, Laura
    Women in medicine: An encyclopedia / Laura Windsor
        p. ; cm.
Includes bibliographical references and index.
        ISBN 1–57607-392-0 (hardcover : alk. paper)
    1. Women in medicine—Encyclopedias.
        [DNLM: 1. Physicians, Women—Biography. 2. Physicians,
Women—Encyclopedias—English. 3. Health Personnel—Biography. 4.
Health Personnel—Encyclopedias—English. 5. Medicine—Biography. 6.
Medicine—Encyclopedias—English. 7. Women—Biography. 8.
Women—Encyclopedias—English. WZ 13 W766e 2002]   I. Title.

R692 .W545 2002
610' .82 ' 0922—dc21

                                                    2002014339

07 06 05 04 03 02   10 9 8 7 6 5 4 3 2 1

ABC-CLIO, Inc.
130 Cremona Drive, P.O. Box 1911
Santa Barbara, California 93116-1911

This book is printed on acid-free paper ∞.

Manufactured in the United States of America

For Mom

Contents

Women in Medicine

Contents

Contents

Contents

Foreword

In any arena there is a need for compiled data to delineate milestones, identify pathfinders and leaders, and document the progress. Laura Lynn Windsor has done just that for the issues surrounding women in the profession of medicine. This work should be of assistance to those writing or speaking on the topic of women in medicine and, while the work is comprehensive in data covered, it serves as well as a timely update on recent additions.

As the material is reviewed, it is noteworthy that while some may argue that women have achieved equity, a substantial number of the entries represent the last quarter of the twentieth century and virtually all of the entries represent barely a century of effort. Although there is work yet to be done, perhaps there is encouragement in so much already accomplished, challenged and conquered—dreamt of, then realized.

Throughout these pages, Ms. Windsor has done a nice job of identifying important mentors and the impact of previous pioneers on the subsequent generations. Although the primary role of this encyclopedia may be compilation of data for historical research purposes, there may well be those who will turn its pages and find encouragement for their own dreams—mentors not yet met who can bridge across time to encourage a young lady to reach further, dream bigger, and then just do it!

Although women who aspire to a role in medicine may be appreciative of those who came before, clearly our patients and communities have much for which to be grateful as well. From scientific discovery that changed lives to commitment to public health and well-being, women have raised standards, created new understanding, and touched lives. Ms. Windsor is to be applauded for creating an encyclopedia that includes so much humanity amidst its data and facts.

Nancy W. Dickey, M.D.

Preface and Acknowledgments

I hold it a noble task to rescue from oblivion those who deserve to be eternally remembered.

—Pliny the Younger

As a reference librarian for more than fifteen years, I was surprised to find no one-volume reference work on women in medicine. There are many out-of-print books on women and the medical profession, as well as some current, more general books on women and science, but it is certainly time to make room for a reference book focused on women in medical science. Despite often-hostile work environments, women have contributed to phenomenal progress in many fields, especially in the last half of the twentieth century. I know this volume will fill a void in my library, and I hope others find it useful as well.

This work compiles biographies of a number of women who throughout history have made a significant impact on medicine. They have demonstrated tremendous talent and insight in caring for the sick; in advancing research on numerous diseases such as cancer and AIDS; and in establishing and running hospitals, colleges, and government agencies. They contributed impressive intellectual gifts and great organizational skills to many medical specialties, serving as role models for women today who desire to become physicians in a profession still dominated by men. This encyclopedia focuses on women physicians, nurses, and researchers in particular but also includes related entries on institutions, medical terms, and social issues relevant to women in medicine.

The volume is arranged alphabetically and includes cross-references where appropriate. Each biographical entry concentrates on the woman and her accomplishments as opposed to a long litany of discrimination she faced in male-dominated institutions. It seems that the hardships faced by women along the way are well documented and do not need to be a focal point in each entry. However, specific incidents are mentioned if they had a significant impact on the woman's medical career.

I attempted to include women from outside North America and Western Europe, although information was often scant. Many of these women broke new ground and should be recognized as pioneers who forged ahead where there were no mentors or role models. Those who left positive legacies were certainly not forgotten in their own countries.

The entries "Mission Work" and "Wars and Epidemics" examine two areas where women found fewer barriers to their participation in medicine. The "Barriers to Success" entry looks at women's overall struggle to achieve in medicine, and the "Public Health and Women" entry examines a twentieth-century window of opportunity for women.

Even societies that resisted conversion to a new faith often accepted medical help from women missionaries. In some cases, cultural norms allowed only women physicians for female patients. During wartime and epidemics, women advanced medical procedures around the globe as they responded to calls for additional practitioners or served disadvantaged populations. Despite these ostensible steps forward, when the crisis was past and social norms were reinstated, women were again subject to limited opportunities.

Women of color have encountered even more obstacles in pursuing medical careers. There is a dearth of information on women of diverse ethnic backgrounds in medicine. Some valuable references do exist, among them Staupers's *No Time for Prejudice: A Story of the Integration of Negroes in Nursing in the United States* (1961); Morais's *History of the Negro in Medicine* (1969); Sammons's *Blacks in Science and Medicine* (1990); and Hine's *Black Women in America* (1993) and *Facts on File Encyclopedia of Black Women in America* (1997). The "Women of Color in Medicine" entry explores some of the obstacles faced by women of color. I hope in the years to come there will be more scholarship and information devoted to the historical significance of contributions of men and women of all races and ethnicities.

This project has reaffirmed my belief that very little information can be found on the internet for free, and the most abundant and reliable information still occurs in books, in microfilm sets that captured historical documents before they disappeared, on old opaque cards, and in print indexes that may never be converted to electronic format. However, the internet was very useful in providing access to a myriad of electronic databases upon which the scholarly world relies, such as ABC-CLIO's *Historical Abstracts* and *America: History and Life,* the Web of Science, OCLC's databases, various women's studies databases, numerous newspaper databases, university catalogs around the world, legal databases, the ERIC site, *PsychInfo, MEDLINE, CINAHL,* and *Health and Wellness Center,* to name just a few. Other helpful reference sources were *American National Biography, Dictionary of American Medical Biography, Dictionary of National Biography,* and *Dictionary of Scientific Biography,* along with standard country-specific encyclopedias such as *Who's Who* and biography databases—*BGMI, Biography Index, New York Times Obituaries Index,* and *Palmer's.*

Current literature on women in medicine is limited to the broader topic of science in general with selected women in medicine included, such as Rossiter's *Women Scientists in America: Struggles and Strategies to 1940* (1982); Kass-Simon and Farnes's *Women of Science* (1990); Sammons's *Blacks in Science and Medicine* (1990); Bailey's *American Women in Science* (1994); Shearer and Shearer's *Notable Women in the Life Sciences* (1996); McGrayne's *Nobel Prize Women in Science* (1998); Proffitt's *Notable Women Scientists* (1999); Ogilvie and Harvey's *Biographical Dictionary of Women in Science* (2000); and Haines's *International Women in Science* (2001).

Some standard sources that are now out of print but are nonetheless quite useful are Hurd-Mead's *A History of Women in Medicine from the Earliest Times to the Beginning of the Nineteenth Century* (1938), Lovejoy's *Women Doctors of the World* (1957), Morantz-Sanchez's *Sympathy and Science* (1985), and Alic's *Hypatia's Heritage* (1986). Stille's *Extraordinary Women of Medicine* (1997), Kent's *Women in Medicine* (1998), and Hunter's *Leaders in Medicine* (1999) are very good juvenile books with a select number of the more well-known women in medicine.

We do have a fair amount of material in letters written by women practitioners before 1950. Gelbart's *The King's Midwife: A History and Mystery of Madame du Coudray* (1998); Morantz-Sanchez's *Conduct Unbecoming a Woman: Medicine on Trial in Turn-of-the-Century Brooklyn* (1999), which chronicles the life of Mary Amanda Dixon Jones; and Comfort's *The Tangled Field: Barbara McClintock's Search for the Patterns of Genetic Control* (2001) are three examples of excellent current biographies.

A number of biographies are very good, but many are out of print. There is an obvious reason for the lack of biographies and autobiographies on women. Men who contributed to the medical field normally had faculty status at universities with a bit of time to write about their accomplishments and personal life; these biographies have been very valuable to those of us interested in the history of medicine. Most women in medicine, however, have not had the leisure to write memoirs. With few exceptions prior to the twentieth century, many were not allowed to have their own laboratories or any academic rank, and even today most women nurses, physicians, and other health care workers are too busy working a long day and then, in many instances, caring for a family.

Acknowledgments

Acknowledging all of the libraries around the world that assisted with this project would take numerous pages. Many of the entries would not have been possible without the help of librarians in the United States who supplied interlibrary loan materials and librarians in other countries who forwarded information from local publications.

I'd like to express my deepest appreciation to these and other people who work in libraries.

I know that many writers acknowledge the phenomenal progress librarians have made as a profession. As a librarian, I know how hard it has been to achieve this progress. Catalogers are the heart of the library system. I found things I never knew existed by simply using the library catalog. Everyone who works to process and keep items in order, whether they are books, microfilm boxes, photos, or journals, saves patrons a tremendous amount of time in accessing the libraries' treasures. Subject-specialist librarians who can put their hands on information without looking in any catalog or index are invaluable. Patrons over the years who have challenged me with hard questions have helped make me a better librarian, able to find sources that didn't come to mind right away. I hope librarians keep working as hard as they do to make resources like this one possible.

Laura Lynn Windsor

Introduction

Nature has given women so much power that the law has very wisely given them little.

—Samuel Johnson, 1892

Women as Natural Healers

From the earliest of times, women have been the natural nurturers, healers, and soothers of those in pain. Taking care of husbands, parents, children, or friends, they have been the tirelessly caring individuals, often charged by men to heal the sick in the home. It was only natural that they eventually desired more medical knowledge in order to do more, be more, and feel more confident in their endeavors.

In ancient times midwives were the norm, and for centuries distances between birthing mothers and a traditional health care institution were far too great to even consider another health care provider. This situation changed very slowly; even today, the majority of the world's population live in rural areas. Only in the eighteenth century, when physicians began to feel threatened by midwives, did laws requiring licenses and the regulation of midwives' activities become a reality.

With these requirements came women's realization that they could advance beyond the restrictions with a better education. They encountered many problems with obtaining the education they were suddenly required to have, but they persevered.

Women's Leadership Abilities

Those of us who look at the history of women in medicine see that women have also been demonstrating leadership abilities for centuries. King Louis XV respected Angelique du Coudray enough to commission her in 1759 to train midwives all over France, Florence Nightingale organized medical staff in order to treat soldiers on the battlefields of Scutari during the Crimean War, and Elsie Inglis organized and ran the Scottish Women's Hospitals in World War I.

Many of the women in this volume attained leadership abilities through dealing with the challenges of their profession. Nancy Dickey, the first female president of the AMA; Antonia Novello, who became the first female surgeon general of the United States; and Gro Harlem Brundtband, who is the first woman to head the World Health Organization (WHO), are outstanding examples of what women have come to achieve.

Social and Economic Forces Affecting Women's Careers

From the earliest times to the present, forces besides gender have played a part in women's long struggle to succeed. In relatively recent times, increased awareness of social problems and public health—an awareness in large part brought about by women in the medical field—have created opportunities for women to work in their chosen professions.

As industrialists built factories that transformed working conditions, crime, poverty, pollution, and disease grew with the further expansion of large urban areas. Social-settlement houses such as Toynbee Hall in London, Hull House in Chicago, and the Henry Street settlement in New York City were the beginnings of social activism by both men and women. Women physicians and nurses such as Alice Hamilton and Lillian Wald saw the tremendous needs of the poor and put their training, care, and concern into action. Wald, who founded the Henry Street Settlement, also formed the Visiting Nurses Service in New York City, which served as a model for many other cities. Both Hamilton and Wald believed that each person had a right to adequate nutrition, housing, and working conditions. Like many other women who had gained a medical education, they utilized their skills to serve the poor and make cities better places for the growing urban population. "Women volunteers saved the American city at the turn of the twentieth century by converting religious doctrine and domestic ideology into redemptive places that produced social order at a critical moment in the nation's development" (Spain 2001, 237).

Influenced by Jane Addams, one of the founders of Hull House in Chicago, Hamilton became a resident at Hull House for many years, tending to individuals as a nurse, physician, baby-sitter, housekeeper, and teacher. She witnessed firsthand the health problems created by industry and authored some of the first reports on the unsatisfactory working conditions for men, women, and children in factories. She lobbied for occupational health and safety. With the sweeping social-settlement movement, many "educated middle-class women who joined the movement were given a chance to move beyond the traditional confines of the home and to enter the working world in positions of leadership, achieving a level of equality with their male colleagues" (Barbuto 1999, ix).

Even by the early twentieth century, the medical community was still hesitant to hire women physicians at hospitals and clinics no matter how good their training was. As the government became involved in social services, regional and national public health organizations created jobs for women. Many women, such as Sara Josephine Baker, found their calling in the public health sector.

As women moved into the workforce, they became empowered. They wanted the option of working outside the home with equal pay and the right to vote. They organized to gain a voice in a changing world. They formed clubs, societies, and regional and national organizations to advance women's status and to meet the need for social services. Religious groups also played a role in working to help the homeless and poor.

Since so many of the early female physicians were relegated to working with the poor, they saw firsthand the abuse many industrial workers, especially women and children, experienced. Their work to increase awareness led to labor unions that worked for reforms in the length of the workday, restrictions on child labor, and better working conditions.

Changing economies worked both for and against women in the workplace. The dual-income family began to seem desirable in order to bring about better living conditions. However, many felt women were taking jobs away from men, especially during the Depression in the United States. The work women did during the war years as physicians and nurses did not carry over to peacetime. They came home to their countries and were not offered work.

In 1932 in the United States, the National Economy Act limited federal civil service to one member of the family. Thus many women had to leave government jobs. In Great Britain, the National Insurance Act reduced women's roles in the workplace. William Beveridge, the British economist, "was aware of the value of married women's unpaid work, and wives and husbands were treated differently under the National Insurance Act of 1946. Single women were treated like men, but married women were normally exempted from the work related provisions and insured as housewives" (Siim 2000, 93). Women physicians, despite their education and skill, had to play minimal roles when it came to working for a wage.

The birth-control movement also had a large impact on women. As public health nurses such as Margaret Sanger saw the toll frequent childbirth was taking on mothers, they begin to feel that more information about sex education and contraception was needed. They fought on through numerous roadblocks in the way of legislation and societal resistance. The Comstock Act of 1873 was a major setback for health care providers wishing to provide birth control in the United States, and birth control wasn't even discussed in medical schools until 1937. "In 1928, the timing of ovulation was established medically, but the safe interval for intercourse was mistakenly understood to include half the menstrual period" (CDC 2000, 326). By 1933, however, family size had declined in the United States. When more women were able to learn about methods for limiting childbirth, they realized a career was a viable option for them even if they had chosen to marry and have a family.

The Unrecognized Heroes—Men
An encyclopedia on women and medicine would not be complete without a word about the many men who have taken risks to mentor women whose potential was evident and to encourage spouses, daughters, students, and colleagues to pursue what many of their friends felt was a waste of time. Society owes a debt to men such as Samuel Blackwell, who felt his daughters should have the same good education as his sons; Dr. William Osler, who encouraged Maude Abbott even after she was relegated to a museum of defective hearts following the denial of a faculty position; and Dr. Alan Whipple, who encouraged Virginia Apgar to go into anesthesiology instead of surgery. Such men exercised a great deal of foresight and genuine concern.

Even male medical students had to adapt to situations that were uncomfortable. Unlike in many other professions infiltrated by women, males in medical education had to deal with sharing with women discussions and demonstrations on topics considered taboo in mixed company: anatomy, reproduction, sex. Some objected to the presence of women in their institutions, but others were accepting, particularly in Europe, where many women sought additional training after obtaining their degrees elsewhere. Emily Blackwell, Eva Salber, and Mary Putnam Jacobi are just a few of the women who sought more clinical training after their initial medical degree. They were able to gain that experience in Europe.

Even if most men were unwilling to take on the role of caregiver for their children, it is important to remember that many women did not accept men as adequate in that role. "Not until the founding of the National Organization for Women in 1966 did a major group contend that men and women should share responsibility for paid work, child rearing, and housework" (Burstein and Bricher 1997, 161). Acceptance of men as caregivers required an adjustment by both men and women.

More men have recognized the importance of a woman's role as wife, mother, and wage earner as living expenses have increased (Gabor 1995, 46). More are accepting of shared parental responsibilities. In many countries, government, educational, and corporate organizations are addressing the importance of adequate childcare.

Women Extraordinaire
The social, cultural, and legal problems women encountered in obtaining higher education and medical training have been well documented over the past several decades. Many had to obtain a medical education outside their own country and learn in totally inadequate facilities and on the battlefield. Elizabeth and Emily Blackwell and many other early physicians served the poor and homeless because no one believed a woman could do the job of a physician. Many early women physicians were relegated to nursing because no one would hire them. May Edward Chinn performed biopsies in secret in order to help diagnose tumors, and Mary Mahoney became a private-duty nurse because hospitals would not hire black nurses in the 1870s.

These and other women who preceded and followed them found opportunities to contribute. Some, such as Elizabeth Garrett Anderson and Elizabeth Blackwell, worked within traditional arenas to further their education and obtain their objectives. Others, such as Sophia Jex-Blake, fought the general injustice they accurately perceived or went to extremes: James Barry impersonated a man for an entire lifetime in order to practice her skills.

Over the years, nurses have soothed, washed, fed, visited, and cared for numerous individual patients in a day. Today, they are expected to have the highest standards and certifications. From the late nineteenth and early twentieth centuries, they have risen from basic helpers to well-educated professionals, thanks to the work of the early pioneers in nursing education. Lillian Wald and Annie Goodrich were exceptional professionals who raised public awareness and the status of nurses.

Female physicians, nurses, and researchers are like other professionals in that they teach along the way whether or not teaching was their initial objective. Those who see a need within the profession and have the organizational and administrative skills take on a primary role as educator. Elizabeth Blackwell founded a hospital and medical college so that other women physicians could gain clinical experience. Ann Preston, Emeline Cleveland, and Margaret Craighill all contributed substantially to women's medical education. Women desperately needed additional opportunities during the past two centuries because it was very difficult or impossible for them to gain admission to male colleges, nurses were subject to higher expectations and needed more rigorous training, and, most important, women needed the collective voice that could be realized only if they were a part of higher education and related professional organizations.

Both male and female medical missionaries are one of the most overlooked groups of physicians. These missionaries were bold and dedicated. Once educated, they worked with limited medical facilities but in many instances obtained great success. Ida Scudder founded the Vellore Hospital and Medical College, Catharine Mabie educated natives in the Congo on the importance of good hygiene, and Anna Dengal was tireless in treating the poor in India. Society owes an immeasurable debt to the women nurses, researchers, educators, and physicians in this volume. Frances Kelsey's refusal to allow thalidomide on the drug market, Alice Hamilton's copious statistics on workers suffering from industrial pollution, and Dame Annie Jean Macnamara's search

for another strain of polio all led to better health and a better society.

Virginia Apgar's score system for infants has been in use for nearly fifty years. Maude Abbott became the leading expert on congenital heart disease during her lifetime. Elsie Inglis and her fellow women physicians traveled around war-torn Europe to mend the wounded during World War I. Adelaide Hautval treated sick Jewish women in Nazi concentration camps. He Manqiu used sticks and dirt because she didn't have pencil and paper and found her laboratory cadaver in the field during the Red Army's long march in 1935. All these women had heart, determination, character, and a desire to heal the sick.

References: Barbuto, Domenica M., *American Settlement Houses and Progressive Social Reform: An Encyclopedia of the American Settlement Movement*, Phoenix, AZ: Oryx Press (1999); Burstein, Paul, and Marie Bricher, "Problem Definition and Public Policy: Congressional Committees Confront Work, Family, and Gender, 1945–1990," *Social Forces* 76:1 (September 1997): 135–168; Centers for Disease Control (CDC), "Achievements in Public Health, 1900–1999: Family Planning, *JAMA* 283, no. 3 (19 January 2000): 326ff.; Gabor, Andrea, "Married, with Househusband," *Working Woman* 20:11 (November 1995): 46–50; Johnson, Samuel, *The Letters of Samuel Johnson, with Mrs. Thrale's Genuine Letters to Him*, vol. 1, no. 157, Oxford: Clarendon Press (1952); Lorber, Judith, "Why Women Physicians Will Never Be True Equals in the American Medical Profession," in Elianne Riska and Katarina Wegar, eds., *Gender, Work, and Medicine: Women and the Medical Division of Labour*, London: Sage (1993); Siim, Birte, *Gender and Citizenship: Politics and Agency in France, Britain, and Denmark*, New York: Cambridge University Press (2000); Spain, Daphne, *How Women Saved the City*, Minneapolis: University of Minnesota Press (2001); Yedidia, Michael J., and Janet Bickel, "Why Aren't There More Women Leaders in Academic Medicine? The Views of Clinical Department Chairs," *Academic Medicine* 76, no. 5 (May 2001): 453–465.

A

Abbott, Maude Elizabeth Seymour
1869–1940

Despite a private and public fight, Maude Abbott was not allowed to attend McGill University for medical study because of her gender. Nevertheless, she became one of the earliest experts in congenital heart disease, paving the way for future women medical professionals in Canada.

She was born on March 18, 1869, at St. Andrews, near Montreal. Her father left the family before Maude was born, and her mother died from tuberculosis just seven months after the birth. Maude's grandmother adopted and raised her and her sister, Alice.

Her grandmother was of strong character and had been through much grief. She had lost all nine of her children early in their lives, eight to tuberculosis. Her husband also predeceased her by several years. She educated the girls at home during most of their early years; Maude had a great desire to attend school with other girls and a burning need to learn, which was fulfilled when she attended high school.

Maude enrolled in McGill University on a scholarship and graduated with a B.A. in 1890. By this time, she knew that she wanted to be a physician, but McGill refused to allow a woman to enter its medical program. She fought this decision with letters to the faculty and even in public, but to no avail. She settled on going to nearby Bishop's College. Many students, as well as some professors, resented a woman in their ranks, and

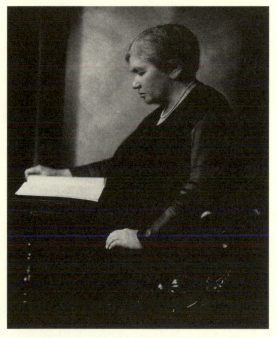

Maude Elizabeth Seymour Abbott (U.S. National Library of Medicine)

her willingness to work so hard was an irritation to some. Fellow students sometimes hid her case reports, and many students even applauded when professors announced they had to attend meetings on keeping women out of the college. However, she looked back with great appreciation on her days at Bishop, where she won the senior anatomy prize and the chancellor's prize for her excellent work on the final examination and where she obtained her M.D.

Upon graduation in 1894, she traveled abroad to work in various clinics in Vienna, Zurich, Edinburgh, and London, where she worked with established physicians who came to appreciate her work. At this time, her ambition was to return to Montreal and obtain a faculty position at McGill.

Abbott's first duties when she returned to Montreal were in the Royal Victoria Hospital. It was here that she began research in cardiology and pathology with Dr. Charles Martin and Dr. J. G. Adami, respectively. Soon thereafter, one of the most influential men in her life, Dr. William Osler, encouraged her to reorganize the pathology museum at McGill. This endeavor led to immense advancement in the medical knowledge of the heart.

Much of the pathology museum was made up of postmortem specimens, many of which showed signs of cardiac defects. Abbott studied the various hearts and their defects and wrote a piece for Osler on congenital heart disease. In this work, she specified cyanotic and acyanotic categories, then a useful distinction.

At the same time, she began to be very involved in the overall operation of the museum and in promoting the use of cadavers in anatomy classes in medical schools. She created the International Association of Medical Museums (now called the International Academy of Pathology), an organization she remained active in for the next thirty years.

In 1919 Abbott underwent successful surgery for an ovarian tumor. While continuing her work at the museum during World War I, she took on the responsibility of editing the *Canadian Medical Association Journal*. After Osler's death in 1919 she began the monumental project of compiling a memorial bulletin of the International Association of Medical Museums. That famous work, *Bulletin No. IX*, eventually became known as the Osler Memorial Volume, a very well-received book of over 600 pages that took six years to complete and contributed to the knowledge of heart disease.

She was now gaining respect for her scientific knowledge and diligence. She was offered a position at the University of Texas as an acting professor of pathology during World War I and as an associate professor thereafter. However, she remained in Canada, as her loyalty was always with McGill.

Abbott earned only a small income in her position at the museum and still longed for a faculty position. It wasn't to come until she received an honorary L.L.D. from McGill in 1936. In the meantime, she had done enough research to begin her monumental work, the *Atlas of Congenital Cardiac Disease*.

Abbott's *Atlas*, just over sixty pages, included excellent plates labeled clearly, a comprehensive index, diagrams interspersed throughout the work, explanations of various heart problems, and acknowledgments of all who had contributed to the project. She had accumulated much of the knowledge for this project through diagnosing heart specimens at the request of clinicians all over the continent who recognized her as the world authority on congenital heart disease. Although Abbott tried to retain her faculty position beyond retirement age, McGill forced her to retire in 1936. Subsequently, her reputation in the medical community now secure, she lectured around the country. She received numerous awards and accommodations during her lifetime, including being named a fellow of the New York Academy of Medicine.

Abbott's deep interest besides pathology was medical history. She wrote on the history of nursing, the history of medicine in Quebec, and the history of the medical faculty at McGill. Abbott never married. After her grandmother died in 1890, her only family was her sister, Alice, who depended on Maude for financial support. In 1898, Alice came down with diphtheria and lost much of her mental capacity. Maude, typically unselfish in all her relationships, tried in various ways to help her sister, but despite her efforts and an operation, Alice never recovered. Maude continued to care for her sister, planning outings when Alice was doing well. They both lived in St. Andrews all of their lives.

Maude tended to be accident-prone. Although she had worn glasses since she was a young girl, many of her close friends felt her accidents were due to the fact that she was very nearsighted and tended to walk with her head down. In Montreal, she collided with an automobile and two streetcars. In New York City, she was hit by a taxi. None of these accidents, however, caused her serious harm. Abbott died on September 2, 1940, from a cerebral hemorrhage. She propelled the field of cardiology from the pathology table toward actual treatment for the living.

References: Abbott, Maude E., *Atlas of Congenital Cardiac Disease*, New York: American Heart Association (1936); MacDermot, Hugh Ernest, *Maude Abbott: A Memoir*, Toronto: Macmillan (1941); Roland, Charles G., "Maude Abbott, MD, 'Madonna of the Heart,'" *Medical and Pediatric Oncology* 35, no. 1 (July 2000): 64–65.

Abouchdid, Edma
1909–1992

Edma Abouchdid was the first woman in Lebanon to obtain a medical degree. She founded the Lebanese Medical Feminine Association and was active in family planning.

Abouchdid was born in São Paulo, Brazil. She wanted to be a doctor at the age of fifteen. Because girls at that time did not usually seek higher education, she had to convince her father, also a school principal, that she should not follow the usual course of waiting for the appropriate suitor.

Abouchdid graduated from the American University in Beirut in medicine in 1931. She was the first Lebanese woman to do so. From 1936 to 1945 she worked at the Royal Hospital in Baghdad. From 1945 to 1948 she traveled to the United States to do graduate work at Johns Hopkins, Duke, and Columbia. When she returned to her homeland, she joined the faculty of the American University in Beirut as professor of clinical gynecology and obstetrics.

There, she founded an infertility clinic as well as the Lebanese Medical Feminine Association. She received numerous awards, most notably the Medal of the Equestrian Order of Saint Sepulchre of Jerusalem for chivalry, which had been reserved for male recipients. She served on many national and international committees and in 1969 founded the Lebanese Family Planning Association.

Abouchdid lived during a time of tremendous change in Lebanon. Massive human losses during the Balkan Wars and World War I pushed women into occupations that had traditionally been dominated by men in Abouchdid's region. During the two world wars, women physicians with the American Women's Hospital Service as well as with other Foreign Service initiatives worked in Lebanon. Abouchdid attended a conference in New York in 1953 and expressed gratitude for the many American women physicians who had spent time in Lebanon working and encouraging others who wanted to enter the profession. She died of heart failure on October 11, 1992.

References: Jurdak, Hania, "The Late Adma Abu Shdeed: AUB's First Woman Doctor," *AUB Bulletin* 35, no. 2 (March 1993): 12–13; Lovejoy, Esther Pohl, *Women Doctors of the World*, New York: Macmillan (1957); *Who's Who in Lebanon 1988–89*, Beirut: Publitec (1988).

Acosta Sison, Honoria
1888–1970

The first female physician in the Philippines, Honoria Acosta Sison was a specialist in obstetrics and gynecology at the University of the Philippines. She educated many in pelvimetry for Filipina women and introduced low cesarean section to the Philippines.

She was born on December 30, 1888, in Calasiao, Pangasinan. Her mother's death when she was only two years old resulted in her being raised by her father and grandparents in Dagupan. She attended Santissimo Rosario Convent in Lingayen for a brief period before attending a normal school run by Americans. She was one of only 10 students out of 375 who passed the government examination upon completing high school. Thus she was sent to the United States for further study in 1904. She went to Philadelphia to attend Drexel Institute and Brown Preparatory School before entering the Women's Medical College of Pennsylvania and graduating in 1909 with her M.D.

There, she worked for a year in the maternity hospital before returning to the Philippines to work.

In the Philippines, she worked as an assistant in obstetrics at St. Paul's Hospital before obtaining a position at the University of the Philippines in the department of obstetrics and gynecology. Women were not well accepted in the field at this time, but Acosta Sison persevered and eventually, in 1942, earned the rank of professor and head of the department. (Her husband, Antonio Sison, served as dean of the College of Medicine and director of the Philippine General Hospital.) Like many women physicians, she managed the duties of career, wife, and mother. Two of her three children also became physicians.

Acosta Sison published extensively in the field of obstetrics and gynecology and received many honors over the years, including a presidential medal for medical research. Ten years after her death in 1970, the Philippines issued a stamp in her honor.

References: Agris, Joseph, "Honoria Acosta Sison: Pioneer Gynecologist and Obstetrician," *Journal of Dermatologic Surgery and Oncology* 6, no. 3 (March 1980): 178; Kyle, Robert A., et al., "Honoria Acosta-Sison," *JAMA* 246, no. 11 (11 September 1981): 1191; Lovejoy, Esther Pohl, *Women Doctors of the World*, New York: Macmillan (1957).

Alexander, Hattie Elizabeth
1901–1968

Hattie Alexander was a pediatrician and microbiologist who contributed to lowering the number of infant deaths from influenzal meningitis. She was also one of the first researchers to discover that bacteria can be resistant to antibiotics and thus contributed to the theory that DNA held the key to many diseases.

Alexander was born on April 5, 1901, in Baltimore, Maryland, to William Bain Alexander and Elsie May Townsend. She was only an average student while attending Western High School in Baltimore but went on to attend Goucher College in Tow-son, Maryland. Alexander seemed much more interested in sports than studies while there but did study bacteriology and physiology and graduated with an A.B. degree in 1923. Her degree enabled her to obtain a job with the U.S. Public Health Service as a bacteriologist. Three years later she worked with the Maryland Public Health Service. The experience gained in these two jobs prompted her to apply for admission to medical school at Johns Hopkins. There, more mature and focused, she was an excellent student, obtaining her M.D. degree in 1930.

Her first internship was in pediatrics at Johns Hopkins Hospital. The second was at Babies Hospital, which was part of Columbia-Presbyterian Medical Center. During these internships she witnessed the devastating effects of bacterial meningitis, which seemed to afflict so many infants and was at the time fatal.

In searching for a better treatment for influenzal meningitis, a common form of bacterial meningitis, Alexander began to build on a successful antipneumonia serum developed at the Rockefeller Institute by Kenneth Goodner and Frank Horsfall Jr. By the 1940s the mortality rate for bacterial meningitis had dropped significantly in the United States. She continued her work, experimenting with combinations of antiserums, sulfa drugs, and eventually antibiotics, finding a cocktail that nearly eliminated fatalities.

Alexander was one of the first to discover that some strains of bacteria seemed resistant to treatment. With this realization, she focused on the genetic makeup of bacteria and its importance in understanding resistance to antibiotics. Her findings also strengthened the theory that DNA held the key to so many diseases. Later she turned her attention to viruses, particularly the poliovirus and its RNA, and assisted others at Columbia in this research.

Alexander published numerous papers and received much recognition over the years. She was the first woman to be elected president of the American Pediatric Society. Her skepticism as a teacher, along with her stern, formal manner and insistence on accuracy, challenged residents and students alike. Dr. Alexander underwent a radical mastectomy late in life and later died from liver cancer on June 24, 1968, in New York City.

References: *American National Biography,* New York: Oxford University Press (1999); Christy, Nicholas P., "Hattie E. Alexander 1901–1968," *Journal of the College of Physicians and Surgeons of Columbia University* (online journal) 17, no. 2 (Spring 1997), http://cpmcnet.columbia.edu/newsjournal/archives/jour_v17n2_0002.html (accessed May 19, 2002); McIntosh, Rustin, "Hattie Alexander," *Pediatrics* 42, no. 3 (September 1968): 544.

Ali, Safieh
ca. 1900–?

Very little is known about Safieh Ali. She was born in Turkey, educated in Germany, and was the first female doctor in her country. Although Ali was unable to receive medical training in Turkey because women were not allowed in medical school at the time she pursued her training, she apparently was one of the first women to benefit from the Turkish reforms of the 1920s and 1930s to stimulate economic growth. Improving women's education played a part in this program. Soon after the reforms in the country started, the medical school at the University of Istanbul allowed women to enter.

In 1924, Ali attended the 1924 London Conference of the Medical Women's International Association. As the first female physician from Turkey, she attracted much attention from the press and from very well-known women physicians of the time who also attended the conference.

References: Lovejoy, Esther Pohl, *Women Doctors of the World,* New York: Macmillan (1957); "Medical Women's International Association," *London Times* (15 July 1924): 17f.

Alvord, Lori Arviso
1959–

The first Navajo female surgeon, Lori Alvord was born as Janette Lorraine Cupp in Tacoma, Washington. Her young mother and father raised her and her two younger sisters on a Navajo reservation in New Mexico. They lived in poverty with most in the community speaking only their native tongue. Lori felt she didn't quite belong because her mother was white and her father was a full-blooded Navajo.

She did well in high school and wanted to attend college:

> My college plans were modest; I assumed I would attend a nearby state school. But then I happened to meet another Navajo student who was attending Princeton. I had heard of Princeton but had no idea where it was. I asked him how many Indians were there. He replied, "Five." I couldn't even imagine a place with only five Indians, since our town was 98 percent Indian. Then he mentioned Dartmouth, which had about fifty Indians on campus, and I felt a little better. Ivy League was a term I had heard, but I had no concept of its meaning. No one from my high school had ever attended an Ivy League college. At my request, my high school counselor gave me the applications for all the Ivy League schools, but I only completed Dartmouth's because I knew there were fifty Indians there. (Alvord 1999, 26)

She was accepted at Dartmouth and graduated cum laude in 1979. After looking for work in New Mexico, she decided to pursue her fascination with the human body. She attended Stanford and obtained her medical degree in 1985. She then went to New Mexico and served Native Americans as a physician and surgeon at the Gallup Indian Medical Center.

Alvord is currently a professor of surgery and the associate dean for student and minority affairs at Dartmouth's Medical

School. As an educator and physician, she strives to incorporate Navajo ways of healing into Western medicine, believing that caring, culture, and tradition have a place in the healing process. "As a physician, teacher, and mother, she hopes to weave together two worlds that have so much to offer each other" (Mangan 1999, A12).

She married Jon Alvord and changed her name to her grandmother's maiden name of Arviso, thus becoming Lori Arviso Alvord. She has two children.

References: Alvord, Lori Arviso, "Navajo Surgeon Combines Approaches," *Health Progress* 80, no. 1 (January–February 1999): 26; Alvord, Lori Arviso, and Elizabeth Cohen Van Pelt, *The Scalpel and the Silver Bear,* New York: Bantam Books (1999); Mangan, Katherine S., "Enlisting the Spirit in Medical Treatment," *Chronicle of Higher Education* 45, no. 42 (25 June 1999): A12.

American Medical Women's Association
1915–

The American Medical Women's Association (AMWA; known as the MWNA, Medical Women's National Association, until 1937) was founded in 1915. Even though the American Medical Association seated its first woman in the same year, many women physicians felt that a male-dominated organization would not address their concerns. They established the AMWA to share these mutual concerns and to learn from one another. Also, since many women physicians of the time worked in isolation, the organization would serve to draw women doctors into the larger medical community and to give them a voice in this community. Bertha Van Hoosen was the AMWA's first president. The organization did not include minorities and medical students until after 1940.

In June 1917, the AMWA formed the War Service Committee, which operated as the American Women's Hospital Service. Although the War Department refused the or-

ganization's request to allow women physicians, the American Red Cross did accept the offer of assistance. Thus the AMWA's involvement in caring for civilian casualties of war abroad became indispensable.

Women missionaries and others working abroad in the aftermath of World War I alerted the organization to the enormous need for physicians in many parts of the world. The AMWA's physicians traveled abroad and set up clinics and hospitals, many in cooperation with U.S. agencies and with foreign aid agencies overburdened with providing medical care to those in need.

During the Great Depression in the early 1930s, the AMWA helped with caring for the sick and underfed in the United States. It also set up care units for hurricane victims in Florida and health care, including education, for pregnant women in rural areas of the Carolinas, Tennessee, Kentucky, and Virginia. Many qualified male physicians joined it in these efforts.

In 1940 the AMWA tried once again to gain commissions for female physicians, but neither the AMA nor the army and navy surgeon general supported the change. In 1943, the demand for physicians was so overwhelming because of World War II that objections were withdrawn. Dr. Margaret Craighill was the first woman to receive a commission. She joined the Army Medical Corps as a major on April 16.

Today, the AMWA focuses on varied issues ranging from funding for female medical students to public health care in rural areas. It continues to play a major role in promoting women as physicians worldwide.

See also: American Women's Hospitals; Craighill, Margaret D.; Van Hoosen, Bertha **References:** Lovejoy, Esther Pohl, *Women Physicians and Surgeons: National and International Organizations,* Livingston, NY: Livingston Press (1939); More, Ellen Singer, *Restoring the Balance: Women Physicians and the Profession of Medicine, 1850–1995,* Cambridge, MA: Harvard University Press (1999).

American Women's Hospitals
1917–

Created by the American Medical Women's Association in 1917, American Women's Hospitals (AWH) provided care for numerous wounded civilians and soldiers during World War I. Women physicians concerned about the overwhelming casualties sustained by the United States and its allies now had a way to contribute to care for the sick and wounded on the battlefront.

Despite the organization's early financial challenges, over 1,000 women physicians registered for service before the end of the year. With help from the American Committee for Devastated France, the AWH established its first hospital on July 28, 1918, in the village of Neufmoutiers, Seine-et-Marne. The hospital treated both civilians and soldiers. Well after the war, hospitals and their staffs were still desperately needed in some parts of the world to cope with widespread disease.

In 1923, Greece experienced a crisis as refugees with typhus and smallpox poured into the country. Greece asked for help from the AWH, which set up a quarantine station and delousing plant on Macronissi Island near the coast of Greece. There, the AWH treated over 10,000 refugees. The organization is currently associated with the American Medical Women's Association and operates nine clinics in the United States and abroad.

References: Lovejoy, Esther Pohl, *Women Physicians and Surgeons: National and International Organizations*, Livingston, NY: Livingston Press (1939).

Andersen, Dorothy Hansine
1901–1963

Dorothy Andersen identified cystic fibrosis as a disease in 1935. After completing an internship in surgery in Rochester, New York, at Strong Memorial Hospital, she was unable to obtain a residency in her preferred field, surgery and pathology. Thus her discovery was the result of being forced because of her gender to turn her attention to medical research.

Born in Asheville, North Carolina, on May 15, 1901, Andersen was an only child. Her father, Hans Peter Andersen, worked for the YMCA and died when she was thirteen. Her mother, Mary Louise (Mason) Andersen, died in 1920. By this time the family had moved to Johnsbury, Vermont, where Dorothy attended St. Johnsbury Academy. Dorothy worked her way through Mount Holyoke College and upon graduation started medical school at Johns Hopkins School of Medicine. She received her M.D. in 1926.

Andersen taught for a year after graduation at the Rochester School of Medicine and then interned in surgery at Strong Memorial Hospital. Unable to find employment as a physician, she obtained a position at Columbia University's College of Physicians and Surgeons as an assistant in pathology. She later began a doctoral program and received her doctor of medical science degree in endocrinology.

In 1938 she published her research on cystic fibrosis, and this achievement launched her into research related to this disease for the next twenty-five years. In order to pursue this path, she obtained additional training in pediatrics and chemistry, and obtained her doctorate in medical science from Columbia University in 1935. Andersen served Babies Hospital at the Columbia-Presbyterian Medical Center as both a pathologist and a pediatrician. She also contributed during her career to the field of cardiac abnormalities and embryology. She was asked to teach cardiology during World War II, when physicians were becoming interested in open-heart surgery.

A determined and dedicated physician, Andersen sometimes irritated others by intruding in areas where she was not an expert. She was also seen as a bit sloppy in appearance and was a chain smoker who rarely bothered to tap the ashes off her cigarettes. Her sense of humor and hard work were, however, appreciated by many who knew her.

Andersen never married. She underwent surgery for lung cancer in 1962 and died from the disease on March 3, 1963. She is best remembered for her work on cystic fibrosis.

References: Damrosch, Douglas S., "Dorothy Hansine Andersen," *Journal of Pediatrics* 65, no. 4 (October 1964): 477–479; McMurray, Emily J. *Notable Twentieth-Century Scientists*, Detroit: Gale (1995).

Anderson, Charlotte Morrison
1915–

Charlotte Anderson was an Australian physician and a pioneer in pediatric gastroenterology. With the publication of *Paediatric Gastroenterology* in 1975, she established herself as a leading authority in the field.

Anderson was born on March 12, 1915. She received her early education at Mont Albert Central School and Tintern girls' grammar schools in Victoria. She worked as a resident biochemist for five years at the Baker Medical Research Institute before receiving her medical degree from the University of Melbourne in 1945. She later worked as a resident medical officer at the Royal Melbourne Hospital and the Birmingham Children's Hospital.

She was first offered a laboratory position at the Royal Hospital for Women, where she had worked with a rubella vaccine, but she "knew she did not wish to return to pure science and lose contact with sick people, particularly children. What she wanted was the opportunity to investigate disorders of largely unknown cause in a clinical context" (Allen 1996, 40). She thus chose to work in a children's hospital.

Anderson served as professor of pediatrics and child health at the University of Birmingham from 1968 to 1980, and from 1982 until 1991 was a researcher at the Gastroenterological Research Unit at Princess Margaret Hospital for Children.

Her 1975 *Paediatric Gastroenterology* compiled much research in the new specialty in one place in collaboration with numerous physicians from various countries. The book is highly informative with numerous diagrams, photos, and extensive bibliographies.

Anderson never married. She is retired and lives in Australia.

References: Allen, Nessy, "A Pioneer of Paediatric Gastroenterology: The Career of an Australian Woman Scientist," *Historical Records of Australian Science* 11, no. 1 (June 1996): 35–50; Anderson, Charlotte M., and Valerie Burke, eds., *Paediatric Gastroenterology*, Oxford: Blackwell Scientific (1975); *Who's Who in Australia*, Melbourne: Information Australia (1998).

Anderson, Elizabeth Garrett
1836–1917

Elizabeth Anderson was the first British woman to become a physician. . . . She was a pioneer in medical education for women in England through founding a hospital, helping to found a medical school for women and serving as its dean, and becoming the first woman to be a member of the British Medical Association.

Born in London, Elizabeth, along with her siblings, was soon moved to Aldeburgh, Suffolk, where her father, Newson Garrett, and mother, Louisa, raised a large family. Elizabeth was the second oldest of ten. Her older sister was Louisa and after Elizabeth came Dunnell, who died at six months. Following were Newson, Edmund, Alice, Agnes, Millicent, Sam, Josephine, and George. Her father became a rather successful businessman and believed all his children should have an adequate education.

For a time their mother educated Louisa and Elizabeth; following that, according to Elizabeth, was a rather boring ordeal with a governess. By the time Elizabeth was thirteen, her father had decided to send the girls to the Boarding School for Ladies, run by Miss Louisa Browning.

Although Elizabeth at first preferred playing outdoors to school, she learned to love books and reading and became a very capable writer.

From 1851 to 1857, she, with her sister Louisa, helped at home and otherwise led a rather carefree life. Elizabeth did continue to educate herself, focusing on arithmetic

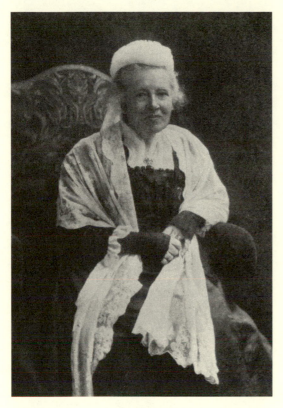

Elizabeth Garrett Anderson (U.S. National Library of Medicine)

and Latin and sometimes utilizing the help of her brother Newton's tutor. During this time, Elizabeth became heavily influenced by other women, among them British suffragist Emily Davies, who felt that intelligent women should pursue careers. Louisa married in 1857. Elizabeth thus took on more responsibilities at home and became even more discontented.

In 1858 the *Englishwoman's Journal* came out and brought the organized women's movement into her life. In the next year she attended a lecture given by Dr. Elizabeth Blackwell and met her later in the evening. Blackwell spoke of the needs of women and children; Elizabeth's other mentor, Davies, had grown up as a clergyman's daughter, seeing firsthand the conditions of tenements in industrial towns. She knew women were suffering because they could not dare ask a male physician to attend to them. Elizabeth asked her father for finan-

cial support to study medicine, and he eventually agreed.

Since no British medical school accepted women, Anderson first worked as a nurse at Middlesex Hospital to see if she was up to the task and to learn as much as possible. Her work led to an invitation to observe patients in the out-clinics of T. W. Nunn, the dean of the medical school at University College. Some doctors, especially the house physician, Dr. Willis, were also willing to help her in private. She realized she needed more physics, chemistry, anatomy, and physiology and took a room to herself at the hospital for intense reading and study.

During winter 1861 while making rounds with the medical students, Anderson answered a visiting physician's question correctly after none of the students responded. Soon thereafter, several students drew up a petition objecting to her admittance to the school. They threatened to leave if she was allowed to continue on with them in lectures and rounds of the hospital. In spite of an offer from her parents to make an endowment to the school for female applicants, the hospital decided against allowing women to attend hospital lectures in the future.

Feeling strongly that she should stay in England and open the doors of medical education for British women, Elizabeth decided to study for the licentiate of the Society of Apothecaries (LSA), which did not stipulate in its charter that applicants had to be male. After she obtained this degree, less prestigious than the M.D., in 1865, the society changed its requirements, and Elizabeth's was the only woman's name on its medical register for the next twelve years.

In 1866, Anderson opened a dispensary for women and children, filling a void in health care for the poverty stricken of the city. No one really objected because a cholera epidemic was spreading over the city. Attitudes changed toward her over the years, and when she obtained an M.D. degree from the Sorbonne in Paris in 1870, medical students cheered.

Elizabeth and James Skelton Anderson developed a strong, trusting relationship while he ran her campaign for the School

Board of London. She was overwhelmingly elected and married James on February 9, 1871.

Elizabeth continued to practice medicine, and her husband, like her father, supported her career. Her dispensary became the New Hospital for Women and Children in 1872. Both its reputation and staff grew. Elizabeth became an able surgeon at this hospital, performing its first ovariotomy. She performed several other gynecological surgeries during her time at the hospital but later said that surgery was one of the most trying of all medical roles for her.

Anderson had her first child, Louisa, in July 1873 and enjoyed being a mother. She continued to work and wanted English-women to know that having children did not eliminate the possibility of a career. She did, however, make the difficult decision to step down from an honorary position at Shadwell Children's Hospital, where she had worked so hard with Nathaniel Heckford to raise money. He had died at the early age of twenty-eight; Elizabeth and his wife, who now ran the hospital, did not get along well.

Her second child, Margaret, was born in 1874. At the same time, she added more room to the New Hospital for Women, and Sophia Jex-Blake, now the leader for medical education for women, established the London Medical College for Women with Elizabeth's help. Elizabeth taught at the college and supported it despite turbulent early years and numerous differences of opinion with Jex-Blake. In 1875, Anderson lost her fifteen-month-old daughter, Margaret, to meningitis. Another child came in 1876, and Elizabeth continued to work at the hospital and teach at the college. She became dean in 1883 and served for twenty years. She died on December 17, 1917. She was the first woman physician in England, the first woman to obtain an M.D. degree in France, and the first woman dean of a medical school. By the time she retired, she had helped raise the London Medical College for Women to new heights as the College of London University.

See also: Blackwell, Elizabeth; Jex-Blake, Sophia Louisa

References: *Encyclopedia of World Biography*, Detroit: Gale (1999); Hume, Ruth Fox, *Great Women of Medicine*, New York: Random House (1964); Manton, Jo, *Elizabeth Garrett Anderson*, New York: Dutton (1965).

Angwin, Maria Louisa
1849–1898

Maria Angwin was the first licensed woman doctor in Nova Scotia. She was born on September 21, 1849, in Blackhead, Conception Bay, Newfoundland. The daughter of a Methodist minister, Thomas Angwin, and Louisa Emma Gill, Maria had four brothers and two sisters, Elizabeth and Phillippa. Both her mother and Phillippa died early of dysentery.

Her father was transferred to Nova Scotia in the 1850s and settled at Dartmouth in 1865. The next year she attended the Wesleyan Ladies Academy, which was part of Mount Allison College in Sackville, New Brunswick. Maria graduated in 1869 with a liberal arts degree and decided on medical school, having been greatly influenced by reading about the Blackwell sisters. No schools in Canada accepted women, however, and she had four brothers who also needed financial support for an education.

Angwin began teaching in Dartmouth after attending the Normal School at Truro. She didn't like teaching, but by living at home with her family she was able to save enough money for medical school. In 1879 she entered the Women's Medical College at the New York Infirmary for Women and Children, which had been established by the Blackwell sisters in 1868.

Upon graduation she served as an intern assistant physician for a year in Boston at the New England Hospital for Women and Children. She then left for London to attend clinics at the Royal Free Hospital.

After returning to Nova Scotia, in 1884 she obtained her license to practice medicine there. She practiced in Halifax, focusing on the urban poor. Angwin was a very active member in the Woman's Christian Temperance Union. She also was a proponent of equal education for women and spoke at any opportunity on women's health, children's well-being, and the rights of women to seek a career instead of, or in addition to, carrying out the duties of marriage and child rearing. She traveled to New York City late in 1897 for postgraduate work. Although she was ill when she returned to Halifax, she expected to resume her practice. She underwent minor surgery while visiting in Ashland, Massachusetts, and died suddenly afterward.

See also: Blackwell, Elizabeth

References: Johnston, Penelop, "Look Back Doctor: Nova Scotia's Amazing Dr. Maria Angwin," *Medical Post* 35, no. 15 (20 April 1999), http://www.medicalpost. com/mdlink/; Kernaghan, Lois, "Angwin, Maria Louisa," *Dictionary of Canadian Biography*, vol. 12, *1891–1900*, Toronto: University of Toronto Press (1990).

Apgar Score System
1952

The Apgar score system became widely used to evaluate the health of newborns after Virginia Apgar published her proposed test in 1953. APGAR is the acronym for the test's measurements: A = appearance, P = pulse, G = grimace, A = activity, and R = respiration. Two points are given for each of these five areas, with a score of seven meaning the newborn is healthy. If the infant scores below seven, the test is repeated every five minutes until a score of seven is attained. An extremely low score alerts the attending physician that something is wrong.

Virginia Apgar, who was an anesthesiologist and worried that infants were not promptly examined after birth, developed the score. More attention in her day was given to the mother. She felt that if there were a quick test available, infant deaths and problems that developed soon after birth could be avoided. The test is still widely used around the world.

See also: Apgar, Virginia

References: *Encyclopedia Britannica Online 2000*, http://www.britannica.com.

Apgar, Virginia
1909–1974

Virginia Apgar is best known for developing the Apgar score system, which helps determine the health of infants immediately after birth. This method, developed in 1952, became widely accepted and put into practice and medical school textbooks very quickly after it was published in 1953. It is still used around the world.

Virginia Apgar was born in Westfield, New Jersey, on June 7, 1909, to Charles Emory and Helen May Clarke Apgar. She had two brothers, Charles, who died of tuberculosis in 1903, and Lawrence. Her father was an automobile salesman. He had a love of science, devoting his spare time to astronomy and electrical experiments. The rest of the family was also interested in science, and in music. Virginia played the violin and was involved in symphonies and orchestra events all her life, even making her own instruments.

She graduated from Westfield High School in 1925 and then attended Mount Holyoke College, supplementing her scholarships by waiting tables and working in the library. She was also very athletic and enjoyed sports, especially tennis, as well as being in the college orchestra and reporting for the college newspaper.

In 1929, she earned her B.A. with a major in zoology and a minor in chemistry. Having always wanted to be a physician, she went on to medical school at Columbia University's College of Physicians and Surgeons. In 1933 she obtained her medical degree and proceeded to a surgical internship at Presbyterian Hospital. Following advice that she should consider the relatively new field of anesthesiology, she attended the University of Wisconsin and then went to Bellevue Hospital in New York City to become certified as an anesthesiologist.

Apgar had always intended to be a surgeon, but Dr. Alan Whipple advised that it would be difficult for a woman to support

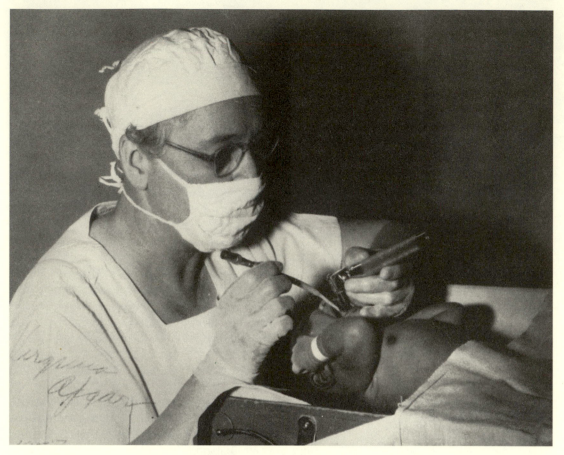

Virginia Apgar (U.S. National Library of Medicine)

herself as a surgeon, especially during the depression. He encouraged her to specialize in anesthesiology because there was a great need for better methods, and at the time, few physicians were specializing in the field.

In 1938 and for the following eleven years, Apgar worked at Columbia-Presbyterian Medical Center as head of the division of anesthesiology. She taught, did research, and continued as a practitioner. During her time there, her workload increased dramatically because so many men left to join the armed forces before and during World War II, and she fought very hard for adequate compensation for her work, even threatening to resign her position at one point. She remained adamant about equal pay for women until her death. In 1949 she became the first female at Colum-

bia to hold the rank of full professor. She held that position until 1959.

It was as a practitioner that Apgar became concerned about quickly ascertaining newborns' physical status. Having seen many heart and lung disorders that she felt could have been prevented with immediate examination, she wanted a simple test that even a delivery-room nurse could administer.

Apgar developed her score system by determining what needed to be checked immediately following the birth of an infant. Her system has been invaluable in preventing further damage from birth abnormalities. She first presented her method in 1952 at the Annual Congress of Anesthetists.

The Apgar score system did more than just help the infants. It also better prepared new physicians and interns to handle a situation in which the infant needed immediate resuscitation or other emergency care. She also researched anesthesia agents, believing that local anesthesia rather than general anesthesia was always preferable for infants. She quit using one of her favorites, cyclopropane, after research fellows under her found that the agent suppressed their immune system.

Honesty about mistakes, without which there could be no learning, was of utmost importance to her, and she emphasized honesty to her students. During her surgical residency, when few admitted any wrongdoing if an infant died, she secretly entered the morgue to check a dead infant after being unable to obtain an autopsy permit. She discovered that a small artery had been clamped and that she had done it. She immediately admitted her mistake to the surgeon.

In 1959 Apgar went to Johns Hopkins University to work on a master's degree in public health. She had become increasingly interested in doing research on birth defects. While she was there, the National Foundation–March of Dimes asked her to head its new division of congenital malformations. Although she felt she was not yet qualified, she determined to learn on the job. She also felt she could go no further in anesthesiology at Columbia. She had become interested in genetics as well, so she finished her master's degree and took the position in 1960. She stayed with the March of Dimes for the rest of her career, becoming vice-president and director of basic research in 1967 and senior vice-president of medical affairs in 1973.

Apgar was also extremely dedicated to alleviating deformities and ailments before birth. She was very concerned about prenatal care, the effects of radiation on the fetus, and nutrition for pregnant women. She coauthored a book in 1972 with Joan Beck called *Is My Baby Alright?*

She was a much sought-after speaker and was invited frequently to speak at conferences and meetings. Although she eventually won international recognition, she remained an unassuming and modest woman.

She walked and talked very fast, loved challenges, and felt women were liberated the day they were born; they just had to be better at what they did to succeed in a man's world or profession. She was unbiased regarding gender, race, and religion.

Apgar died on August 7, 1974, at Columbia-Presbyterian Medical Center in New York City, where she had trained and worked for so many years. She was inducted into the Women's Hall of Fame in 1995.

References: Apgar, Virginia, "A Proposal for a New Method of Evaluation of the Newborn Infant," *Current Researches in Anesthesia and Analgesia* 32 (July–August 1953): 260–267; Calmes, Selma Harrison, "Virginia Apgar: A Woman Physician's Career in a Developing Specialty," *Journal of the American Medical Women's Association* 39, no. 6 (November–December 1984): 184–188; Duffin, Jacalyn, "Apgar, Virginia," *American National Biography*, New York: Oxford University Press (1999); James, L. Stanley, "Fond Memories of Virginia Apgar," *Pediatrics* 55, no. 1 (1975): 1–4; Ogilvie, Marilyn B., *Biographical Dictionary of Women in Science: Pioneering Lives from Ancient Times to the Mid-20th Century*. New York: Routledge (2000); Wyly, M. Virginia, "Apgar, Virginia," *Dictionary of American Biography, Supplement 9, 1971–1975*, New York: Scribner's (1994).

Ashby, Winifred Mayer
1879–1975

Winifred Ashby was the first person to determine the life span of erythrocytes (red blood cells). Her "Ashby method" is included in many hematology books. The technique involves mixing different types of red blood cells in patients and following those cells over time to observe the disappearance of different cell types. She concluded that human red blood cells can circulate in the body for up to 110 days. Prior to her work, it was thought that they survived only two to three weeks. Many disputed her findings initially, but over time her conclusions were found to be accurate. Her work went largely unnoticed until the 1930s.

Ashby was born in London, England, on October 13, 1879. She was the daughter of George Mayer and Mary-Ann Brock Ashby. She moved with her family to Chicago when she was fourteen years old. She attended Northwestern University and also the University of Chicago, obtaining a B.S. in 1903. She earned an M.S. two years later at Washington University in St. Louis and from there went to the Philippines to study malnutrition.

When she returned to the Midwest, she taught physics and chemistry in Berwyn, Illinois, and Maryville, Missouri. From 1914 to 1916 she carried out laboratory work at Rush Medical College and Illinois Central Hospital in Chicago. In 1917 she began a fellowship in immunology and pathology at the Mayo Clinic, during which time she developed her method for determining the life of erythrocytes.

She attended the University of Minnesota and received her Ph.D. in 1921. She remained at the Mayo Clinic until 1924, then took a job at St. Elizabeth's Hospital in Washington, D.C., where she worked in the bacteriology and serology laboratories and supervised numerous activities. She retired in 1949 to Lorton, Virginia.

Ashby died from a cerebrovascular accident on July 19, 1975, at the age of ninety-five.

References: Fairbanks, Virgil F., "In Memoriam: Winifred M. Ashby, 1879–1975," *Blood* 46, no. 6 (December 1975): 977–978; Kass-Simon, G., and Patricia Farnes, *Women of Science: Righting the Record*, Bloomington: Indiana University Press (1990); Parry, Melanie, ed., *Chambers Biographical Dictionary*, Edinburgh: Chambers (1997); *Who Was Who in America with World Notables: Volume VI, 1974–1976*, Chicago: Marquis Who's Who (1976); Wintrobe, Maxwell M., *Blood, Pure and Eloquent: A Story of Discovery, of People, and of Ideas*, New York: McGraw-Hill (1980).

Aspasia
A.D. 200

Aspasia was a Greco-Roman whose writings on obstetrics and gynecology were considered a major contribution to medical practice in the Greco-Roman world. Her writings survived over 1,000 years until Trotula's works became widely used.

Because Aetios of Amida wrote about her in the sixth century B.C. and quoted from her extensively in his *Tetrabiblon*, she is considered to be one of the most knowledgeable of the time on female diseases. Aetios was a physician who attended to Justinian I, the Byzantine emperor.

Most of her writings concern pregnancy, the determination of fetal positions before birth, and herbal treatments for some conditions. She also performed surgery and made the early observation that the mental health of the mother plays a part in a healthy birth and the health of the child.

References: Shearer, Benjamin F., and Barbara S. Shearer, *Notable Women in the Life Sciences: A Biographical Dictionary*, Westport, CT: Greenwood Press (1996).

Avery, Mary Ellen
1927–

Mary Ellen Avery discovered the reason behind respiratory distress syndrome (RDS) and helped develop a treatment for the condition. Infants with RDS cannot develop enough pulmonary surfactant to coat their lungs in order for them to breathe easily. In many instances, this condition is fatal. Avery's work has saved thousands of premature infants around the world.

Avery was born on May 6, 1927, in Camden, New Jersey, to William Clarence Avery and Mary Catherine Miller Avery. She has one sister.

Avery was influenced early by a neighbor, Emily Bacon, who was a doctor and a professor at the Women's Medical College of Pennsylvania and took Avery on rounds at the hospital. Avery's parents both encouraged her to pursue the career of her choice.

She attended Wheaton College, where she majored in chemistry and graduated summa cum laude in 1948. She then went to Johns Hopkins University School of Medicine to obtain her M.D. degree. Soon after receiving her M.D. in 1952, Avery developed tuberculosis. She was sent to Trudeau Sanitarium for a year but left after just a few days because she didn't think bed rest for a year could possibly help. She recovered at home and, during her illness, began to read more about tuberculosis and other lung ailments.

During her days at Harvard on a research fellowship, she discovered RDS firsthand in the autopsy room. She spent a lot of time there studying newborn infants who had died of RDS, a condition no one then understood. In order to learn more about lung function, she began work with Dr. Jere Mead at Harvard.

Together they discovered that a foamy substance called pulmonary surfactant was lacking in newborns who had died of RDS. Avery realized that this substance was of great importance for newborns to breathe normally. She also discovered that glucocorticoid hormones assisted with lung development; they are now given to pregnant women who are at risk for premature delivery.

Avery feels that research findings must be disseminated to a wide audience as quickly as possible. She is a strong advocate for basic medical service to children of economically depressed countries, evidenced by her involvement in UNICEF.

Avery has served in various faculty roles over the years. She worked at Johns Hopkins until 1969, then took a position at McGill University in Quebec as professor of pediatrics at Children's Hospital. In 1974 she began work as the physician in chief at Boston's Children's Hospital while serving as professor of pediatrics at Harvard. She has written extensively on newborns, received numerous awards, and been a very busy speaker abroad. She has left a permanent mark on the field of pediatrics.

References: Bailey, Martha J., *American Women in Science: 1950 to the Present*, Santa Barbara, CA: ABC-CLIO (1998); *Contemporary Authors Online,* Detroit: Gale (2000); *Notable Twentieth-Century Scientists Supplement,* Detroit: Gale (1998); Shearer, Benjamin F., and Barbara S. Shearer, *Notable Women in the Life Sciences*, Westport, CT: Greenwood Press (1996).

B

Bacheler, Mary Washington
1860–1939

The degradation of women in India in the late nineteenth and early twentieth centuries motivated the Free Baptists to move into the mission field there. Mary Bacheler, an active medical missionary in India, carried out their work for decades.

Bacheler was born in New Hampton, New Hampshire, on February 22, 1860. Her father was a medical missionary and had returned with his wife for the birth of Mary, the ninth of ten children. In 1866, leaving the other children in the United States, Mary's mother took Mary to India for the first time. There she got an early look at her father's work in treating the Indians in and around Midnapore.

In the late nineteenth century in India, many women were not allowed to permit a man to examine them if they had an ailment, and thus many of them suffered from poor health. Medical missionary women like Bacheler often were able not only to cure the women of their ailments but also to thereby establish trust and win converts to the faith.

An earlier development had given the Free Baptist missionaries access to Indian women. In February 1866, the Hindus began to allow outside women into the zenanas, the female part of the household. Missionary women of the time were allowed in some instances to gather with Hindu women and teach various domestic practices as well as crafts. Some Free Baptist supporters were disappointed that this type of outreach did not bring about many conversions, but Mary was certain that the younger ones might eventually benefit from the missionaries' religious teachings. In the meantime, they were helping to educate young women, a practice that initiated an expectation in Indian society.

In 1883 Mary returned to the United States for seven years, much of that time being spent at the Women's Medical College of the New York Infirmary for Women and Children, where she graduated with her M.D. degree in 1890. She returned to Midnapore and the Brown Dispensary to work with her father. At one point they were seeing over 3,000 patients a year. Mary traveled often to homes, as many women were now willing to let a female physician see to their needs. Her popularity grew so fast that after her parents left in 1892, she became totally immersed in health care and ministering to the people. After several years, she suffered a complete breakdown and had to return to the United States. Her parents both died soon thereafter. Her health regained, Mary returned to India and her work in 1903.

During the next three decades she worked in various roles as assigned by the Free Baptists. She oversaw an orphanage, tended to administrative duties, and was tough on new missionaries, insisting they be better acquainted with the Bible. She herself enjoyed telling Bible stories while she tended to the ill. She also was a tireless advocate of women's and children's health care.

She retired in 1933, left India for the last time in 1936, and died in the United States on November 5, 1939. Her friends and patients in India were still receiving Christmas presents from her when they learned of her death.

References: Bickers, Robert A., and Rosemary Seton, eds., *Missionary Encounters: Sources and Issues,* Richmond, Surrey: Curzon Press (1996); Congdon-Martin, Elizabeth W., "Mary Washington Bacheler, M.D.: Enlisted for Life," *American Baptist Quarterly* 12, no. 3 (1993): 271–282.

Bain, Barbara
1932–

Barbara Bain developed the mixed leukocyte culture (MLC), which is essential in determining bone marrow and organ compatibility for transplants. She discovered that combining the blood lymphocytes of two different people results in the activation of the lymphocytes. The amount of in vitro activation is an indication of how compatible one set of cells is with the other. Researchers determine the degree of activation from the amount of DNA synthesis that has occurred over five or six days.

Bain was born in Montreal, Quebec, on May 8, 1932. She attended McGill University and received B.S. and M.S. degrees in 1953 and 1957, respectively. In 1965 she obtained her Ph.D. in experimental medicine. She developed MLC while at the Royal Victoria Hospital as a graduate student. She currently is a professor at St. Mary's Hospital Medical School, Department of Haematology, London.

Her current research focuses on sickle cell disease, leukemia, genetics, and the role of ethnicity in blood-related health issues.

References: *American Men and Women of Science 1998–99,* New Providence, NJ: Bowker (1999); Kass-Simon, G., and Patricia Farnes, *Women of Science: Righting the Record,* Bloomington: Indiana University Press (1990).

Baker, Sara Josephine
1873–1945

Sara Baker was a physician and public health administrator in the early twentieth century. She became an authority on the

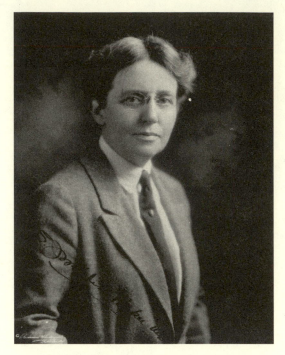

Sara Josephine Baker (Underwood & Underwood/ U.S. National Library of Medicine)

welfare of poor women and children and served in various government and organizational roles to assist those who needed care the most. She was one of the first women to become involved in social medicine and the first woman to obtain a Ph.D. in public health from New York University's Bellevue Hospital Medical School.

Baker was born November 15, 1873, in Poughkeepsie, New York. Her father, Orlando Daniel Mosher Baker, was a lawyer, and her mother, Jenny Harwood Brown, was one of the first to graduate from Vassar College. Baker had intended to go to Vassar as well, but her father and brother died unexpectedly when she was sixteen. She decided not to accept a scholarship to Vassar, as her mother wanted; instead she set her sights on a medical career.

Her mother was not very encouraging but still supportive. In 1894 Baker began her studies at the Women's Medical College of the New York Infirmary for Women and Children, which had been founded by Elizabeth and Emily Blackwell. It was the only medical school in New York that accepted women. She then turned down an opportunity to intern at the New York Infirmary because she wanted to work in a large general hospital. However, since none of them took women interns, she settled on Boston's New England Hospital for Women and Children, whose staff included many very well-trained women physicians.

In Boston, Baker also cared for outpatients of the hospital who lived in the slums, in time realizing that she had found her life-work. She took a practical view of her mission, concluding that someone had to deal with the effects of an unjust society.

She attempted private practice among the poor but realized she could not make a living. Then, after she had worked briefly as a medical examiner for an insurance company, New York City's Health Department hired her in 1907 to head the Bureau of Child Hygiene. It was here that she began her contributions to public health. She could see that giving the poor medical treatment was not enough; legislation, regulations, and staff adequately trained to work with the population would be necessary. Because of her efforts in training midwives, New York City achieved the lowest infant mortality rate of any large city.

Baker was a feminist, a lesbian, and an active suffragist. She associated with many influential and unconventional women throughout her life; most of these women were members of the Heterodoxy Club, founded in 1912. Members met to discuss mutual concerns, women's rights, and how to handle the inequality women were facing professionally.

Baker felt it was important to have the public image of an exceptional professional in order to make improvements in public health. By continually focusing, without racial prejudice, on the plight of mothers and children, she was able to influence political leaders on their behalf; it was difficult for a politician to be against mothers and children.

She authored many books and articles and retired to Bellemead, New Jersey, where she had a farm and lived with her partner, Ida Wylie, the novelist, and Louise Pearce, a physician. She died of cancer on February 22, 1945, in New York City.

References: Baker, Sara Josephine, *Fighting for Life,* New York: Macmillan (1939); Morantz-Sanchez, Regina, "Baker, Sara Josephine," *American National Biography,* vol. 2, New York: Oxford University Press (1999); *Notable Twentieth-Century Scientists,* Detroit: Gale (1995).

Balfour, Margaret Ida
18?–1949

Margaret Balfour was a physician very active in organizing activities in connection with the Medical Women's International Association and the Women's Medical Service in India. She was a leader in foreign medical services and became an expert on Indian medical care and facilities as well as worked in many African countries. Her prolific correspondence and other writings during the early twentieth century alerted many in the world to the unhealthy environments in many countries, particularly to the needs of women and children in India and Africa. She also was indispensable in organizing medical education for women in India and Africa. Her book *The Work of Medical Women in India* was a source on many aspects of Indian social and cultural life. It also documents the progress that had been made to date and has good statistics on female practitioners.

Balfour was born in Edinburgh, the daughter of Robert Balfour. Little is known about her early life and education except that she did attend Edinburgh University. Her interests in medicine focused on the health of women, particularly when pregnant, and of children in Asia.

References: Balfour, Margaret I., and Ruth Young, *The Work of Medical Women in India,* London: Oxford University Press (1929); Lovejoy, Esther P., *Women Doctors of the World,* New York: Macmillan (1957); *Who Was Who, 1941–50,* "Balfour, Margaret Ida," London: A & C Black (1951); *Who Was Who among English and European Authors, 1931–1949,* "Balfour, Margaret Ida," Detroit: Gale (1978).

Barnes, Alice Josephine
1912–1999

The first woman to become president of the British Medical Association, Barnes spent her life as a gynecologist and obstetrician trying to improve the health of women and infants.

Born in Sheringham, Norfolk, England, on August 18, 1912, to a minister and a gifted pianist, she determined early in her life that she wanted to become a doctor. She went to Oxford High School and later won a scholarship to Lady Margaret Hall, a women's college at the University of Oxford, where she earned her master's degree in 1937.

After World War II began, many male physicians were called into the military and their absence enabled her to obtain a position at the Samaritan Hospital in 1939. She worked delivering babies and caring for people injured in the Nazi bombings of London, and earned her M.D. at University College Hospital Medical School in 1941.

She married Dr. Brian Warren in 1942 and they started a family, eventually having three children. She continued working as a physician at various hospitals in London and managing a private practice while raising her children. She became a well-known gynecologist and obstetrician, and as her reputation grew, so did requests for her to serve on various governmental and organizational committees.

She investigated the effectiveness of the Abortion Act (1967), concluding that it did more good than harm. She also worked to determine the appropriate conditions for conducting experiments on embryos. One of the most memorable things Barnes did was to save the Elizabeth Garrett Anderson Hospital from closure during the 1970s. She earned the position of president of the British Medical Association in 1979 because her colleagues, most of them male, felt she was a tremendously productive and ethical physician.

Barnes retired from private practice in 1995 but continued to be interested in medical affairs. She became a Dame Commander of the Order of the British Empire (DBE) in 1974. Outside of work she enjoyed traveling, cooking, and music. She died on December 28, 1999.

References: "Dame Josephine Barnes," *Times* (29 December 1999): 19; Haines, Catharine M. C., and Helen Stevens, *International Women in Science: A Biographical Dictionary to 1950*, Santa Barbara, CA: ABC-CLIO (2001).

Barriers to Success

Many obstacles hindered women from success in the medical field. Key areas of difficulty were cultural and societal expectations, education, and laws and religion. Despite having the desire and intelligence needed, many women had to fight for the education required and the acceptance of society.

Until the late twentieth century, it was exceptional for a woman to be encouraged to study a science discipline such as medicine. Most societies had a traditional view of women as homemakers and childbearers, and most women were raised from an early age with these expectations in mind. Very few were bold enough to set out to become physicians. Many who did so had physician fathers or relatives that piqued their interest in medicine or a related discipline.

The notion that women were not up to the same tasks as men was put forth by many men during the women's rights struggles of the late nineteenth century, when women were pressing for more options than just domestic careers. In his controversial book *Sex in Education; or A Fair Chance for the Girls*, Edward H. Clarke, M.D., a former Harvard University professor, proposed that women should not be allowed to study with men. "Identical education of the two sexes is a crime before God and humanity, that physiology protests against, and that experience weeps over" (Clarke 1873, 127). He also felt that women would do themselves harm by exerting undo energy during menstruation and could permanently damage their reproductive organs. This view was shared by many.

Throughout history, the gender issue has

been problematic. Even in the late 1600s and 1700s, when wet nurses and governesses increasingly served the upper classes of Europe, women did not find encouragement. "Women's desires to engage like men in productive lives free of the cares of parenting came into conflict with growing beliefs that those nations were strongest which had the largest population" (Schiebinger 1989, 218–219). Governments believed that the high infant mortality rate could be lowered only by educating women on infant care and having them take care of their own young.

Margaret Cavendish spoke for many in the seventeenth century when she wrote that "women's brains are simply too 'cold' and 'soft' to sustain rigorous thought" (Schiebinger 1989, 2). This view has continued to evolve and wear different faces.

"The alleged defect in women's minds has changed over time: in the late eighteenth century, the female cranial cavity was supposed to be too small to hold powerful brains; in the nineteenth century, the exercise of women's brains was said to shrivel their ovaries. In our own century peculiarities in the right hemisphere supposedly make women unable to visualize spatial relations" (Schiebinger 1989, 2). Over the centuries, many educated men and women have held such views.

Many colleges and universities constantly turned females away simply because they were women. A few women were able to gain admission to appropriate medical colleges, but such admissions were rare even after Elizabeth Blackwell was admitted to Geneva College in 1847 in the United States. Many women were able to find the education they wanted only when new occupations materialized. Physiology, for example, was considered an appropriate area for women because it involved public hygiene and required work in the cities and public schools. Since such work was not seen as in men's domain, physiology became part of the curriculum in many women's colleges in the late nineteenth century in the United States.

Many women were able to do research and publish during the late nineteenth and early twentieth centuries even if they held no academic position. This was possible in disciplines that required no laboratory work. Few women that managed to achieve an appropriate education were equally successful in acquiring the academic position that would have given them access to adequate facilities for research in certain clinical areas. They were nevertheless productive in writing about others' findings, researching the literature of their fields, and using their own observations and practices, particularly in Russia, the United States, and Great Britain. The major focus of their studies during this time was pathology, neurology, physiology, and anatomy.

There appeared to be only four U.S. schools—"Michigan, Chicago, and Cornell, and Bryn Mawr College" (Creese 1998, 135) —that trained a meaningful number of women for medical careers in the late nineteenth and early twentieth centuries. Also of note is Johns Hopkins University, which accepted an endowment for its medical school in 1889 on the condition that it admit women as well as men. In other countries, educational institutions changed even more slowly.

Many people were against coeducation of any kind, particularly in medicine. Others felt women were not physically up to the task. Still others argued that women should be educated as physicians only if they attended women's colleges. Women felt that the public needed to be assured they were being trained as well as men and that some women's schools would produce—in fact they sometimes did produce—substandard physicians. The Blackwells' New York Infirmary for Women and Children and Jex-Blake's Edinburgh School of Medicine for Women accomplished the task of providing exemplary training for women physicians.

Based on the premise that a woman had to achieve extraordinary training in order to enter a man's domain, the Blackwells strove for standards higher than those required by the traditional medical schools of the time. The curriculum that evolved at the New York Infirmary provided more clinical experience than was available in the traditional schools. Women trained there were also much more likely to be more experienced with female difficulties during pregnancy and early-birth difficulties than their male counterparts.

Women who wished to be physicians had another problem besides education. Even if they could find a school willing to admit and train them, who would want a woman physician, and where would they practice? This concern still applies today for many women physicians around the world. Most women who were pioneers in education, including Elizabeth Blackwell, had a hard time winning patients in private practice, and many hospitals did not accept women physicians. Numerous women eventually died in debt or poverty because their practice was limited to those who couldn't afford medical care or they provided care in their own homes for donations. Thus a woman physician's qualifications became meaningless because no one in the traditional establishment wanted women in the profession.

Countless women died because they did not feel it was appropriate to allow males to examine their bodies. Nuns would not allow an examination by a male. Perhaps this attitude led to so many women becoming interested in obstetrics and gynecology. Even some men saw that women might be better than men in this field, as well as better at dealing with children's ailments.

Laws and regulations in many countries were restrictive regarding who could obtain medical degrees or certification. In many countries the legal system and the church or religious beliefs were intertwined, as in seventeenth-century England. Women were not restricted from being licensed as surgeons, for example, but from the few records that exist, it would appear that women had to prove quite superior to their male counterparts in order to be approved by the church. Records show documentation of extraordinary detail for the few women who managed to gain a license. In seventeenth-century England, licensing "was a barrier which prevented women from standing on an equal footing with their male counterparts" (Evenden 1998, 212).

In Eastern Europe, more women were able to enter the profession, particularly in Russia. There, most men entered other areas of study, and a degree in medicine did not carry the prestige it did in other countries. Except for Chile and Brazil, Latin American countries were slow to let women enter the profession. A decree by the Chilean government in 1877 allowed women to take examinations for a profession as long as they were trained just like men. Chile was well ahead of many countries.

In Asia circumstances varied greatly by country. In Japan a long and strong tradition of women as housekeepers and mothers was crucial. Medical schools for women now exist, but change came about very slowly. China, in contrast, has been very supportive of women seeking a career in medicine. India has a high number of women physicians, and a huge percentage in obstetrics and gynecological care. Many Indian women will allow only a female to examine them, and this attitude is well accepted.

In the Islamic world, change for women has been slower due to cultural and religious beliefs and laws. However, since the end of World War II a few women have been able to enter the medical profession. Within Africa, poverty rather than restrictions against women is the problem. There are few facilities for training and working as well as a lack of skilled teachers for basic science courses. Australian universities accept women, but medical degrees have typically taken six years to attain and thus some females are discouraged early on by their parents.

The effects of two world wars—widows needed to find a way to support their families, and countries needed women physicians to fill in for male medical doctors that went to war or to replace those who were killed—led some people to see the advantages of preparing women for careers. Societies also began to see the benefit of a dual-income household, especially when domestic help became more readily available and affordable in many countries.

Despite progress, however, there are still those who feel women physicians will never have equality with men, particularly in the United States.

There is a "glass ceiling" on women physicians' upward mobility. They are kept from top-level positions, I will argue, through the subtle process of a kind of colleague boycott—not keeping them out entirely, but not including them in ways that allow them to replace the senior members of the medical community. This process is the "Salieri phenomenon"— a combination of faint praise and subtle denigration of their abilities to lead which delegitimates women physicians' bids to compete for positions of great authority. The reason men are so reluctant to allow women into the inner circles, I contend, is their fear that if too many women become leaders, the profession will "tip" and become women's work—and men will lose prestige, income and authority. (Lorber 1993, 63)

Others disagree and feel economics will dictate the need for more women physicians because of the growth in the field of health care.

Research has revealed what obstacles are most troublesome for women in the medical field, including in academia. "The chairs we interviewed painted a broad tableau of factors constraining women's advancement to leadership positions in academic medicine, and they identified three sources of barriers: historical developments (e.g., shortage of women in the pipeline), broad social forces (e.g., gender roles and socialization patterns affecting women's status), and the expression of these forces in the medical environment (e.g., sexism in recruitment and promotion practices, a shortage of effective mentors for women)" (Yedidia 2001). The fact that the male-dominated American Medical Association elected a woman, Nancy Dickey, as its president in 1997 suggests that more women can achieve leadership roles with administrative power.

See also: Wars and Epidemics; Women of Color in Medicine
References: Bowers, John Z., "Women in Medicine," *New England Journal of Medicine* 275, no. 7 (18 August 1966); Burstein, Paul, and Marie Bricher, "Problem Definition and Public Policy: Congressional Committees Confront Work, Family, and Gender, 1945–1990," *Social Forces* 76, no. 1 (September 1997): 135–168; Clarke, Edward H., *Sex in Education; or A Fair Chance for the Girls*, Boston: J. R. Osgood (1873); Creese, Mary R. S., *Ladies in the Laboratory? American and British Women in Science, 1800–1900*, Lanham, MD: Scarecrow Press (1998); Evenden, Doreen A., "Gender Differences in the Licensing and Practice of Female and Male Surgeons in Early Modern England," *Medical History* 42 (1998); Gabor, Andrea, "Married, with Househusband," *Working Woman* 20, no. 11 (November 1995): 46–50ff.; Lorber, Judith, "Why Women Physicians Will Never Be True Equals in the American Medical Profession," in *Gender, Work, and Medicine: Women and the Medical Division of Labor*, edited by Elianne Riska and Katarina Wegar, London: Sage (1993); Rossiter, Margaret W., *Women Scientists in America: Struggles and Strategies to 1940*, Baltimore, MD: Johns Hopkins University Press (1982); Schiebinger, Londa, *The Mind Has No Sex? Women in the Origins of Modern Science*, Cambridge, MA: Harvard University Press (1989); Walsh, Mary Roth, *Doctors Wanted: No Women Need Apply: Sexual Barriers in the Medical Profession, 1835–1975*, New Haven, CT: Yale University Press (1977); Yedidia, Michael J., and Janet Bickel, "Why Aren't There More Women Leaders in Academic Medicine? The Views of Clinical Department Chairs," *Academic Medicine* 76:5 (May 2001): 453–465.

Barringer, Emily Dunning
1876–1961

Emily Barringer was the first female ambulance surgeon in New York City and the first female physician to work as an intern at a New York City hospital. She was born September 27, 1876, in Scarsdale, New York, to Edwin James Dunning and Frances Gore Lang. At eight she found her calling when she helped her mother after the birth of her sixth child. "I truly believe that it was at this time that the great desire was born in me to help the sick and suffering which later was to lead me into medicine" (Barringer 1950, 28).

Emily's family suffered financial reverses when she was still a child, and her mother felt her daughters needed an education so that they could support themselves. Emily thought about becoming a nurse, but after listening to a lecture by Mary Putnam Jacobi, she realized a medical profession was possible. She graduated from Cornell University in New York and proceeded to the Medical College of the New York Infirmary for Women and Children. She received her medical degree in 1904 and married a fellow medical student, Benjamin Stockwell Barringer.

Before receiving her medical degree, she wanted to intern at a large hospital, but women physicians were not allowed in these facilities. She took hospital exams and did well but was refused any appointment until 1903, when she went to work at Gouverneur Hospital in New York City. She had worked to lobby the mayor, who was in support of women holding physician positions if they did well on standard examinations.

Several male physicians tried to force her to resign, but because of her good and efficient work, she had support from the rest of the hospital staff and eventually from the residents of New York City.

She worked at other hospitals, specializing in gynecological surgery and later in venereal diseases. She was also active in various organizations involved in providing medical services during World War I, particularly those that worked to provide ambulances in Europe. During World War II she had a large hand in promoting women's rights, particularly their right to commissions in the military. Barringer lobbied both the president and Congress for over a year on the legislation that made it possible for women to be commissioned into the military and receive the same benefits as men. In 1943, President Franklin D. Roosevelt signed into law the Sparkman Act, which was supported by U.S. senator John Jackson Sparkman of Alabama.

Barringer answered thousands of ambulance calls and encountered birth and death:

Between these two irrevocable markers, the beginning and the end, I was to see every phase of human activity and human emotion, the full gamut of life. I was to see heroism, devotion, loyalty, hard work and honest labor, illness in every form, poverty, hunger, cold; pitiless cold in winter, unbearable heat in summer, in the old tenements reeking with overcrowded humanity; crime in every form, robbery, murder, rape; insanity, alcoholism in all stages; I was to meet the budding gangster, the prostitute and to visit dives where the underworld held out and one reeled under the nauseous opium-laden air. Industrial accidents little understood in those days came my way; men suffering "the bends" or strange deaths from monoxide poisoning, before preventive measures were established. (Barringer 1950, 149)

Barringer did much to set an example not only for women who wanted to be medical practitioners but also for women who had to fight in order to use their skills and talents in the service of others. She died on April 8, 1961, in New Milford, Connecticut.

References: Barringer, Emily Dunning, *Bowery to Bellevue: The Story of New York's First Woman Ambulance Surgeon*, New York: W. W. Norton (1950); German, Lisa Broehl, "Barringer, Emily Dunning," *American National Biography*, vol. 2, New York: Oxford University Press (1999).

Barry, James
1795–1865

James Barry's story is incredible in that she masqueraded as a man all her life, her gender revealed only at her death. She entered the British army disguised as a man in 1813 after being educated at the Edinburgh School of Medicine. She shied away from her classmates for obvious reasons. As a woman, she would not have been allowed to study at the university, let alone to practice as a physician. During her forty-year career, she rose to the rank of inspector-general in the Army Medical Department.

Little is known about her early life except that she intended early on to become a physician and made excellent marks in school. As an army surgeon she was well respected. She served at Malta and the Cape of Good Hope beginning in 1816. She spent unusually long hours with lepers and blacks, to the consternation of some colleagues who felt such work was unimportant. She is known to have dueled, had a very hot temper, and been sent home occasionally due to various breeches of military conduct. She was five feet tall with a slight frame and a high-pitched voice

Unsubstantiated rumors circulated after her death—that she was possibly a hermaphrodite, that she was in love with another army surgeon. It was discovered that she had borne a child, about whom nothing is known. She is remembered in South Africa, where she served the destitute and practiced preventive medicine decades before such work was regarded as important.

References: Harrison, Robert, "Barry, James," *Dictionary of National Biography, Volume I,* London: Oxford University Press (1973); *Notable Women Scientists,* Detroit: Gale (2000); Rose, June, *The Perfect Gentleman,* London: Hutchinson (1977).

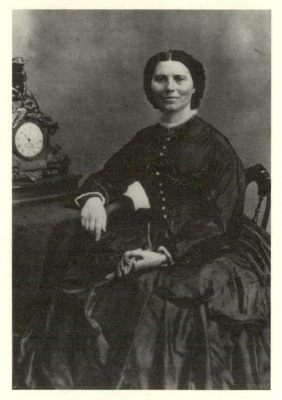

Clara Barton (National Archives/U.S. National Library of Medicine)

Barton, Clara
(Clarissa Harlowe)
1821–1912

Clara Barton is well-known for her nursing abilities during the American Civil War. Her leadership abilities and organizational skills enabled her to bring disaster nursing to the forefront of her profession, found the American Red Cross, and lead that growing organization into public-relief efforts all over her country.

Born in Oxford, Massachusetts, on December 25, 1821, she was the youngest of five children of Steven and Sarah Stone Barton. Both humanitarian and patriotic, her parents were a great influence on her. She

enjoyed learning and problem solving and early on studied math, chemistry, Latin, philosophy, and history.

When she was eighteen she began teaching, an occupation she enjoyed. When she was thirty, she enrolled in the Liberal Institute of Clinton, New York. She completed her studies and returned to teaching in New Jersey. She later moved to Washington, D.C., and obtained a position in the patent office.

When the Civil War broke out, Barton started helping on her own with just a few people donating money or supplies. It was easier during the beginning of the war, before other organizations had a handle on the tasks, to get to battle victims, and she became a dependable and indispensable relief worker in the early going.

Once the war was over, she took on the huge job of identifying for the government missing soldiers and those who had died. She also saw to properly marking their graves. President Lincoln was very supportive of this effort. Her biggest job during this time was marking the graves at the infamous Anderson Prison in Georgia, officially Camp Sumter. It was one of the largest prisons during the Civil War, and Union soldiers died daily due to lack of food and health care and overcrowding.

Dorence Atwater wrote to Clara Barton at the end of the war when he learned that she wanted to find missing soldiers and mark graves appropriately. He had been a prisoner at Andersonville whose job it was to record the deaths of Union soldiers for Confederate records. He secretly made his own copy of the record, fearing that the original might be lost. He took his copy with him upon discharge and with the information he obtained Clara Barton's help in identifying thousands of graves and marking them properly.

Most of Barton's work during this period was in Annapolis and Washington, D.C., but she also traveled extensively, speaking to audiences about her work. She considered writing a book about all she had seen during the war but decided instead to give lectures in order to earn a living. She attended lectures given by other women in order to observe and hone her skills. Audiences responded positively, and she found the income sufficient to travel and support herself. She lectured throughout the Midwest and New England until her voice failed from exhaustion and nervous prostration. She was advised to go to Europe for rest and went to Switzerland in 1869. As she recovered, she became very interested in the International Red Cross and its treaty of humanitarian assistance to all who needed it in times of war. Barton was astonished that the United States had not signed this treaty.

She worked in Europe with some of the Red Cross volunteers during the Franco-Prussian War. After returning to the United States, she worked for years to persuade government officials that the United States should join the International Red Cross. The American Red Cross finally became a reality on May 20, 1881.

Barton urged President James Garfield to become president of the American Red Cross because in other countries, presidents served as leaders of the organization. President Garfield instead nominated Clara Barton. She took office and served for the next twenty-three years, leading the organization to relief efforts in many areas.

Barton was praised during the early years of the American Red Cross, and she maintained a small, efficient organization. Her leadership was vital because she had gained the respect of thousands of people who knew of her humanitarian nature and work. However, the organization grew far too large for a single woman to lead. After the Spanish-American War many saw the need for reorganization. Barton, now nearing eighty years of age and feeling the proposal a personal insult, disagreed.

President Roosevelt told her he could no longer be an officer of the Red Cross with such unrest surrounding the idea of reorganization, and a disheartened Barton resigned on June 16, 1904. She refused the move to make her honorary president for life with an adequate salary. She retired to Glen Echo, Maryland, outside of Washington, D.C., which was her home. She continued to be interested in some of the women's issues of the time and continued correspondence with friends and writing in her diary. She died on April 12, 1912, and was buried in Oxford, Massachusetts.

References: Barton, William E., *Life of Clara Barton, Founder of the American Red Cross*, Boston: Houghton Mifflin (1922); Bullough, Vern L., Olga Maranjian Church, and Alice Stein, *American Nursing: A Biographical Dictionary*, New York: Garland (1988); Snodgrass, Mary Jane, *Historical Encyclopedia of Nursing*, Santa Barbara, CA: ABC-CLIO (1999).

Bassi, Laura Maria Caterina
1711–1778

An Italian anatomist, Bassi was an unusually talented woman from a family that afforded her a university education, an educational opportunity rare for women of the time period.

Born October 29, 1711, in Bologna to Giuseppe Bassi and Rosa Cesari Bassi, she was educated early in the home and tutored by the family physician. One of the family friends was Cardinal Lambertini (became Pope Benedict XIV in 1740), who felt Bassi had a gift that should be demonstrated to the public. After she had impressed many professors with her intellectual giftedness in the arts and sciences, Cardinal Lambertini told her she would be allowed to pursue a university education.

She earned a Ph.D. around 1732 from the University of Bologna and then lectured as a professor. Her main areas of study were anatomy and physics. She married Giuseppe Verati on February 6, 1738, and they had several children. She continued teaching at the university and at home. Bassi serves as an exception to traditional roles of women of her day. She died in 1778 in Bologna.

References: Ogilvie, Marilyn, and Joy Harvey, eds., *The Biographical Dictionary of Women in Science*, New York: Routledge (2000).

Bayerova, Anna
1852–1924

Anna Bayerova was the first Czech woman physician. She attended college in Switzerland, as no Czechoslovakian college allowed women to enroll for a medical degree. She graduated in 1881 from the University of Bern. She also completed studies in Dresden and Paris. She practiced in Baden and at a children's hospital in Bern and served as a state physician beginning in 1892 in Bosnia-Herzegovina.

While serving in Bosnia-Herzegovina as a state physician, she dealt with inadequate facilities and her own poor health. Prior to 1892, very little had been accomplished in the field of health care. Her duties included attending to the many needs of Muslim women and children. From 1900 to 1909 she worked in several sanatoriums in Switzerland and Prague. She authored a book in 1923 on women as physicians.

References: *Ceskoslovensky Biograficky Slovnik.* Prague: Academia (1992); Navratil, Michal, *Almanach Ceskych Lekaru,* Prague: Náklaem Spisovatelovým (1913); Necas, Ctibor, "Prvni Uredni Lekarka V Bosnen," *Casopis Matice Moravske* [Czechoslovakia] 102, nos. 3–4 (1983).

Biheron, Marie Catherine
1719–1786

Marie Biheron was a talented anatomist in France. She gained considerable recognition during her lifetime for her wax models, which she made to overcome the lack of cadavers for use in studying the human body. Her anatomically correct models were used a great deal to teach both male and female students who had an interest in medicine or midwifery.

What we know about Biheron comes from writings of her contemporaries. She was born in Paris, and her father was an apothecary. Madeleine Basseport, a talented illustrator, was her teacher. Biheron never divulged her secrets in making the models she sold; some didn't believe they were wax because they didn't melt when heated. She was invited by royalty on more than one occasion to display her models or to lecture, and she was a well-respected anatomy teacher.

References: Ogilvie, Marilyn, and Joy Harvey, eds., *The Biographical Dictionary of Women in Science: Pioneering Lives from Ancient Times to the Mid-20th Century*, New York: Routledge (2000); Schiebinger, Londa, *The Mind Has No Sex? Women in the Origins of Modern Science*, Cambridge, MA: Harvard University Press (1989).

Blackwell, Elizabeth
1821–1910

Elizabeth Blackwell was the first woman to attend medical school and become a physician in the United States. She was a pioneer in opening doors that had been closed to women for centuries. She championed med-

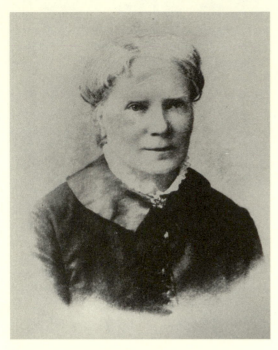

Elizabeth Blackwell (U.S. National Library of Medicine)

ical education for women, helped found the New York Infirmary for Women and Children, and served the medical profession with high ethical standards.

She was born February 3, 1821, in Counterslip near Bristol, England, to Samuel Blackwell and Hannah Lane. Her father had a very heavy influence on his family. He supported women's rights, was against slavery, and encouraged all his children to be active in society. He was also very religious, and Elizabeth participated in Bible study and daily prayers. She had eight surviving siblings: Anna, Marianne, Samuel Charles, Henry Browne, Emily, Ellen, John Howard, and George Washington. Three children died in infancy.

Illiteracy was at an all-time high in England. Samuel Blackwell was a Dissenter, and as such his children were barred from the Church of England schools, which were much better than any of the others. An excellent tutor, Samuel brought his children up to study the same subjects together and had high expectations, making no distinctions in this regard between his sons and his daughters. Elizabeth would always concur with her father's view on educating both men and women.

The Blackwell family left for the United States in 1832 after the local sugar refinery burned down and their financial situation became bleak. Samuel was determined to introduce the vacuum-pan sugar-refining process, showing that it would alleviate the need for slavery. Thus they sailed for New York and a new start. They were met with a cholera epidemic that had left the city deserted. Once it was over, he acquired a place for a refinery.

In the United States, the family associated with the Quakers, but Samuel was still very open about most social events. While Hannah worried about preparing her daughters for marriage, Elizabeth thought about career plans. Samuel suffered financially during the Great Panic of 1837 and the depression that followed. He sold the sugar refinery and shortly thereafter took Elizabeth and her younger siblings to Cincinnati for a fresh start.

Samuel bought a mill near the Ohio River but realized quickly that the depression had affected the entire country. He did little business. Soon thereafter, his health declined, and he died of bilious fever in August 1838. Many of the children began to work to support the family; Elizabeth began to teach. She was moved by the more liberal thinkers of the time, such as Catherine Beecher and Horace Mann. She was restless but continued to teach until a dying friend told her she would be a good physician. After studying on her own with a physician in Charleston and later Philadelphia, she decided to apply to medical school. She was turned down by twenty-eight colleges and finally accepted by Geneva College in New York. The faculty there had put the matter to the male students; they decided to allow her entrance, although many agreed as a joke, feeling that a female would alleviate any boredom. In the beginning few months at Geneva College, Blackwell was ostracized and stared at as she walked to and from her classes, but students and staff soon adjusted to her presence. She became absorbed in her studies and looked forward to being a surgeon. She graduated in 1849 with outstanding grades and became the first female physician in the United States.

For practical medical experience, Blackwell set her sights on Paris. She was able to study at clinics in England and eventually in Paris at La Maternité. She was not accepted as a physician, however, but only as an aide. She observed the French physicians as they delivered babies in all kinds of circumstances, and learned equally from her twelve-hour days in the wards and from the lectures on midwifery. It was at La Maternité that she let her feelings be known about using animals for experiments. Throughout her life, she fought vivisection at every turn, a stance that at this time was in the minority.

On November 4, 1849, she contracted ophthalmia, from a baby she had helped operate on that morning. After losing sight in her left eye, she tried several cures. Eventually, however, an infection set in and she had the left eye removed and a glass eye inserted. Her right eye remained unaffected, and she resigned herself to giving up surgery and pursuing general medicine or research. She consulted with family members concerned about her outlook and her future and worked to be able to read and write well again. Two of her sisters, Marianne and Ellen, wrote to Elizabeth at this time in support of the women's rights movement. Elizabeth, who had managed to garner some support and encouragement in a man's world, felt her sisters were in an antiman movement and didn't support their views. She saw no common thread between women's rights and education.

During her two years in Europe, Blackwell had met Florence Nightingale, whose views on the importance of sanitation had profoundly influenced her. In her later life she worked to educate people on proper hygiene for good health.

Blackwell returned to the United States ready to practice medicine. She and her sisters had won a writing contest, and she used the $100 to set up an office, furnishing it herself. Society wasn't ready for a female physician, however, and Elizabeth suffered from loneliness and depression.

She resorted to giving physical education lectures to girls, and eventually lectured on several subjects for a fee. She also met Ann Preston, who later founded the Women's Hospital of Philadelphia (1861). They encouraged each other in their prospective endeavors. Many Quaker women came to hear her, and even some men. They were impressed at her knowledge and convinced that her views on the importance of hygiene were not to be taken lightly. This work eventually led to her being accepted in the medical community. Quaker women and children also began to come to her office for treatment. Her practice grew as she worked both day and night.

She continued to keep in touch with her family and to prepare public lectures. Some prominent New Yorkers eventually came to support her, such as Horace Greeley and many Quaker men of the day. Elizabeth's sister Emily was at the same time enduring the frustrations Elizabeth had experienced earlier. Medical schools were rejecting her because she was a woman and she very much wanted Elizabeth's support, which she received through correspondence. They grew much closer when Emily visited New York in 1852.

It was not long before Rush College in Chicago accepted Emily as a medical student. She completed her studies while Elizabeth continued to expand her medical practice. Elizabeth tried again to work at a dispensary in New York but was told a lady doctor would not do. In 1853, she opened her own dispensary in a poor section of town in order to attend to poor women and children.

It was here, in the slums and unsanitary tenement buildings near Tompkins Square, that she saw the effects of unsanitary conditions. She began lecturing mothers about cleanliness and seeing that their children spend more time outdoors to benefit from fresh air. When she later moved into a house, she was still receiving abusive, anonymous letters for approaching the subject of hygiene with anyone who would listen.

Emily visited over a few summers to get practical experience at Bellevue Hospital as well as help Elizabeth with her patients. They worked well together and learned from each other, and Elizabeth sometimes despaired as to her future when Emily was away. In October 1854, she decided to adopt a daughter. Katharine Barry, a seven-year-old Irish child, became her daughter and treasured lifelong companion. Over the years, Katharine was Elizabeth's accountant, secretary, and housekeeper as well.

In that same year, Emily obtained her medical degree from Western Reserve College. Elizabeth was still in New York and met Marie Zakrzewska, a Pole who had been working as a midwife in Germany. She had been told to see Elizabeth Blackwell if she was interested in getting a medical degree. The timing was good, as Blackwell was in need of an assistant and at the same time could help Zakrzewska qualify for entrance into Western Reserve College.

At this time, Blackwell already had her sights set on opening her own hospital. With Marie's arrival, she felt she could count on three women in her endeavor: herself; Emily, who was getting very good clinical experience in Europe; and Marie when she graduated from medical school. Her private practice was still yielding a small income. She had moved her dispensary to a better location, and she obtained a charter to operate a hospital. Setbacks postponed her plans. In 1855 she had to close the dispensary for a time in order to transform it into the hospital she wanted, and she had difficulty raising the needed funds. She continued lecturing the public on sanitation and informing those who would listen of her plans. She continued to receive information on medical advances from Emily, information that she incorporated into her public lectures.

The first to help in her campaign for a hospital were her fellow Quakers, who raised money through their sewing skills. The money came very slowly at first, but when Marie got out of medical school with her diploma, she traveled in support of the cause and was also successful in raising money from some influential New Yorkers. Elizabeth and Marie bought a house to turn into a hospital. Emily went to England to further her studies, and when she returned, the three were ready to embark on their project.

On May 12, 1857, in honor of Florence Nightingale's birthday, the New York Infirmary for Women and Children officially opened with Dr. Marie as the resident physician, Dr. Emily as the surgeon, and Dr. Elizabeth as director. Within a month the beds were filled with patients from all backgrounds and speaking many different languages.

Troubles still lay ahead. Elizabeth continued her lectures for the money they continued to bring in. The infirmary was saved from burning down when the wind happened to change direction. A patient died of puerperal fever, and the relatives formed a mob outside, threatening the physicians and claiming the death was their fault. A similar incident occurred when a patient died from a ruptured appendix. This time a male physician who had been consulted on the case quieted the mob. Over time, people began to trust these women doctors.

One of Elizabeth's noble causes was to give female physicians fresh out of medical school a chance for some clinical practice, an opportunity that was rare in the United States when she had graduated from medical school. The infirmary thus became the great opportunity for many women physicians who had graduated from the New England Female Medical College in Boston and the Women's Medical College of Pennsylvania in Philadelphia, respectively. Elizabeth, Emily, and Marie held clinics for these new graduates, and later began training nurses. Blackwell was very particular about qualifications for the nurses' training program.

Although other members of their family were firmly behind the women's movement, Elizabeth and Emily remained distant from the cause, refusing to become a haven for the movement. They focused on establishing sound medical practices to prove themselves to the public. As the infirmary became well grounded and funded after a year of doubts, Blackwell looked to England, where she'd been asked to speak on women's progress in the medical field in the United States. She decided she could contribute to the cause of medical education for women in England, a contentious issue there. In 1859, she became the first woman in Great Britain accredited as a physician. Several prominent people, including Lady Byron, wanted Blackwell to stay in England and begin a teaching hospital there. Blackwell thought the idea was premature and wanted to go back to the United States and continue her work as a medical-education reformer.

She visited France and some of the mental institutions to which Dorothea Dix had drawn so much attention. She also visited Florence Nightingale, now ill but working toward her plans for the future Nightingale Training School for Nurses at St. Thomas's Hospital. Blackwell became a much-requested speaker on women's medical care and medical education. She was well respected also among poor mothers who needed her guidance.

On her return to New York, Blackwell found that Zakrzewska had left the infirmary to take a position in Boston only to find it didn't meet her expectations. She thus eventually founded the New England Hospital for Women and Children in 1862 and did very well in private practice.

The infirmary was still successful. Elizabeth and Emily obtained new quarters for the hospital and began making some headway financially. Elizabeth was not as interested in practicing medicine as in lecturing and educating the masses about hygiene. She also was ready to plan for adding a medical college for women to the hospital. The trustees of the infirmary were strongly supportive of this effort.

The plans for a medical college had to be postponed when the Civil War broke out. Elizabeth and Emily had both opposed slavery since their early days with their father and offered their infirmary in support of the Union's cause. They set about to prepare as many women as possible for the nursing field. They sent women who seemed suited for training to their infirmary, Bellevue, or New York Hospital. They would then go to Washington, where Dorothea Dix was the superintendent of nurses.

Elizabeth followed the progress of the war with great interest. Mary E. Walker, a surgeon, impressed her by managing to get to the front because of her rank of lieutenant in the army. Walker was captured at one point but was exchanged for a man fairly quickly. Both Blackwell sisters were working long hours at the infirmary as well as being involved with the Women's Central Relief Association, which met frequently at Cooper Union.

The Union Conscription Act of 1863, which made it possible for rich draftees to buy their way out of the federal army for $300 (leaving the burden of service to freed slaves and immigrants), caused riots in New York. The Blackwells were shocked by white patients' demands that black patients be excluded from the infirmary. Their infirmary, like orphanages and churches, served as a place for blacks to hide from the torture inflicted by some whites. The infirmary somehow survived the threats of destruction during the four-day period of the Draft Riots, which also were fueled by Northerners' fears that blacks who had been freed would take their jobs.

Elizabeth corresponded a little during this time with Elizabeth Garrett Anderson, who had received her apothecary license in England. Blackwell had inspired Anderson when she lectured in England, and Blackwell was gratified that progress was taking place in that country.

With the end of the Civil War, Blackwell realized that women had earned some recognition for their contributions in the medical field. Women still found it difficult, however, to find schools and hospitals that would accept them. She also felt that even long-established medical schools did not offer adequate academic and clinical training. She devised an educational curriculum for her infirmary that was extremely regimented with three years of medical schooling as the minimum in addition to rigorous clinical training. The trustees asked for a college charter and the college officially opened its doors in 1868.

Medical advances at the time included inoculations for some diseases. In opposition to most of her colleagues, however, Blackwell refused to support some kinds of inoculation. She was influenced in this view by the fact that a baby she had vaccinated had died. As she noted, "Although I have always continued to vaccinate when desired, I am strongly opposed to every form of inoculation of attenuated virus, as an unfortunate though well-meaning fallacy of medical prejudice" (Blackwell 1895, 240).

The infirmary began to be held in high regard as graduates obtained positions at prestigious colleges. The women's movement was also beginning to open new doors for women. At the same time, the struggle was continuing in England, and it was here that Elizabeth felt she could contribute to the cause. Upon arriving in England in 1869, she became very involved in social and moral reforms. She became very disturbed about the disparity between the wealthy and the poor, which drove her to continue education in public hygiene and the prevention of disease. She was well ahead of her time in seeing the worth of prevention as opposed to cure, her battle cry for the rest of her life.

While she continued her lectures, she formed the National Health Society in England, which began promoting public health and hygiene issues. Blackwell also took an interest in three other women who were in her field: Elizabeth Garrett Anderson, Sophia Jex-Blake, and Mary Putnam, who had taken her medical degree and was currently working at the infirmary in New York. Blackwell encouraged them all, corresponding all her life with women who needed her support.

Elizabeth's mother died in 1870, and although most of her remaining family was still in the United States, Elizabeth felt she was beginning to put down roots in England. She heard from Emily that the infirmary was doing very well and growing. She became an advocate of Christian Socialism because she believed the practice of medicine could cure many social ills. At this point, she considered health issues political in terms of benefitting the whole human race. She also believed that physical ailments could stem from mental distress.

She herself had health problems for several years, particularly in the 1870s. She struggled with this and finding the best climate in which to live was difficult, so she led a rather nomadic life. During this time, though, she felt she could reform through writing. Her book *Counsel to Parents on the Moral Education of Their Children in Relation to Sex* at first did not find a publisher, but she persisted. The book was eventually published and went through several editions. Blackwell also was appointed professor of gynecology at the London School of Medicine for Women in 1875. She continued to teach off and on there until 1907.

In 1878 she and her daughter traveled to France, and on return to England, they found a suitable house on the English Channel at Hastings. Her health improved, and she continued to campaign for public hygiene and moral reform. Numerous family members, friends, and physicians, as well as many male and female medical school students in England and graduates of her infirmary in New York, were guests in her new home.

Two of Blackwell's sisters, Marianne and Anna, came to live near her in England. They were both suffering from failing health. At this time, Elizabeth set out to free the local government of corruption, an effort that on occasion stirred up both Tories and Liberals. She also tried to have the brothels closed because of unsanitary conditions.

During the 1880s and 1890s, she was unwavering in fighting for her causes, and she wrote extensively from her lectures as well as kept up her correspondence. In the 1890s, some of her friends died. Then in 1900, her sister Anna died, followed in 1901 by Samuel and Ellen.

She did visit the United States again and saw that Cornell had absorbed her college in 1899; the infirmary was still growing and thriving. She was very pleased at the progress women had made in the medical field. As Dr. Cushier wrote of both Blackwells late in life, "What we should never forget is that the dignity, the culture, and the high moral standards which formed their character, finally prevailed in overcoming the existing prejudice, both within and outside the profession. By their standards, the status of women in medicine was determined" (Ross 1949, 291).

Blackwell returned to England knowing she would probably never see her friends or family in the United States again. In 1907 she fell down some stairs and became an invalid shortly thereafter. Her daughter was with her most of the time in her final days. She died on May 31, 1910, in Hastings.

See also: Anderson, Elizabeth Garrett; Blackwell, Emily; Jex-Blake, Sophia; Nightingale, Florence; Zakrzewska, Marie Elizabeth

References: Blackwell, Elizabeth, *Pioneer Work in Opening the Medical Profession to Women: Autobiographical Sketches*, London: Longmans, Green (1895); Ross, Ishbel, *Child of Destiny: The Life Story of the First Woman Doctor*, New York: Harper (1949); Snodgrass, Mary, *Historical Encyclopedia of Nursing*, Santa Barbara, CA: ABC-CLIO (1999).

Blackwell, Emily
1826–1910

Emily Blackwell obtained her M.D. from Western Reserve College in 1854 and founded the New York Infirmary for Women and Children with her sister, Elizabeth Blackwell. Often overshadowed by her older sister, Emily nevertheless was an excellent surgeon, physician, and educator of medical students. She enjoyed practicing medicine much more than Elizabeth; the two worked well together.

Emily was born February 3, 1826, in Counterslip near Bristol, England, to Samuel Blackwell and Hannah Lane. Her father had an important influence on her. He supported women's rights, was against slavery, and encouraged all his children to be active in society. He was also religious, studying the Bible and participating in daily prayers.

Being a Dissenter meant that Samuel Blackwell's children were not allowed to attend the Church of England schools, which were considered the best in the country. Aware of the high illiteracy rate and wanting all his children to have a good education, he decided to tutor them himself. Emily and her eight siblings were brought up by their father to study the same subjects together. He expected the same high standards from both the boys and the girls. Emily, like Elizabeth, felt the way her father did.

The Blackwell family left for the United States in 1832 when Emily was only five years old. Samuel suffered financial losses in New York, and in 1844, the family moved to Cincinnati, Ohio. There, the family associated with the Quakers, but Samuel was still very open about most social events. While Hannah worried about preparing her daughters for marriage, Emily, again like Elizabeth, thought about a career.

Emily was shy and timid but was very much influenced by her older sister and wanted to follow in her footsteps. She applied to several medical schools and was turned down by eleven before Rush Medical College in Chicago accepted her. She was unable to complete her degree there because the state medical board did not agree with Rush's decision to admit a woman to the school. Emily finished her studies at Western Reserve College in Cleveland; this school had just begun allowing women into its medical program.

She traveled to Europe to train with Sir James Young Simpson, who saw no reason that women should not practice medicine. From him, she gained invaluable experience in gynecology and obstetrics. He was also impressed with Emily's talent as a surgeon. She then attended clinics elsewhere in Europe to gain more experience.

When she returned to New York in 1856, she was ready to help Elizabeth and Dr. Marie Zakrzewska with the New York Infirmary for Women and Children, where she worked as a surgeon. The three collaborated well, and the beds filled quickly with patients.

After initial financial and other challenges, the infirmary thrived. Many female physicians just out of medical school came to gain clinical experience. Elizabeth, Marie, and Emily arranged clinics for the new students and later started training nurses.

Emily, like her sister, did not want the infirmary to become a center for the women's rights movement. Their most important objective was to establish sound medical practice and prove themselves to the public. In this stance, they were sometimes challenged by family members supportive of the movement. For example, two of her brothers were very active in the women's movement. Henry had married the feminist Lucy Stone, and Samuel was married to Antoinette Louisa Brown, the first ordained minister in the United States.

The infirmary survived the Civil War, and the three doctors obtained a college charter, their ultimate goal, in 1868. Elizabeth, who saw herself as a reformer and speaker on public hygiene, left for England in 1869, and Emily took the initiative in the infirmary.

Emily threw herself into her work for the next thirty years. She served as a teacher and administrator as well as a surgeon. She ran the infirmary and the medical school, strengthening the curriculum, until the school merged with Cornell in 1899.

Emily realized that the obstacles for women in medicine were not all within the education community: "Their troubles begin when they graduate. The walls are as high as ever when it comes to internships or hospital posts. Much as we have gained, it will take more than one generation to demonstrate to the full our scientific and social value" (Ross 1949, 281).

She retired in 1900, spending most of her retirement time going back and forth between her home in New Jersey and her summer cottage in Maine. She shared a house with her longtime partner, Dr. Elizabeth Cushier, who had been trained at the infirmary. Blackwell developed enterocolitis and passed away on September 7, 1910, shortly after her sister Elizabeth died.

See also: Blackwell, Elizabeth; Zakrzewska, Marie Elizabeth

References: Blackwell, Elizabeth, *Pioneer Work in Opening the Medical Profession to Women: Autobiographical Sketches*, New York: Source Book Press (1970); Ross, Ishbel, *Child of Destiny, the Life Story of the First Woman Doctor*, New York: Harper (1949).

Blanchfield, Florence Aby
1882–1971

Florence Blanchfield served as superintendent of the Army Nurse Corps (ANC) during both world wars and became the first woman to be regularly commissioned into the U.S. Regular Army in 1947. She worked diligently over the years to gain for women military nurses' status and recognition equal to that of male nurses.

Born in Shepherdstown, West Virginia, on April 1, 1882, she was one of eight children of Joseph Plunkett Blanchfield, a stonemason, and Mary Louvenia Anderson Blanchfield, a nurse. She wanted to be a nurse early in life. She was educated in both public and private schools in Walnut Springs and Oranda, Virginia. She attended the Southside Hospital Training School for Nurses in Pittsburgh, Pennsylvania, and graduated in 1906.

She then went to Baltimore and worked as a private-duty nurse while attending Dr. Howard Kelly's Sanitarium and Johns Hopkins University. In 1907 she supervised the operating room at Southside Hospital and the next year at Montefiore Hospital. She also worked at Suburban General Hospital in Bellevue, Pennsylvania, and later was the supervisor of nurses. In this capacity she was a leader in getting an approved school of nursing.

She took leave from the hospital during World War I to answer the call for army nurses. After serving in France, she returned briefly to Bellevue and then went back into the ANC in January 1920. At the time, nurses could gain in rank but did not receive the same pay as or have equal authority with males.

Blanchfield served in numerous locations throughout the United States and abroad. In 1935, after a tour of duty in China, she settled in Washington, D.C., and held a number of positions at the ANC over the next twelve years. Nurses in the corps usually entered as a second lieutenant and remained at that rank their entire career. Blanchfield, however, received a promotion in 1939 and held the rank of captain when she worked in the capacity of assistant to the superintendent, at that time Julia Flikke. Both women saw the need to expand the ANC, particularly with the outbreak of World War II in Europe.

Blanchfield also wanted to gain permanent status for the ANC within the army. The best way to do this was to gain commissions in the regular army for women. After a sustained effort, in 1942 both Flikke and Blanchfield received temporary commissions as colonel and lieutenant colonel, respectively. It took ten years and a congressional bill, however, before they received adequate pay.

Blanchfield was appointed superintendent of the ANC upon Flikke's retirement in 1943. She concentrated on strengthening the ANC and providing adequate clinical experiences for nurses who would serve in wartime. She also moved nurses closer to soldiers on the battlefield to make sure they received immediate care after being injured and changed the nursing uniforms to combat fatigues when appropriate.

Blanchfield continued to fight for full military rank during the war, and in 1947 the Army-Navy Nurse Act gave women nurses equal status in the military with equal pay and promotion possibilities. It also created the ANC within the regular army. On July 18, 1947, General Dwight D. Eisenhower commissioned Blanchfield as a lieutenant colonel in the army.

She communicated over the years with nurses in the field in order to learn about their experiences and thus improve training for army nurses. Partly due to her efforts, special training programs grew in anesthesia, neuropsychiatric nursing, air evacuation, obstetrics, and pediatrics, among others. Blanchfield retired from active duty in 1947 after twenty-nine years of service. She never married and in her later years lived in Arlington, Virginia, with a sister and brother-in-law. She died at Walter Reed Medical Center on May 12, 1971, from atherosclerotic cardiac disease and was buried with full honors at Arlington National Cemetery in Virginia.

References: Bullough, Vern L., Olga Maranjian Church, and Alice Stein, *American Nurs-* *ing: A Biographical Dictionary*, New York: Garland (1988); Sherrow, Victoria, *Women and the Military: An Encyclopedia*, Santa Barbara, CA: ABC-CLIO (1996).

Bocchi, Dorothea
1390–1436

Dorothea Bocchi was a well-respected professor of medicine and philosophy at the University of Bologna. Appointed to succeed her father, she taught at a time in Italy when women were afforded the same educational opportunities as men. In the fourteenth century, Italy led the world in the field of medicine.

References: Hurd-Mead, Kate Campbell, *A History of Women in Medicine from the Earliest Times to the Beginning of the Nineteenth Century*, Haddam, CT: Haddam Press (1938).

Boivin, Marie Anne Victoire Gillain
1773–1841

Marie Anne Boivin was a French midwife whose publications on childbirth and pregnancy became very popular textbooks in France and Germany. She invented a new pelvimeter and a vaginal speculum and was the first to listen to a fetal heart using a stethoscope.

Born in Montreuil and educated by nuns, she married Louis Boivin in 1797. After her husband died early in the marriage, leaving her with one daughter, she continued her medical training with Madame Lachapelle until she earned her degree and then went to Versailles. When her daughter was killed, she returned to work at the Hospice de la Maternité in Bordeaux with Lachapelle, her good friend and teacher. She and Lachapelle stressed that midwives should be trained and licensed and know how to handle difficult pregnancies.

In 1827 Boivin received an honorary M.D. from the University of Marburg, Germany. Her goal had been to obtain a French med-

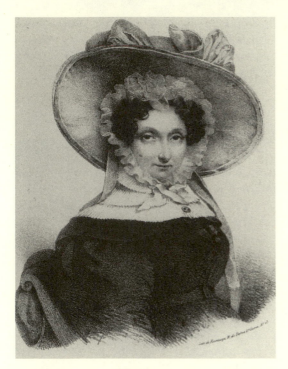

Marie Anne Victoire Gillain Boivin (de Fonrouge/ U.S. National Library of Medicine)

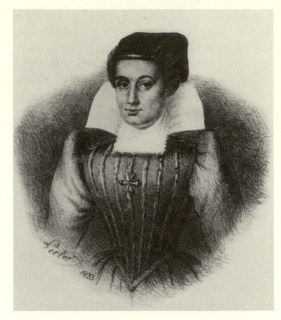

Louise Bourgeois (Leclos/U.S. National Library of Medicine)

ical degree, but she could not obtain admission to the Academy of Medicine in Paris. She died in poverty.

References: Hurd-Mead, Kate Campbell, *A History of Women in Medicine from the Earliest Times to the Beginning of the Nineteenth Century,* Haddam, CT: Haddam Press (1938); Ogilvie, Marilyn, and Joy Harvey, eds., *The Biographical Dictionary of Women in Science: Pioneering Lives from Ancient Times to the Mid-20th Century,* New York: Routledge (2000).

Bourgeois, Louise
1563–1636

Louise Bourgeois was an obstetrician and gynecologist as well as a surgeon in France. Her work *Observations,* published in 1610, was a landmark contribution to the knowledge of childbirth.

Born in Hainault at Mons of well-to-do parents, she married an army surgeon and had three children. She stayed with her par-

ents in Paris when her husband served during wartime. When Paris was devastated by troops of Henry of Navarre (later King Henry IV), her family's property was totally destroyed, and Louise had to take work as a seamstress. Disliking the work, she decided to become a midwife, training with Ambroise Pare, a gifted surgeon and very knowledgeable in the field of obstetrics.

At this time in France, prospective midwives had to pass a licensing examination. Bourgeois passed her exams and obtained her diploma on November 12, 1598. She achieved early success, with members of the aristocracy becoming some of her patients. Eventually she achieved the title of Royal Midwife after attending to three births of Queen Marie de Medici. The first baby, in 1601, later became King Louis XIII.

(Initially King Henry IV had wanted another midwife, but the Queen rejected her because she had delivered for his mistresses.)

After King Henry IV was murdered and Queen Marie de Medici no longer needed midwife services, Bourgeois continued to practice her profession among the aristocracy. She lost some credibility when a fever took the life of the Duchesse de Montpensier. Following this event, her practice declined and she spent much of the rest of her life writing her book *Observations*. She died in 1636.

References: Hatcher, John, "Mme Louise Bourgeois—Royal Midwife and Remarkable Character," *Midwives Chronicle and Nursing Notes* (January 1971); Hurd-Mead, Kate Campbell, *A History of Women in Medicine from the Earliest Times to the Beginning of the Nineteenth Century*, Haddam, CT: Haddam Press (1938); Ogilvie, Marilyn, and Joy Harvey, eds., *The Biographical Dictionary of Women in Science: Pioneering Lives from Ancient Times to the Mid-20th Century*, New York: Routledge (2000).

Britton, Mary E.
1858–1925

Mary Britton was the first black female physician in Kentucky, serving both blacks and whites in the Lexington area. She attended Berea College and taught for a while in Lexington. She was better known for her writing in newspapers throughout the eastern United States.

Britton was born to Henry and Laura Britton in 1858. Her father was half-Spanish and half-Indian; her mother was born of a white slave owner and a slave mistress. She was one of the first free blacks to graduate from college and pursue a career after the American Civil War of 1861–1865. Her older sister, Julia, was a gifted teacher and musician who became the first black teacher in Berea.

Britton taught school for a while before deciding on a medical career. She trained at Battle Creek Sanitarium in Michigan, which had been established as a health-reform institute by the Seventh Day Adventists. She also studied at the American Missionary Medical College in Chicago, graduating in 1903. She became a proponent of alternative medicine, vegetarianism, hydrotherapy, massage, metaphysics, and phrenology. She was an effective speaker on women's rights and a prominent and respected black woman leader of the times. She died in 1925.

References: Lucas, Marion Brunson, *A History of Blacks in Kentucky*, vol. 1, Frankfort: Kentucky Historical Society (1992); Wade-Gayles, Gloria, "Britton, Mary E.," *Black Women in America: An Historical Encyclopedia*, vol. 1, Brooklyn, NY: Carlson (1993).

Brown, Dorothy Lavinia
1919–

Dorothy Brown is the first black female in the American South to become a surgeon. Her work in general surgery and education has forged a path for future generations of black female physicians and surgeons.

Born in Philadelphia on January 7, 1919, she was taken by her mother to an orphanage in Troy, New York. She stayed there for the next twelve years. During this time, her mother tried several times to take her back, but Dorothy ran away each time to return to the Troy orphanage. After her tonsils were removed when she was five, she decided to become a doctor. She attended school in Troy and, when she was fifteen, went to live with foster parents Samuel and Lola Redmon.

She graduated at the top of her high school class and went on to earn her A.B. degree in 1941 from Bennett College in Greensboro, North Carolina. Her time there was difficult because even though she had a scholarship from the Women's Division of the Methodist Church, college administrators didn't feel she was a suitable candidate for their school. They discouraged her from taking science courses and from going to medical school, believing teaching would suit her better. After graduation she worked at the Rochester Army Ordinance Department during World War II and then entered medical school at Meharry Medical College in Nashville, Tennessee.

She obtained her M.D. degree in 1948 and then served a one-year internship at Harlem Hospital. In order to become a surgeon, she went back to Nashville to complete a five-year residency at Meharry and Hubbard Hospitals. She became an assistant professor of surgery in 1955 and in 1959 became the first black female surgeon to become a fellow of the American College of Surgeons.

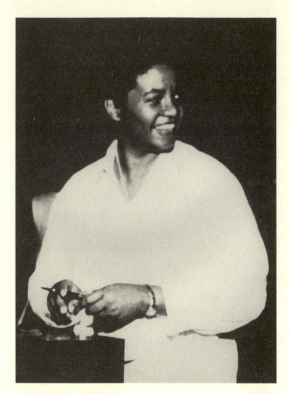

Dorothy Lavinia Brown (Meharry Medical College/U.S. National Library of Medicine)

mons, Vivian Ovelton, *Blacks in Science and Medicine,* New York: Hemisphere (1990).

Brown, Edith Mary
1864–1956

Born on March 24, 1864, in Whitehaven, Cumbria, England, Brown became a physician who helped found the North India School of Medicine for Christian Women in Ludhiana.

Edith developed an interest in medicine and missions because her older sister was a missionary. She earned a degree at Cambridge University and taught science in order to earn money to further her education with a medical degree. She studied medicine in London and gained her certification in Scotland in 1891, as women could not be certified in England at the time.

She immediately went to India and was shocked at the condition of health care in that country. She worked to educate and heal women and children, and became increasingly interested in educating midwives. Eventually she saw a need for a medical school for Indian women and set about organizing one with several cooperating societies, including the Baptist Zenana mission. The North India School of Medicine for Christian Women opened in 1894.

After only two years, the government recognized the college and its importance to the country. In 1931 Brown was made Dame Commander of the Order of the British Empire (DBE) for her meritorious work. Brown retired to Kashmir in 1941 and died in Srinagar on December 6, 1956. The school continued to thrive, beginning to train men in 1951, and awarding medical degrees by 1953.

In 1956, a young pregnant girl offered Brown her baby, and Brown became the first single woman to adopt a child (Lola Denise) in Tennessee.

Brown served as chief of surgery at Riverside Hospital in Nashville from 1960 to 1983. She also built up her own private practice despite skepticism about black female physicians. In 1966, Brown served in the Tennessee legislature for a two-year term, becoming the first black woman to earn such an honor in Tennessee.

She has received many awards and honorary degrees and is a fellow of the American College of Surgeons. She is also a life member of the National Association for the Advancement of Colored People (NAACP).

References: "Bachelor Mother," *Ebony* (September 1958); *Notable Black American Scientists,* Detroit: Gale Research (1998); Organ, Claude H., and Margaret M. Kosiba, *Century of Black Surgeons: The U.S.A. Experience,* Norman, OK: Transcript Press (1987); Sam-

References: Haines, Catharine M. C., and Helen Stevens, *International Women in Science: A Biographical Dictionary to 1950,* Santa Barbara, CA: ABC-CLIO (2001); Murray, Jocelyn, "Brown, Edith Mary," *Biographical Dictionary of Christian Missions,* New York: Macmillan (1998).

Brown, Rachel Fuller
1898–1980

Along with Elizabeth Hazen, Rachel Brown was responsible for discovering the first antifungal antibiotic that could be used safely on humans. This biomedical discovery was considered by most to be the most important since Sir Alexander Fleming discovered penicillin in 1928. She and Hazen subsequently donated all their royalties from the patent to scientific research, making a huge financial contribution to science.

Brown was born on November 23, 1898, in Springfield, Massachusetts. Her father, George Hamilton Brown, worked in real estate and insurance. Her mother was Annie Fuller. When she was very young, the family moved to Webster Groves, Missouri, just outside of St. Louis. She had one younger brother, Sumner Jerome, and when her father left the family in 1912, her mother returned to Springfield and worked to support them. Brown graduated from high school and went on to attend Mount Holyoke College, where her education was funded by Henrietta Dexter, a close friend of her grandmother's. Brown later paid Dexter back for the loan.

Her primary interest had been history, but she developed an interest in chemistry at Holyoke and double-majored in history and chemistry, receiving her degree in 1920. She then obtained a master's degree in organic chemistry from the University of Chicago. After graduating, she worked for three years at the Frances Shimer School near Chicago, teaching physics and chemistry.

Unsatisfied with teaching, she returned to the University of Chicago to work on her Ph.D. in organic chemistry with a minor in bacteriology. She completed her studies short of her oral exams in 1926 and went to work for the New York Department of Health's Division of Laboratories and Research in Albany, New York. It was in Albany that she met Dorothy Wakerley, her lifetime companion. Brown did not obtain her degree until seven years later.

Brown's work at first focused on the bacteria that cause pneumonia; this work helped lead to a vaccine for the disease. Later she worked on the causes of syphilis. Her long-distance collaboration with Hazen (Brown was in Albany and Hazen in New York City), an expert on fungus, began in 1948. Penicillin had been discovered and was able to cure many infections, but fungal infections were a serious problem.

In 1950 Brown and Hazen discovered the first antifungal agent that could be used safely on humans. E. R. Squibb and Sons developed the method for mass production of the agent, called Nystatin, and it became available to the public in 1954.

Nystatin proved to have many uses. It can be used to treat Dutch elm disease and fight molds in foods and was used after a flood in Italy to save priceless artworks.

Brown received numerous awards in her lifetime. She was also a sought-after speaker who lectured on antibiotics and cautioned against their unnecessary use. When she retired in 1968, she had served the state of New York for forty-two years and had taken only two sick days. She died on January 14, 1980, at her home in Albany.

See also: Hazen, Elizabeth Lee
References: Baldwin, Richard S., *The Fungus Fighters*, Ithaca, NY: Cornell University Press (1981); *Notable Twentieth-Century Scientists*, Detroit: Gale Research (1995); Vare, Ethlie Ann, and Greg Ptacek, *Mothers of Invention: From the Bra to the Bomb: Forgotten Women and Their Unforgettable Ideas*, New York: Morrow (1988).

Brundtband, Gro Harlem
1939–

Known more as a politician and environmentalist, Gro Harlem Brundtband is the first woman to head the World Health Organization (WHO), based in Geneva, where she is concerned with raising public awareness of international health issues and bringing the alleviation of poverty to the forefront of WHO's goals.

In 1998 she was elected to the World Health Assembly after being nominated by the executive board of WHO.

She was born in Oslo, Norway, April 20, 1939. Her father, Gudmund Harlem, was a physician, political activist, and major influence in her life. She married Arne Olav and had four children. She earned her medical degree in 1963 from the University of Oslo and in 1965 added a master of public health degree from Harvard University.

Brundtband was a physician for ten years in the Norway Public Health System. She served as a medical officer at the Norwegian Directorate of Health and later with Oslo's Board of Health. Her work included cancer prevention and childhood diseases. She became the director of health services for Oslo's schoolchildren while raising a family of her own.

At age forty-one, Brundtband became prime minister of Norway, a position she held for over ten years. She is the first female to hold the post and the youngest in Norway's history. In her memoirs, *Dramatic Years*, she criticizes the Norwegian health service for being too slow to import drugs that could help alleviate psychological illnesses like that of her manic-depressive son, Joergen, who committed suicide in 1992.

References: Borchert, Thomas, "Norway's Former Premier Puts Son's Suicide at Center of Memoirs," *Deutsche Presse-Agentur* (24 November 1998); Kaiser, Jocelyn, "WHO Gets New Head," *Science* 279, no. 5351 (30 January 1998); WHO home page, http://www.who.int/.

Budzinski-Tylicka, Justine
Late nineteenth century

Justine Budzinski-Tylicka became one of the first female physicians in Poland. She received her medical training at the University of Paris and returned to Poland to work in her country's clinics and hospitals. She advocated birth control and was against legalized prostitution. She was a strong supporter of women's rights.

References: Lovejoy, Esther Pohl, *Women Doctors of the World*, New York: Macmillan (1957).

C

Calverley, Eleanor Jane Taylor
1887–1968

Eleanor Calverley was the first woman physician to work in Kuwait. A medical missionary, she gained the trust of Arab women who were forbidden to see male physicians.

Calverley was born in Woodstock, New Jersey, on March 24, 1887; her parents were William Lewis and Jane Long Hillman Taylor. She was educated in the public schools of New Haven, Connecticut, and later attended the Women's Medical College of Pennsylvania, obtaining her medical degree in 1908.

She married Edwin E. Calverley, a missionary and preacher, on September 6, 1909, and together they trained for work in Arabia. They traveled to Kuwait in 1911, and she opened a small dispensary connected to her home so that Kuwaiti women, among others, could seek medical care. "We saw both wealth and poverty among the Arab and Persian populations of Kuwait. Some Persian families were rich; but there were others, recently immigrated from Persia, who had no homes except the sand beside a boat drawn up on the shore. Their only protection was a curtain of sacking, fastened above them to the side of the boat and pegged down into the sand. Freed African slaves, deprived of their former masters' support, were also often destitute. Of such we could not require any fee for medical service" (Calverley 1958, 74).

She and her husband spent many years in Kuwait. In 1919 a women's hospital opened there under her leadership. She had three daughters: Grace, Elisabeth, and Eleanor. Calverley died on December 22, 1968, in Hartford, Connecticut.

References: Calverley, Eleanor T., *My Arabian Days and Nights*, New York: Crowell (1958); *National Cyclopedia of American Biography*, vol. 57, Clifton, NJ: James T. White (1977).

Canady, Alexa Irene
1950–

Alexa Canady is the first female African American in the United States to become a neurosurgeon. She has held various teaching positions over the years and is currently the director of neurosurgery at Children's Hospital of Michigan.

Born in Lansing, Michigan, on November 7, 1950, Canady was the second oldest in a family of four and the only girl. Her father, Clinton Canady, was a dentist, and her mother, Elizabeth Hortense Golden, worked in various educational occupations and was the first black elected to the Lansing Board of Education. She was a Fisk University graduate and fostered a love for learning in Alexa and her three brothers.

Alexa did well in school and graduated from high school with honors. She then went on to the University of Michigan to major in mathematics. She soon discovered she did not have a commitment to the subject despite good grades. She participated in a minority health-careers program at Michigan and worked with Art Bloom, a pediatrician and geneticist, and decided to pursue a career in medicine.

She graduated with a B.S. in 1971 and entered medical school at the University of Michigan with the initial intention of becoming an internist. She earned her M.D. in 1975 and proceeded to the Yale New Haven Hospital for an internship in 1975–1976. She was later admitted to the Department of Neurosurgery at the University of Minnesota and became the first black female resident there.

In 1981 she continued her resident training under Luis Schut at the University of Pennsylvania and the Children's Hospital of Philadelphia.

She returned to Michigan in 1982 to take a position with the Henry Ford Hospital in Detroit as both a teacher and a neurosurgeon. In 1987 she became the director of neurosurgery at Children's Hospital of Michigan and has received much credit for making the hospital's neurosurgery department one of the best. She married George Davis in 1988. Canady credits affirmative action and other programs emanating from the civil rights era in helping her to achieve her goals. She mentors young people of color in following the profession of their choice.

References: Lanker, Brian, *I Dream a World: Portraits of Black Women Who Changed the World*, New York: Stewart, Tabori, and Chang (1989); *Notable Twentieth-Century Scientists*, Detroit: Gale Research (1995); Rich, Mari, "Canady, Alexa," *Current Biography* 61 no. 8 (August 2000): 11–15.

Chevandier Law of 1892

Passed in France, the Chevandier Law of 1892 was intended to keep unlicensed physicians from practicing medicine. It gave exception to mothers of families as long as they practiced medicine in the home. Public schools were also allowed to teach women basic hygiene and first aid techniques. As a result of the law, conflicts arose over "domestic" and "professional" medicine. Some male physicians of the day objected that the law would encourage women to practice medicine without a license outside of the home. The French Republic, however, was concerned about depopulation and the health of its citizens. The government determined that better health care from birth was more advantageous than stimulating an increase in births and set out to define in an amended law which aspects of health care women could legally practice in the home.

References: Lacy, Cherilyn, "Science or Savoir-Faire? Domestic Hygiene and Medicine in Girls' Public Education during the Early Third French Republic, 1882–1914," *Proceedings of the Annual Meeting of the Western Society for French History* 24 (1997): 25–37.

Chinn, May Edward
1896–1980

May Chinn was one of the first black female physicians in New York City. Her work in early cancer detection helped in the development of the Pap smear. She was the first black female to graduate from Bellevue Hospital Medical College and the first black female physician to intern at Harlem Hospital. After her internship, she was denied privileges at all hospitals until 1940. She persisted on her own and by the time of her death was a well-respected physician.

Born in Great Barrington, Massachusetts, on April 15, 1896, Chinn was the only child of William Lafayette Chinn and Lulu Ann Evans. Her father had escaped from slavery on a Virginia plantation when he was eleven years old, and her mother was born on an Indian reservation near Norfolk. She grew up in New York City, where her mother sent her to boarding school.

After developing osteomyelitis, Chinn had to leave school and lived with her mother on the estate of a wealthy white family, where her mother worked. While being treated for the disease, she studied and developed an interest in music through attending concerts with the white children of the family. She later gave piano lessons to youngsters.

Chinn attended Morris High School but dropped out in order to help her family by taking a factory job. Later, with her mother's encouragement, she took a high school equivalency test. She did well and entered Columbia University Teachers' College in 1917. After a year there, she changed her major from music to science. She graduated in 1921 and entered Bellevue Hospital Medical College, where she graduated in 1926. She interned at Harlem Hospital.

After being denied work in hospitals, she opened her own practice near the Edgecombe Sanitarium. In exchange for living and office space, she answered the all-night emergency calls for the group of black physicians who owned her space and the sanitarium. Because she saw so many patients in the advanced stages of cancer, she became interested in cancer research. She also continued her studies, receiving a master's degree in public health from Columbia in 1933. During this time she gained permission to do biopsies at Memorial Hospital under George Papanicolaou, who later developed the Pap smear. Eventually, black physicians who found out about her access to Memorial Hospital began to send biopsy specimens directly to her. Without an official affiliation with Memorial Hospital, she had the work done in secret.

In 1944 she joined the staff of Strang Clinic, a cancer-detection center affiliated with Memorial Hospital and New York Infirmary Hospital. She stayed there twenty-nine years. She became a legend in Harlem as a woman who overcame many racial and gender barriers in order to provide health care to the poor.

References: Clark, Darlene, Elsa Barkley Brown, and Rosalyn Terborg-Penn, *Black Women in America: An Historical Encyclopedia,* Brooklyn, NY: Carlson (1993); Hayden, Robert C., *American National Biography,* New York: Oxford University Press (1999); "May Edward Chinn," http://www.sdsc.edu/ ScienceWomen/chinn.html.

Claypole, Edith Jane
1870–1915

Edith Claypole did early research in infectious diseases in order to distinguish be-

tween tuberculosis and infections that resembled it. Her work in histology and hematology aided future researchers in their explorations.

Claypole was born along with a twin sister, Agnes, on January 1, 1870, in Bristol, England. Their mother died a short time after the births. When her father remarried, he took his new wife and daughters to Akron, Ohio, where he had a teaching job. He had a love of science, and he and his second wife taught the girls at home.

Edith majored in biology and graduated from Buchtel College in Akron in 1892. She went on to Cornell to study for an advanced degree. She taught physiology and histology at Wellesley College in Massachusetts upon graduation and later became interested in pathology and medicine. While in medical school at the University of California (UC) at Los Angeles, she worked for a group of physicians as a pathologist. As a result, by the time she received her M.D. she was knowledgeable about vaccines and bacterial cultures.

She continued her pathology work after graduation, volunteering at the University of California, Berkeley, because she could not find an academic position for pay in 1904. The university offered her a research associate position in 1912, and she was able to use the laboratory facilities there for her research.

She began to study tuberculosis and the bacteria associated with it. The bacteria also caused other infections, and Claypole developed a test that was helpful in determining the differences in infections that afflicted humans.

When World War I broke out, she and others began working on a vaccine for typhoid fever for the British and French troops in Europe. Although she was vaccinated against typhoid, over the course of a few years the exposures to it were so great that she died from it in 1915 at the early age of forty-five.

References: Bailey, Martha J., *American Women in Science: A Biographical Dictionary,* Santa Barbara, CA: ABC-CLIO (1994); Shearer, Benjamin F., and Barbara S.

Shearer, *Notable Women in the Life Sciences: A Biographical Dictionary*, Westport, CT: Greenwood Press (1996).

Cleveland, Emeline Horton
1829–1878

A respected physician and educator, Emeline Cleveland was one of the first female surgeons to remove ovarian tumors. She was the second female dean of the Women's Medical College of Pennsylvania (WMCP) and created new educational opportunities for women while strengthening the curriculum at her college.

Born in Ashford, Connecticut, on September 22, 1829, Cleveland grew up in Madison County, New York. Her parents were Chauncey Horton and Amanda Chaffee Horton. Her father set up a school on their farm, and she received her early education from tutors. Her father died early, and she taught in order to earn money sufficient for a college education.

In 1850 she enrolled at Oberlin College in Ohio and graduated in 1853. Interested in becoming a missionary and a physician, she went to the Female Medical College of Pennsylvania (renamed the Women's Medical College of Pennsylvania in 1867), graduating in 1855. She had married the Reverend Giles Butler Cleveland in 1854; they had both intended a life of missionary work, but his poor health changed their course.

She started a small medical practice near her home in New York and the next year was asked to teach at WMCP. Before long, she became the chair of anatomy and physiology. In 1860 she went to Paris for specialty training at the School of Obstetrics at La Maternité. Because WMCP needed a better setting for its students to gain clinical experience, she also visited various hospitals to learn more about hospital administration. Once Cleveland returned, she became the chief resident of Women's Hospital, which collaborated with the Women's Medical College of Pennsylvania to provide clinical training for medical students. Cleveland also served the college as a professor of obstetrics and gynecology.

Cleveland had a son in 1865. In 1872 she succeeded Ann Preston as dean of WMCP. She resigned two years later due to poor health. She suffered from tuberculosis and died in Philadelphia on December 8, 1878. At the time she was working for the Department of the Insane at Philadelphia Hospital.

See also: Medical College of Pennsylvania; Preston, Ann
References: DeFiore, Jayne Crumpler, "Cleveland, Emeline Horton," *American National Biography*, vol. 5, New York: Oxford University Press (1999); Peitzman, Steven J., *A New and Untried Course: Women's Medical College and Medical College of Pennsylvania, 1850–1998*, New Brunswick, NJ: Rutgers University Press (2000).

Cobb, Jewel Plummer
1924–

Jewel Cobb has contributed to the field of cell biology in her research on how drugs affect cancer and on the skin pigment melanin and the cause of melanoma, an increasing skin cancer. Cobb has also supported numerous programs throughout her career to encourage young students, especially minorities, to enter the science field.

Cobb was born on January 17, 1924, the only child of Frank Plummer, a physician and graduate of Rush College, and Carriebel Plummer, who taught in the public schools. Cobb came into contact with other professionals through her parents, whom she admired. Like her father, she enjoyed science, and she did well in school, often facing racism.

While at the University of Michigan, she encountered more racism in the dormitories and local businesses and transferred to Talladega College in Alabama, where she graduated in 1944. She went on to New York University on a fellowship that lasted six years. There in 1947, she earned a master's degree in cell physiology and in 1950, a Ph.D. She obtained a fellowship from the National Cancer Institute and began her cell research at the Harlem Hospital Cancer Research Foundation.

She held several university positions following her time at the research foundation, first at the University of Illinois Medical School. In 1954 she married Roy Raul Cobb and returned to the Harlem Hospital Cancer Research Foundation. She had a son, Roy Johnathan Cobb, in 1957. She then worked at New York University, Hunter College, and Sarah Lawrence College. During this time she continued in her research on melanoma and in 1960 published a five-year cytological study.

She then went to Connecticut College to become dean and professor of zoology. In 1976 she became dean and professor of biology at Douglass College of Rutgers University. From 1981 until 1990 she served as president of California State University at Fullerton. In all positions she held, she assisted with program development for underrepresented ethnic groups.

References: *Notable Black American Scientists*, Detroit: Gale Research (1998); Shearer, Benjamin F., and Barbara S. Shearer, *Notable Women in the Life Sciences: A Biographical Dictionary*, Westport, CT: Greenwood Press (1996).

Cole, Rebecca
1846–1922

The second black woman in the United States to graduate from medical school and become a physician, Rebecca Cole devoted over fifty years to the health care of women and children during a time when women of any color were not well accepted as physicians. She worked in patients' homes, in the sparsely furnished clinics of the post–Civil War era, and into the twentieth century.

Born on March 16, 1846, in Philadelphia, she had four siblings. She taught school after graduating from the Institute for Colored Youth (currently known as Cheyney University). A year later she entered the Women's Medical College of Pennsylvania, where in 1867 she was the first black to graduate.

She went to work as a visiting practitioner with Elizabeth Blackwell at the New York Infirmary for Women and Children. She had a great interest in helping poor women and children, so Blackwell assigned her to the slum areas of New York City. Cole worked in harsh conditions, teaching women and children proper hygiene and basic medical care, and teaching mothers how to better care for their infants.

After several years she ventured to Columbia, South Carolina, and opened a private practice, later moving to Washington, D.C., to work as the superintendent for the Government House for Children and Old Women. Later she moved back to her birthplace of Philadelphia and opened a practice while coordinating a medical and legal directory for the poor with Charlotte Abby, another physician in Philadelphia. She died on August 14, 1922.

See Also: Crumpler, Rebecca Lee
References: Krapp, Kristine M., ed., *Notable Black American Scientists*, Detroit: Gale Research (1999); Sterling, Dorothy, ed., *We Are Your Sisters: Black Women in the Nineteenth Century*, New York: W. W. Norton (1984).

Comnena, Anna
1083–1148

Anna Comnena ran the huge hospital her father built in Constantinople. He was Alexius I, emperor of the Romans, and thus she was a Byzantine princess and well educated. She taught various aspects of medicine in his hospital as well as practiced medicine in other hospitals and in orphan asylums and attended her father during his last illness. She was an expert on gout.

She is better known for her historical writing, a massive fifteen-volume work about her father's reign titled the *Alexiad*. The work provides insight into the period in which she lived, although some of the chronology is incorrect.

She married Nicephorus Bryennius and, along with her mother, tried to persuade her father, even on his deathbed, to disinherit her brother, John II, in favor of Nicephorus. Her father refused, so after John ascended to the throne, she plotted against him. She failed and had to retire to a convent. This is where she spent the rest of her days and wrote the *Alexiad*.

References: Buckler, Georgina, *Anna Comnena: A Study*, London: Oxford University Press (1929); Hurd-Mead, Kate Campbell, *History of Women in Medicine from the Earliest Times to the Beginning of the Nineteenth Century*, Haddam, CT: Haddam Press (1938); Ogilvie, Marilyn, and Joy Harvey, eds., *The Biographical Dictionary of Women in Science: Pioneering Lives from Ancient Times to the Mid-20th Century*, New York: Routledge (2000).

Comstock Act of 1873

Passed by the U.S. Congress, the Comstock Act of 1873 banned the distribution of literature on birth control. It has been used widely over the years to censor the mails, limit contraceptive information, and prosecute publishers, physicians, social reformers, and women's rights advocates who violate it. The major architect behind the law was Anthony Comstock, a well-known crusader against obscenity, pornography, and literature or personal conduct considered by him to be immoral.

The interpretations of the act have been broad over the years, violating human rights and personal liberties in many instances. Officially called the Act for the Suppression of Trade in, and Circulation of, Obscene Literature and Articles of Immoral Use, it was meant to punish those who

> shall sell, or lend or give away, or in any manner exhibit, or shall offer to sell, or to lend, or to give away, or in any manner to exhibit, or shall otherwise publish or offer to publish in any manner, or shall have in his possession, for any such purpose or purposes, any obscene book, pamphlet, paper, writing, advertisement, circular, print, picture, drawing or other representation, figure, or image on or of paper or other material, or any cast, instrument, or other article of an immoral nature, or any drug or medicine, or any article whatever, for the prevention of conception, or for causing unlawful abortion, or shall advertise the same for sale, or shall write or print, or cause to be written or printed, any card, circular, book pamphlet, advertisement, or notice of any kind, stating when, where, how, or of whom, or by what means, any of the articles in this section hereinbefore mentioned, can be purchased or obtained, or shall manufacture, draw, or print, or in any wise make any of such articles. (*U.S. Statutes* 1873, 598–599)

Violation of the act was a misdemeanor.

Comstock was appointed a special agent of the U.S. Postal Service in order to enforce the law. His methods were extreme, constantly entrapping criminals, prosecuting without mercy, and writing vociferously on the vices of society. He intended to rid society of everything and all pieces of information that could corrupt youth. He abhorred the feminists and women's rights advocates such as Margaret Sanger and persecuted them. Many influential New Englanders, such as Morris Jesup and William E. Dodge, supported him. The law and his efforts inhibited the distribution of birth-control information for women who desired it. It also prevented physicians from distributing contraceptive devices and information. The act is still on the books and continues to be controversial.

References: Foer, Albert A., "Heroes of the First Amendment," *Washington Post*, sec. 10 (16 November 1997): 4; *U.S. Statutes at Large and Proclamations of the United States of America*, vol. 17, *1871–1873*, Boston: Little, Brown: (1873): 598–600.

Conley, Frances Krauskopf
1940–

Frances Conley became the first tenured neurosurgeon in the United States and brought international attention to the gender discrimination she faced for thirty years at Stanford when she resigned her position for several months in 1991. She continues to fight for gender equity in education.

Born on August 12, 1940, in Palo Alto, California, to Konrad Bates and Kathryn McCune Krauskopf, Conley attended Bryn Mawr College for two years and then transferred to Stanford University. She received a B.A. in 1962, an M.D. in 1966, and an M.S. in 1986, all from Stanford. She married Phillip R. Conley in 1963.

A gifted neurosurgeon, Conley rose in the ranks at Stanford and became a tenured associate professor of neurosurgery in 1988. Unwilling to stay after a male colleague she considered sexist was appointed department head, she resigned and charged the university with sexual harassment. Other Stanford women who had been reticent to speak up before Conley went public came forward with similar complaints. Stanford had to seriously study the issues she raised, but never ruled on the matter. In her 1998 book *Walking Out on the Boys,* Conley details the conduct of some of her male colleagues that she considered unethical. She feels women have made very little progress since the 1960s with the exception that more women are in the field.

References: Barinaga, Marcia, "Sexism Charged by Stanford Physician," *Science* 252, no. 5012 (14 June 1991): 1484; Conley, Frances K., *Walking Out on the Boys,* New York: Farrar, Straus and Giroux (1998); Leslie, Connie, and Barbara Kantrowitz, "Showing Its Age," *Newsweek* 118, no. 15 (7 October 1991): 54–58.

Cori, Gerty Theresa Radnitz
1896–1957

Gerty Cori, along with her husband and another researcher, won the Nobel Prize in 1947 in physiology or medicine for their work on sugar and the enzymes that convert glycogen to sugar. The Coris shared the Nobel Prize with Bernardo Alberto Houssay.

Born in Prague on August 15, 1896, Cori was the daughter of Otto Radnitz, a fairly

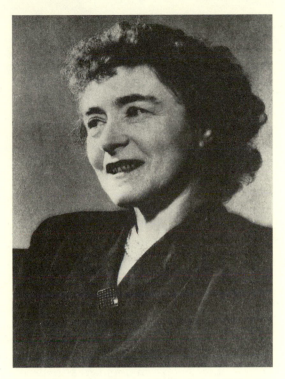

Gerty Theresa Radnitz Cori (U.S. National Library of Medicine)

well-to-do Jewish chemist and businessman who managed sugar refineries. The oldest of three girls, Cori was educated at home before going to a school for girls, graduating in 1912. She studied on her own the subjects required to get into medical school because at that time, although women were allowed to enter a university in Prague, few female schools taught the science and Latin required for entrance.

Her uncle was a pediatrician and encouraged her to go to medical school. She passed the entrance examination in 1914 and received her doctorate in medicine in 1920, the same year she married Carl Cori. Despite the fact that Gerty converted to Catholicism, Carl's parents felt that Gerty's Jewish background would harm Carl's career.

It wasn't long after graduation that both Coris realized the need to go elsewhere to do research. Eastern Europe was still recovering from World War I, and research facilities were not a priority there. Eventually Carl was offered a position at a cancer research institute in Buffalo, New York. Gerty was hired as an assistant pathologist.

Gerty Cori was troubled throughout her professional life by the fact that she was not recognized for her work with her husband. Husband-and-wife teams were becoming more common in the United States, but the husband had the secure, tenured position, whereas the wife held a lower-level position. A female researcher in this situation was secure in her position only as long as she stayed married.

After several years in Buffalo, Carl accepted a position in St. Louis at the Washington University School of Medicine. The Coris moved there in 1931, with Gerty Cori hired as a research associate and Carl as a professor. They had become naturalized American citizens in 1928.

In 1936, the Coris discovered the compound glucose-l-phosphate, also known as the Cori ester. This compound occurs as one of the three steps in the breakdown of glycogen into sugar. They also found that enzymes played a role in the sugar breakdown, and before long they discovered phosphorylase, an enzyme that breaks down glycogen into the Cori ester.

When World War II broke out, most of the men in research had to turn to defense projects, and women scientists were in demand in the universities. Thus in 1944, Gerty Cori attained the rank of associate professor at Washington University. She continued the work on enzymes. When the war was winding down and in response to offers the Coris had received from Harvard and the Rockefeller Institute, Washington University offered Carl a larger biochemistry department to chair with Gerty as a professor. Many scientists were pursuing enzyme research at the time, and by 1947 their department had become the world's foremost center for enzyme study, drawing researchers from around the globe.

Women who came to work with Cori found her both exacting and supportive, especially the latter with women who were wives and mothers like her. She had had a son, Tom Carl, in 1936.

Both she and her husband cared little about who was credited for discoveries as long as the work was based on sound science. Their lab was also unusual in that they did not discriminate when hiring against women, Jews, or other minorities.

On October 24, 1947, the Coris learned of their Nobel Prize, won for their earlier work on synthesizing glycogen in a test tube. "Physiologists had been told for years that large molecules could only be made within living cells. Yet the Coris had executed the first bioengineering of a large biological molecule in a test tube" (McGrayne 1998, 106).

The Coris shared the Nobel Prize with their friend Bernardo Alberto Houssay of Argentina.

Before the couple traveled to Stockholm to receive the award, Gerty found she was suffering from agnogenic myeloid dysplasia, a severe anemia wherein the body does not produce red blood cells and fibrous tissue slowly replaces the bone marrow. For the rest of her life she relied on blood transfusions to live.

The Coris shared their prize money with coworkers. They each gave part of the Nobel lecture, sharing the recognition as they had done their research. Over the next ten years Cori suffered from her illness but continued to do research when she could. She became interested in glycogen-storage diseases in children and identified four that were caused by a missing or defective enzyme.

As time went on she became weaker, and in 1957 she published her last paper. She died at home on October 26, 1957.

References: McGrayne, Sharon Bertsch, *Nobel Prize Women in Science*, New York: Carol (1998); Nobel Foundation, Official Web Site of the Nobel Foundation, 2000, http://www.nobel.se/medicine/laureates/1947/cori-gt-bio.html.

Correia, Elisa
1866–?

Elisa Correia was the first female physician in Portugal. She graduated in 1889 from the University of Coimbra in Portugal.

References: Lovejoy, Esther Pohl, *Women*

Doctors of the World, New York: Macmillan (1957).

Craighill, Margaret D.
1898–1977

Margaret Craighill was the first woman physician to be commissioned into the U.S. Army Medical Corps (1943). Craighill also served as dean of the Women's Medical College of Pennsylvania from 1940 to 1946.

Craighill was born on October 16, 1898, in Southport, North Carolina. She attended the University of Wisconsin and obtained an A.B. degree in 1920 and an M.S. in 1921. She earned her M.D. degree at Johns Hopkins University in 1924. She also graduated from the New York Psychoanalytic Institute in 1952.

During World War II she took a leave of absence from her position as dean of the Women's Medical College of Pennsylvania to serve with the preventive-medicine division of the Army Medical Corps. She surveyed war conditions and reported on the welfare of nurses and other members of the corps. She also worked in the office of the surgeon general as chief of the Women's Health and Welfare Unit. After the war she became a consultant to the Veterans' Administration on the care of women veterans, the first position of its kind.

Craighill eventually turned her attention to psychiatry and attended the Menninger School of Psychiatry as part of its first class, transferring from there to the New York Psychoanalytic Institute. She started her own private practice in Greenwich and New Haven, Connecticut, as well as serving at the Connecticut College for Women in New London as its chief psychiatrist.

She never had children and was widowed twice. Her husbands were Dr. James Vickers and Alexander S. Wotherspoon. She died in her home in Connecticut in July 1977 at the age of seventy-eight.

References: "Dr. Margaret D. Craighill, at 78, Former Dean of Medical College," *New York Times* (26 July 1977): 32; Lovejoy, Esther Pohl, *Women Doctors of the World*, New York:

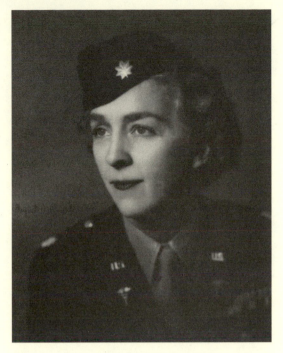

Margaret D. Craighill (U.S. National Library of Medicine)

Macmillan (1957); *Who's Who of American Women*, 5th ed., Chicago: Marquis Who's Who (1968).

Crosby, Elizabeth Caroline
1888–1983

Elizabeth Crosby was recognized in her day as one of the most learned experts on neuroanatomy. She worked well past retirement age and was a prolific writer and researcher. She was the first female full professor at the University of Michigan's Medical School.

Born in Petersburg, Michigan, to Lewis Frederick Crosby and Frances Kreps on October 25, 1888, Elizabeth had a rather normal and happy childhood. She attended public schools and received very good grades. She continued her studies at Adrian College in Michigan, where she obtained her B.S. in 1910. Interested in anatomy, she continued her studies at the University of Chicago, earning a master's degree in 1912 and a Ph.D. in 1915.

She returned to Petersburg to teach, but

after her mother died in 1918 she applied to the University of Michigan in order to pursue her research interests. She gained an instructor position in 1920 and rose through the ranks to become the first female professor in the university's medical school in 1936. While there, she kept to a rigorous schedule of teaching and research. She stayed until 1958.

With the publication in 1936 of the two-volume *Comparative Anatomy of the Nervous System of Vertebrates, Including Man,* she became known as an authority on brain morphology. She had collaborated on the work with C. U. Ariens Kappers and G. Carl Huber before he died in 1934. The book received international recognition.

Although Crosby never married, in 1940 she adopted a daughter, Kathleen, who was from Scotland. Crosby received numerous awards and continued her research well into her later years. She died on July 28, 1983, at her daughter's home in Michigan.

References: Bailey, Martha J., *American Women in Science: A Biographical Dictionary,* Santa Barbara, CA: ABC-CLIO (1994); Haines, Duane E., "Crosby, Elizabeth Caroline," *American National Biography,* vol. 5, New York: Oxford University Press (1999); Shearer, Benjamin F., and Barbara S. Shearer, *Notable Women in the Life Sciences: A Biographical Dictionary,* Westport, CT: Greenwood Press (1996).

Crumpler, Rebecca Lee
1833–?

Rebecca Crumpler was the first black woman to become a physician in the United States. She practiced in Boston after graduating from the New England Female Medical College and later moved to Richmond, Virginia, to treat newly freed slaves following the American Civil War.

Born in Richmond, Virginia, in 1833, she was raised by an aunt in Pennsylvania who worked as a doctor. She worked as a nurse in Massachusetts and then entered the New England Female Medical College to become a doctor. She graduated in 1864.

She wrote a book in 1883 on the care of women and children.

References: Crumpler, Rebecca, *A Book of Medical Discourses,* Boston: Cashman, Keating (1883); Jolly, Allison, "Crumpler, Rebecca Lee," in Darlene Clark Hine, ed., *Facts on File Encyclopedia of Black Women in America,* vol. 11, New York: Facts on File (1997); Sammons, Vivian Ovelton, *Blacks in Science and Medicine,* New York: Hemisphere (1990).

Curie, Marie Sklodowska
1867–1934

Marie Curie, probably the world's best-known woman scientist, was a pioneer in the field of radiation and chemotherapy. She was the first woman awarded a Nobel Prize, in 1903, for her research on radioactivity. Sharing the prize were her husband, Pierre Curie, and Henri Becquerel, who had discovered radioactivity in uranium. She was also awarded a Nobel Prize in 1911 for the previous discovery of polonium and radium and for the isolation of pure radium. She went beyond the study of the element radium to discover a few of its medical uses. It is still widely used for cancer treatment.

Curie was born in Warsaw, Poland, on November 7, 1867, and was the youngest of five children. Her parents were Wladyslaw and Bronislava Boguska Sklodowska, both intellectuals. She did exceptionally well in her schoolwork but suffered from depression during much of her early life. At a very young age, she and her siblings were subjected to Russian oppression: Officials denied students access to the literature of some countries and demanded that students recite their Catholic prayers in Russian and be familiar with certain aspects of Russian history.

When she was nine, she watched as her oldest sister, Sophia, died from typhus. When she was eleven, her mother died from tuberculosis. Curie turned to her father and his books for comfort and encouragement, and after completing school in 1883, she spent time in the country with her uncle Sklodowski. When she returned to Warsaw, she began tutoring, since girls were not allowed to enter universities in Poland.

Curie supported the Polish movement for independence and was active in the underground, or "floating," university, where many youths found fellowship and learned together, having been denied a higher education for one reason or another. Both she and her sister Bronia dreamed of attending a university in France. Because her father's bad investments had left him with little to support the higher education of his children, Curie began working as a governess to finance the move.

Bronia went to Paris first and entered medical school, passing all the required exams by 1890. She encouraged Marie to join her and her husband, Casimir Dluski. Although Marie was reticent to leave her father, she went to France in 1891 and enrolled in physics at the Sorbonne in November of that year. She passed her examination in physics in 1893, then in mathematics a year later. By now she desperately needed an adequate laboratory to continue working and was told to see Pierre Curie, a well-established physicist. Before long they were married and working together. In September 1897 their first daughter, Irene, was born.

Henri Becquerel had discovered radioactivity, a term coined by Marie, and the Curies worked on researching this phenomenon. The world had not taken great notice of Becquerel's discovery because of excitement over Roentgen's discovery of X rays in 1895. By 1898, however, Marie and Pierre had discovered two unknown radioactive elements in uranium—polonium and radium. To prove their discovery, they would need a huge amount of an expensive crude material, specifically pitchblende, and a place to work with it. The Austrian government gave the Curies a ton of pitchblende, and they used an old shed, a dissecting room the faculty of medicine had abandoned, to carry out their four-year attempt to isolate polonium and radium.

Marie had a miscarriage during this period but had a very healthy second daughter, Eve, in 1904. After winning the Nobel Prize in 1903, Pierre assumed a professor

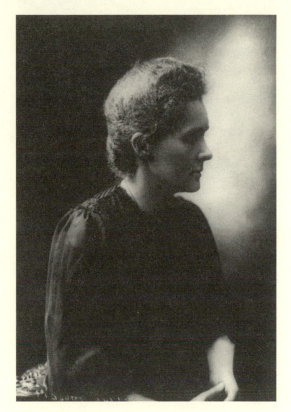

Marie Sklodowska Curie (Library of Congress)

position at the Sorbonne, and she was manager of the Ecole Supérieur de Physique et de Chimie, her husband's laboratory.

On April 19, 1906, Pierre was run over by a large horse-drawn carriage and was killed immediately. Marie was asked to take over her husband's position and lead the work on radioactivity at the Sorbonne. She was the first woman professor there. During the same year, Lord William Thomson Kelvin announced that radium was not an element after all, just a compound of lead and helium. He was mistaken, but Marie Curie could not prove it. She would have to keep working on isolating radium; she accomplished this in 1910.

During this time, a scandal erupted because Curie and a former student of Pierre Curie's, Paul Langevin, also a gifted French physicist and married, had begun seeing each other frequently. The press got wind of their meetings and claimed a foreigner had stolen a French woman's husband. They immediately ended the relationship, Curie realizing she could not have any kind of relationship with a married man.

Also during this time, she received word of her second Nobel Prize, this time in chemistry for the isolation of pure radium. With this award, she became the first to receive two Nobel Prizes.

After World War I broke out, Curie spent much of her time during the following four years organizing an X-ray service to assist in treating wounded soldiers on the front lines and in hospitals. By the time the war was over, 1 million soldiers had been examined. She also began bottling the radon gas from radium into small tubes and sent these to doctors around the world for the treatment of cancerous tumors. By this time, she was experiencing frequent exhaustion.

Although Curie was aware of the benefits of radiation for people with cancerous tumors, it is clear that she was not aware of its harmful effects. She was an avid outdoorswoman who felt that if people were strong and got enough fresh air, they would be fine. She continued in this belief even when lab assistants later died from anemia and leukemia due to overexposure. It wasn't until the 1920s that the public became aware of the damaging effects of exposure to radiation.

After the war, Curie was determined to build a research institute in France. Her Radium Institute at the University of Paris opened after the war but had little in the way of resources because of the depressed postwar economy. She came to change her mind about patenting scientific discoveries, realizing the income could finance further research.

In 1920, she met Missy Meloney, a journalist from the United States with whom she would form a lifelong friendship. Meloney was impressed by Curie's work, and when she learned that Curie's Radium Institute had little to work with, including very little radium, she vowed to help raise funds in the United States. Shortly thereafter, when Curie traveled to the United States with her two daughters, Meloney welcomed her with $100,000 for the Ra-

dium Institute. Also, at a White House ceremony, President Harding presented Curie with the key to a metal box containing radium.

During the 1920s, Curie had numerous symptoms of radiation exposure. She had cataracts and numbness in her fingers from handling radium and suffered fatigue. Marie Curie had trained Irene in radium research and had worked side by side with her during World War I. Irene and her husband, Frederic Joliot, discovered artificial radioactivity, work for which Irene received a Nobel Prize in 1935. Frederic would much later realize that it was dangerous to handle Marie and Pierre's papers, which were still contaminated with radioactivity decades after they died.

Curie tried to burn much of her personal papers before she died in order to gain more privacy. She kept only the love letters from Pierre and a diary. She also tried to organize and prepare for a transition at the Radium Institute, wanting an aide and then Irene to take over.

She was never recognized in France for her work during World War I because many still considered her a foreigner. She was loyal to her native Poland, teaching her daughters Polish at an early age and helping Poland establish its own radium institute.

Curie's health was in continual decline after suffering a broken wrist in 1932 that never healed properly. In May 1934, she was misdiagnosed with tuberculosis. At this point even Curie saw that radiation could be harmful. Eve cared for her almost constantly until Curie died from leukemia on July 4, 1934. She was buried with Pierre in a small cemetery in Sceaux. Many years later, on April 20, 1995, both their remains were moved to the Pantheon, France's memorial to the nation's great men. Marie Curie is the first woman to be buried there based on her own merits.

Today some still question whether Curie deserves so much credit for what her husband may have discovered. It is obvious from her writings and what she said on record that both she and Pierre were very careful to take credit together for the work they shared and give credit to each other as appropriate.

References: Curie, Eve, *Madame Curie: A Biography,* New York: Doubleday (1938); *Dictionary of Scientific Biography,* New York: Charles Scribner's Sons (1971); *Encyclopedia of World Biography,* Detroit: Gale Research (1998); McGrayne, Sharon Bertsch, *Nobel Prize Women in Science: Their Lives, Struggles, and Momentous Discoveries,* Secaucus, NJ: Carol (1998); Pflaum, Rosalynd, *Grand Obsession: Madame Curie and Her World,* New York: Doubleday (1989).

D

Dalle Donne, Maria
1778–1842

Exceptionally talented and intelligent, Maria Dalle Donne was dedicated to eradicating barbaric methods of medical treatment for women. She educated numerous midwives at the University of Bologna; this work was critical because there were few doctors in that day to attend to the rural population, and thus gynecological and obstetric patients depended upon midwives for all necessary care. Dalle Donne did not turn away women who sought education even if they could not afford it. Her uncle, recognizing her extraordinary talent, took her in and educated her. Her tutors were eventually so impressed that they encouraged, and arranged, a demonstration of her skills so that she could obtain a medical degree and earn her own living. She impressed the University of Bologna officials and was admitted to the university, obtaining her degree in philosophy and medicine in 1799.

She became the director of midwives at the university and was highly regarded for her teaching abilities.

See also: University of Bologna
References: Ogilvie, Marilyn, and Joy Harvey, eds., *Biographical Dictionary of Women in Science: Pioneering Lives from Ancient Times to the Mid-20th Century*, New York: Routledge (2000).

Daly, Marie Maynard
1921–

Marie Daly was the first African American to earn a Ph.D. degree in chemistry. Her research focused on the physiological levels of creatine, hypertension, protein synthesis, and atherosclerosis.

Daly was born in New York City on April 16, 1921, to Ivan C. Daly and Helen Page Daly. She had younger brothers who were twins. Her education started in the public schools of Queens, and she then attended Hunter College High School in Manhattan. She did very well in school and had much support from her family, teachers, and friends.

She went on to Queens College and obtained her B.S. in chemistry in 1942. She graduated magna cum laude and was ambitious for a research career. After obtaining a lab assistant position at Queens College, she began the master's program at New York University. She received her master's a year later and remained at Queens College, teaching in the lab and tutoring.

She later entered Columbia University to work on her Ph.D. in chemistry, which she obtained in 1947. She then went to Howard University and taught in the physical sciences, afterward moving on to the Rockefeller Institute for seven years. During this time she was learning a great deal and meeting well-established researchers such as Leonor Michaelis and Francis Peyton Rous.

In 1955 she returned to Columbia University and in 1960, she went to Albert Einstein

College of Medicine. She published many articles on her research involving the synthesis of protein, the relationship between hypertension and cholesterol, and the effects of cigarette smoking. She became an associate professor in 1971 and held that position until she retired in 1986. She married Vincent Clark in 1961.

References: Grinstein, Louise S., Rose K. Rose, and Miriam H. Rafailovich, *Women in Chemistry and Physics: A Biobibliographic Sourcebook*, Westport, CT: Greenwood Press (1993).

Daniel, Annie Sturges
1858–1944

A physician and public health crusader who worked in numerous settlement houses, Annie Daniel set early standards in proper hygiene and sanitation as well as emphasized adequate nutrition and space for families in substandard living conditions. Her practical handling of destitute individuals and patients was a model for students required to visit patients in run-down tenement buildings, crowded shelters, and unsanitary homes.

Born on September 21, 1858, in Buffalo, New York, she was the daughter of John M. Daniel and Marinda Sturges Daniel. Her parents died when she was still a child, and relatives in Monticello, New York, raised her. She had an early interest in biology and entered the Women's Medical College of the New York Infirmary, where she obtained her M.D. in 1879. Elizabeth Blackwell placed Daniel in the Out-Practice Department, which gave her leadership responsibility for persons living in the tenements of New York City.

She would find ensuring better health and circumstances for the poor to be her life's work. Many who lived in tenement buildings during her time were immigrants living in extended families. They earned meager wages and did not always have the education needed for basic health care and a nutritious diet.

By 1889 she was teaching many medical students at the Women's Medical College about the circumstances of the poor.

Eventually health officials came to her for advice, and in 1884 she was appointed to serve with the New York State Tenement House Commission. She investigated child labor in homes and sweatshops and also advocated prison reform.

Daniel never married and died on August 10, 1944, in New York City.

References: Ogilvie, Marilyn, and Joy Harvey, eds., *The Biographical Dictionary of Women in Science: Pioneering Lives from Ancient Times to the Mid-20th Century*, New York: Routledge (2000); Perry, Marilyn Elizabeth, "Daniel, Annie Sturges," *American National Biography*, vol. 6, New York: Oxford University Press (1999).

Darrow, Ruth Renter
1895–1956

Little is known about Ruth Darrow except that she published various research articles on erythroblastosis foetalis, a hemolytic disease of newborns (HDN), and concluded that an unknown fetal antigen caused the disease. She herself was "a mother of several Rh-HDN-afflicted newborns" and "was first to suggest a relationship between maternal sensitization to a fetal blood antigen and subsequent fetal pathology" (Lloyd 1987, 299). She worked in Chicago for a time with the Women and Children's Hospital. Her research led the way for the discovery of the Rh factor and its importance for pregnant women and fetuses.

References: Darrow, Ruth Renter, "Icterus Gravis (Erythroblastosis) Neonatorum," *Archives of Pathology* 25 (1938): 378–417; Kass-Simon, G., and Patricia Farnes, *Women of Science: Righting the Record*, Bloomington: Indiana University Press (1990); Lloyd, Thomas, "Rh-Factor Incompatibility: A Primer for Prevention," *Journal of Nurse-Midwifery* 32, no. 5 (September–October 1987): 297–307.

Dayhoff, Margaret Oakley
1925–1983

Margaret Dayhoff was an early pioneer in molecular biology. She initiated development of the protein sequence database (PSDB), which led her to a great understanding of the evolution of proteins. This database also led to the use of computers in the life sciences. Her series of books, beginning with the 1965 *Atlas of Protein Sequence and Structure,* would prove invaluable to researchers in the field of molecular biology.

Born on March 11, 1925, in Philadelphia, Pennsylvania, she was the daughter of Kenneth W. Oakley and Ruth P. Clark. They moved to New York City when Margaret was ten, and she attended public schools, graduating from high school as a valedictorian. She went on to major in mathematics at Washington Square College, part of the University of New York, and graduated magna cum laude in 1945. In 1948 she received a Ph.D. from Columbia University in quantum chemistry.

Following school, she worked at the Rockefeller Institute and the University of Maryland. In 1959 she took a position at the National Biomedical Foundation, where her interests were in the origins of life and the relationship between protein sequences as well as the role they played in the evolutionary process. Her protein sequence database consisted of sixty-five sequences. She also developed an amino acid similarity-scoring matrix, which was one of the first tools for database searching, comparing protein sequences, and building evolutionary trees. All this work is helpful to scientists researching macromolecules and their structure.

She married Edward S. Dayhoff, a physicist, in 1948, and they had two daughters who became physicians. Dayhoff died on February 5, 1983, in Silver Springs, Maryland, of a heart attack at the age of fifty-seven.

References: Ledley, Robert S., "Dayhoff, Margaret Oakley," *American National Biography,* vol. 2, New York: Oxford University Press (1999); Proffitt, Pamela, ed., *Notable Women Scientists,* Detroit: Gale Research (1999).

Dejerine-Klumpke, Augusta
1859–1927

Augusta Dejerine-Klumpke was an outstanding neurologist who was an early pioneer in treating patients with nervous diseases. She was also the first woman to become a member of the Societé de Neurologie in 1914.

Born in San Francisco on October 15, 1859, Augusta was the daughter of John Gerard Klumpke and Dorothea Matilda Tolle. She received an early education in San Francisco before the family moved to France. She attended the University of Paris and obtained her medical degree in 1889. She worked at La Laribosiére Hospital along with her husband, Jules Dejerine, also a neurologist. They were married on July 11, 1888, and had one daughter, Yvonne Dejerine. Later, they both worked at the clinic for nervous diseases at La Salpêtrière, contributing much to the field.

Because of the many soldiers of World War I who suffered from paralysis, Dejerine-Klumpke opened her own clinic for the purpose of studying that condition. Her work earned her a great deal of distinction and respect. She died in Paris on November 5, 1927.

References: "Dejerine, Augusta Klumpke," *The National Cyclopedia of American Biography,* vol. 31, New York: J. T. White (1944): 404; Haines, Catharine M. C., and Helen Stevens, *International Women in Science: A Biographical Dictionary to 1950,* Santa Barbara, CA: ABC-CLIO (2001).

Delano, Jane Arminda
1862–1919

Jane Delano was the first director and organizer of the American Red Cross Nursing Service. She enabled the organization to provide over 20,000 professional nurses during World War I.

Born in Townsend, New York, on March 12, 1862, Delano was one of two daughters of George and Mary Ann Wright Delano. Her father died in the Civil War, and her

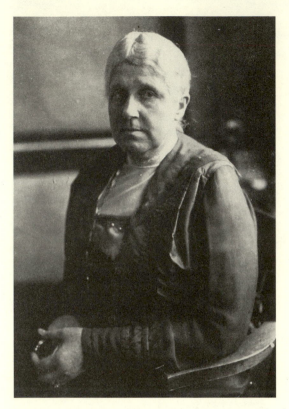

Jane Arminda Delano (American Red Cross/U.S. National Library of Medicine)

home. Delano became the leader of this initiative, replacing the Army Nursing Reserve with the Red Cross Nursing Service. She was very active in recruiting nurses of professional caliber and received many honors over the years for her dedication to the Red Cross.

After World War I ended, Delano went abroad to oversee Red Cross activities in postwar Europe. She suffered from mastoiditis and died in a base hospital in Savenay, France, on April 15, 1919. She never married or had children. She was buried at Arlington National Cemetery in Virginia.

References: Gladwin, Mary E., *The Red Cross and Jane Arminda Delano*, Philadelphia: W. B. Saunders (1931); *Notable American Women 1607–1950*, Cambridge, MA: Belknap Press (1971); Reeves, Connie L., "Delano, Jane Arminda," *American National Biography*, vol. 6, New York: Oxford University Press (1999).

Dempsey, Sister Mary Joseph
1856–1939

Sister Mary Joseph Dempsey played an important role in the growth of St. Mary's Hospital and in its collaboration with the Mayo Clinic. As nurse, hospital administrator, and surgical assistant to Dr. Will Mayo, she contributed to the success of both institutions.

Born in Salamanca, New York, on May 14, 1856, Dempsey was the second of seven children of Irish immigrants Patrick Dempsey and Mary Sullivan Dempsey. Not long after she was born, the family moved to a farm in Olmsted County, Minnesota. Dempsey, christened Julia, and two of her sisters became Franciscan nuns. Julia became Sister Mary Joseph of the Third Order of St. Francis at the age of twenty-two. She trained as a teacher and worked in several schools over the next decade.

A terrible tornado hit Rochester, Minnesota, in 1883, convincing the convent's Mother Alfred that the convent needed a hospital. Dr. William Worrall Mayo agreed to staff the hospital if the sisters of the convent would build it. Mother Alfred felt that Sister Joseph would be a good nurse and

mother remarried. Her sister died in 1883, and thereafter Delano felt the lack of family ties even though she now had four stepsisters. She was educated at Cook Academy in Montour Falls.

In 1884 she attended the Bellevue Hospital Training School for Nurses in New York. She showed unusual skill and proficiency and was chosen early on to attend a mayor. Her observations in the hospital of organization and leadership skills served her well in later years. In 1888 she volunteered to serve during the yellow fever epidemic in Florida. Then she worked in Arizona, organizing a hospital during an epidemic of scarlet fever. Following this, she went to the University of Pennsylvania Hospital and became the superintendent of nurses.

It became very apparent after the Spanish-American War that the Red Cross needed an organized reserve of ready professionals in case of wars or epidemics at called on her to learn nursing and work at the hospital.

In 1889, Sister Joseph became head nurse at the newly created St. Mary's Hospital. A year later she began to work for Dr. Will Mayo as a surgical assistant and in 1892 was the superintendent of the hospital. She was an exceptional administrator who had to deal with financial planning, personnel problems, and the ongoing cooperation with the Mayos' medical practice. St. Mary's went through a period of tremendous growth and change as staff responded to an increasing number of medical discoveries that changed the hospital's procedures and treatments.

Sister Joseph, seeing a great need for nurses, started the St. Mary's Hospital School for Nurses in 1906. She was a stern disciplinarian who emphasized the importance of academic education as well as practical experience and tried to raise the status of nursing as a profession. She died of bronchopneumonia on March 29, 1939, at St. Mary's Hospital.

References: Ogilvie, Marilyn, and Joy Harvey, eds., *The Biographical Dictionary of Women in Science: Pioneering Lives from Ancient Times to the Mid-20th Century*, New York: Routledge (2000); Steller, Robert E., "Dempsey, Sister Mary Joseph," *Notable American Women 1607–1950*, Cambridge, MA: Belknap Press (1971).

Dengal, Anna Maria
1892–1980

Anna Dengal became a well-known medical missionary and founded the Catholic Medical Mission Sisters in 1925. She is said to have had some influence on Pius XI's decision to lift the ban on women in religious work entering the medical field. In 1936, after he had lifted the ban, Dengal's group became a religious congregation. Dengal was born in Steeg, Austria, the oldest of nine children. Her mother died when she was eight, and she went to boarding school in France. She was advised to go into the medical field and of the need for medical mis-

sionaries by a Scottish suffragist, Agnes McLaren. McLaren was a physician and needed more medical missionaries in India. Dengal pursued her premedical studies at Cork University, Ireland, and in 1919 graduated from Queens College Medical School.

In India she worked at St. Catherine's Hospital, treating women and children of all religious backgrounds. She traveled to the United States in 1924 in order to raise funds to form the Catholic Medical Mission Sisters. The sisters trained nurses, midwives, and others for foreign missions. They were the first to provide surgeons and obstetricians for mission work within the Roman Catholic congregations.

Dengal laid out the foundations of mission work in her *Mission for Samaritans* in 1945. She believed missions were a practical way to follow the example of Jesus Christ and the Good Samaritan and to deliver the justice the white race owed to others who were less fortunate. She died in Rome in 1980.

References: Dries, Angelyn, "Dengel, Anna," *Biographical Dictionary of Christian Missions*, New York: Macmillan (1998); Ogilvie, Marilyn, and Joy Harvey, eds., *The Biographical Dictionary of Women in Science: Pioneering Lives from Ancient Times to the Mid-20th Century*, New York: Routledge (2000).

Diaz Inzunza, Eloiza
1866–1950

Eloiza Diaz Inzunza was the first woman in Chile to obtain a medical degree. Graduating from a high school for boys that she had special permission to attend, Diaz went on to the Instituto Nacional in Santiago and graduated in 1881 at the age of fifteen with a bachelor of arts. She then attended the medical school at the University of Chile and spent five years studying before earning a medical degree in 1887. She spent all her career serving women and children. She died on November 1, 1950.

References: Lovejoy, Esther Pohl, *Women Doctors of the World*, New York: Macmillan (1957); Vargas, Tegualda Ponce de, "Women

Doctors of Chile," *Journal of the American Medical Women's Association* 7, no. 10 (1952): 389.

Dick, Gladys Rowena Henry
1881–1963

Gladys Dick, along with her husband, George, were key figures in researching the treatment and prevention of scarlet fever prior to the development of antibiotics during World War II. Their research proved that hemolytic streptococci caused scarlet fever. They were nominated in 1925 for the Nobel Prize in physiology or medicine, although no award was given that year.

Dick was born in Pawnee City, Nebraska, on December 18, 1881. Her father, William Chester Henry, was a banker and grain dealer and also raised horses. Her mother was Azelia Henrietta Edson Henry. Dick was the youngest of three children. The family moved to Lincoln, Nebraska, when she was still a baby. She was educated locally, then attended the University of Nebraska, where she obtained her B.S. degree in 1900. Unable to convince her mother that medicine was an appropriate course of study, she settled for teaching biology in Carney, Nebraska.

She also took graduate courses at the University of Nebraska until her mother agreed to her pursuing a medical career. At that point she entered the medical school at Johns Hopkins University in Baltimore. She worked at Johns Hopkins after her graduation in 1907, then spent a year in Berlin, where her research interests in blood chemistry intensified. After she returned, she went to the University of Chicago in 1911.

It was here that she met George Dick. They were married in 1914, and she worked for a time in private practice while George took a position at McCormick Memorial Institute for Infectious Diseases. Soon she joined her husband in researching scarlet fever.

At the time scarlet fever was a huge problem in North America as well as Europe. The mortality rate was 25 percent, and those children who survived had a great risk of

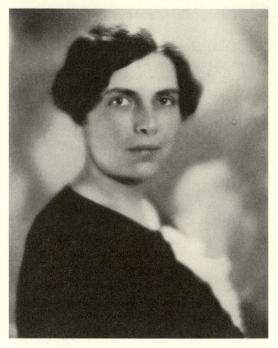

Gladys Rowena Henry Dick (U.S. National Library of Medicine)

being crippled for the rest of their life. After the Dicks' discovery of the agent causing the disease, they developed a toxin and antitoxin preparation and patented it in 1924. Some saw the patent as a move that fostered commercialism and that could hinder research. The Dicks argued that their approach would ensure quality. They later won a lengthy court battle when they brought a lawsuit against a manufacturer for patent infringement and inappropriately preparing the toxin.

Their discovery led to the Dick skin test, which determined an individual's susceptibility to scarlet fever. Once antibiotics became abundant during World War II, their test was no longer needed.

Dick's later research involved polio, and she also was deeply involved in the public health and welfare issue of adoption. She was active in the Cradle Society, an adoption organization in Evanston, Illinois, for many years. She and her husband adopted two children, Roger and Rowena, in 1930.

Dick suffered a stroke on August 21, 1963, and died in Menlo Park, California.

References: Bailey, Martha J., *American Women in Science*, Santa Barbara: ABC-CLIO (1994); *Notable Twentieth-Century Scientists Supplement*, Detroit: Gale Research (1998).

Dickens, Helen Octavia
1909–

Helen Dickens became a specialist in obstetrics and gynecology and was the first African American woman to become a fellow of the American College of Surgeons. She is most noted for her counseling of students in the allied public health and medical fields and as an advocate of education in order to reduce the rate of teen pregnancy.

Dickens was born to a former slave from Tennessee, Charles Dickens, on February 21, 1909, in Dayton, Ohio. She was the oldest of three. Her mother was Daisy Jane Green Dickens. She attended integrated public schools in Dayton. Upon graduation she attended Crane Junior College in Chicago. There, she ignored the racist attitudes of some students and focused on her studies, doing well in her premed courses.

She continued her studies at the University of Illinois, receiving her B.S. degree in 1932. She went on to the university's medical school, graduating in 1934. She interned at Chicago's Provident Hospital and later became a resident in obstetrics. She and others had a desire to go out into the community but did not have the opportunity during their residency. Afterward she was drawn to a Quaker practicing medicine in her home in Philadelphia, Dr. Virginia Alexander. Dickens went to work with Alexander for a while, taking on the entire practice when Alexander left for further education. She stayed for six years until deciding she needed to learn more about obstetrics and gynecology.

Upon learning that the University of Pennsylvania Graduate School of Medicine offered an advanced degree in medical science, she studied there and then went back to Provident Hospital in Chicago for her residency. There, she met Purvis Sinclair Henderson, a resident in general surgery. They married in 1943, and soon thereafter Dick-

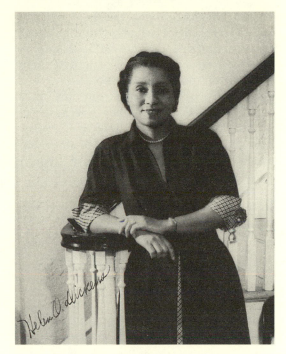

Helen Octavia Dickens (U.S. National Library of Medicine)

ens took a residency at Harlem Hospital in New York City. Henderson returned to his practice in Savannah, Georgia, and they thus had a long-distance marriage.

Dickens completed her residency at Harlem Hospital in 1946. She became certified by the American Board of Obstetrics and Gynecology and in 1948 became director of the Department of Obstetrics and Gynecology at Philadelphia's racially integrated Mercy Douglass Hospital. She would remain there until 1967. In 1950 she became a fellow in the American College of Surgeons.

Henderson eventually went to Pennsylvania and took a residency in neurosurgery at the University of Pennsylvania Medical College. He and Dickens had two children. He died in 1961. Dickens began her relationship with the University of Pennsylvania School of Medicine in 1965. In 1976, she attained the position of professor of obstetrics and gynecology. She currently is professor emerita at the University of Pennsylvania School of Medicine.

Through her many publications on the

subject of teen pregnancy, its prevention and effects, Dickens had a great influence on prevention programs. She has also done extensive research on cancer and sexually transmitted diseases. She also counsels students, particularly women, who are interested in medicine or other science disciplines. She has received numerous awards over the years, including an honorary doctorate from the Medical College of Pennsylvania.

References: *Contemporary Black Biography,* vol. 14, Detroit: Gale Research (1997).

Dickey, Nancy Wilson
1950–

Nancy Dickey was the first female president of the American Medical Association (AMA). Her yearlong term began in June 1998, and during that time she helped create the National Patient Safety Foundation, discussed issues concerning terminal illness and the rights of the patient, and challenged the profession to be more forthright about mistakes.

Dickey was one of seven children. She was born in South Dakota on September 10, 1950, and was raised on a farm. She and her siblings gathered eggs, slopped hogs, and helped with the other farm chores until she was ten and the family moved south. They ended up in Katy, Texas, where Dickey first became interested in medicine. Her parents were very encouraging, but some teachers and others warned against such high ambitions. They urged her to have either a family or a medical career. She was discouraged until she met her future husband, who supported her in pursuing both goals. She studied psychology at Stephen F. Austin State University in Nacogdoches and worked as a nursing aide in the summers. She obtained her M.D. from the medical school at the University of Texas in Houston in 1976. She chose family practice instead of a limited specialty because she felt she would like the diversity. She was a resident in family practice from 1976 to 1979 at Memorial Hospital System in Houston.

She has tackled tough ethical issues, particularly the end-of-life issue, while working within the AMA and as its president. Under her leadership the AMA ethics committee resolved that "honoring the request of terminal patients or their surrogates to discontinue artificial nutrition or hydration was ethical" (Turner 1997, 1).

She also feels that although physicians now have the capability to keep people alive longer, that is sometimes not the ethical choice. She is opposed to physician-assisted suicide but feels that "we do things because we can. We need to think more about whether we should" (Mangan 1997, A10).

Her husband is a football and basketball coach in Bryan, Texas. She has three children and is also active in her community. She was the founding program director for the Brazos Valley Family Practice Program in Bryan and treats patients there on a regular basis. She is also a professor at the Texas A&M University College of Medicine, and serves on staff at St. Joseph's Hospital in Bryan, Texas, and the College Station Medical Center, College Station, Texas. She is currently president of the Health Science Center and vice chancellor for health affairs for the Texas A&M University system.

References: Mangan, Katherine S., "First Female President: Texas A&M Professor Prepares to Lead AMA," *Chronicle of Higher Education* 44 (10 October 1997): A10; Turner, Allan, "Healthy, Irrepressible Perspective: AMA's First Female President Breaks Through Perceived 'Old Boys' Network," *Houston Chronicle* (29 June 1997): 1.

Dix, Dorothea Lynde
1802–1887

Dorothea Dix was an early advocate for the rights of the mentally ill and responsible for bringing state and national attention to the problems of the day in caring for and treating those with mental illnesses. Without a formal education, she symbolizes the value of common sense with her view that mental illness is a medical problem, not a moral one. Because of her efforts there were 123 mental hospitals in the United States in 1880 compared to only 13 in 1843. Without being aware of her influence, she also laid the groundwork—in her *Remarks on Prisons and Prison Discipline in the United States*—for the changes to come in the care and treatment of prisoners. She emphasized the need to educate inmates and give them psychiatric treatment and the need to keep certain types of prisoners separated from others.

Born in Hampden, Maine, on April 4, 1802, Dix was the daughter of Joseph and Mary Bigelow Dix. Her father was a minister. She had two younger brothers, whom she cared for often because her mother was handicapped. Occasionally, she was able to spend time in Boston, where she visited her grandparents and became interested in gaining an education. She was an avid reader and, despite being raised by relatives in her early teens, managed to gain enough education to open a small school. She taught on and off for years until she became interested in the plight of the mentally ill.

Her interest in the well-being of the mentally ill grew out of her astonishment at the cruel and unusual punishment they were receiving in jails and prisons around the country. She had gone to teach a Sunday school class for women prisoners and was shocked to find that some of them were imprisoned only because they were mentally ill. As time went on, she surveyed other institutions and found that most facilities for the insane were entirely inadequate.

She began to bring the problem before the legislatures in many states, using the slavery issue in her arguments. How could abolitionists propose freeing slaves when they couldn't take care of their own mentally ill? Soon many states appropriated funds for proper facilities.

Eventually Dix presented her case at the national level, feeling that federal land should be set aside for a trust whose income would benefit the insane. Congress grappled with this matter for six years, finally passing a bill in 1854. President Franklin Pierce vetoed the bill, saying the states should deal with the problem.

Dix suffered from poor health throughout

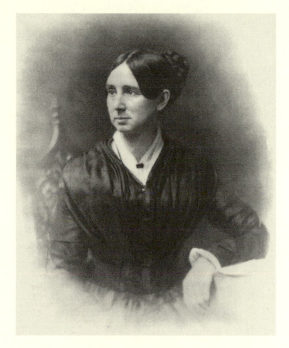

Dorothea Lynde Dix (Library of Congress)

her life but never gave up the fight for the mentally ill. She also volunteered her services during the Civil War and was made the superintendent of army nurses. This was a frustrating role for her because she didn't possess the organizational skills necessary for such a position. Eventually the secretary of war lessened her authority because she was not an effective leader. She continued her service until the war ended.

Following the war, she picked up where she left off, visiting several southern states and lobbying on behalf of various causes, among them prison reform. While visiting the mentally ill in numerous institutions, she also saw firsthand the prison conditions of inmates who were not mentally ill. She advocated better conditions for them.

During Dix's career as a social reformer, she met many influential people, once visiting a welcoming Pope Pius IX in order to describe the conditions in prisons and asylums that existed in Rome.

She never married or had children. She retired to Trenton, New Jersey, and died on July 18, 1887.

References: Marshall, Helen E., *Dorothea Dix, Forgotten Samaritan*, Chapel Hill: University of North Carolina Press (1937); *Notable American Women 1607–1950*, Cambridge, MA: Belknap Press (1971); Snodgrass, Mary Ellen, *The Historical Encyclopedia of Nursing*, Santa Barbara, CA: ABC-CLIO (1999).

Dmitrieva, Valentina Ionovna
1859–1947

Valentina Dmitrieva was one of the early Russian women physicians. She is better known as a revolutionary and writer, but her brief medical career led her to working with the less fortunate during famine and epidemics. Her fiction and memoirs give one of the few early pictures of the desperate situation in Russia toward the end of the nineteenth century as medical providers faced insurmountable odds in trying to help the helpless.

She was born on April 28, 1859, in Voronino, a village in Saratov Province. Her father was a serf, and her mother taught her to read, which she did avidly. She was able to attend high school in Tambov and did well. The family struggled after emancipation and lived a transient life.

She pursued medical training in St. Petersburg, and she also went to Moscow to study obstetrics. She worked as a physician most of 1892–1894, when epidemics and starvation were widespread in Russia. A revolutionary, she spent years in exile in Tver and Voronezh. She wrote an autobiography in 1930, *Tak Bylo: Put Moei Shizni* (The Way It Was), and several of her memoirs depict the seemingly hopeless situation she faced as a physician.

In one village, she wrote, "I could see the whole panoply of destruction wrought by chronic hunger: the ulcers, rashes, bleeding gums, paralysed muscles, and putrefying bones. . . . The crowd straggled after me, staring at me with a mixture of hope and desperation. And I realized my total impotence: all the medicine I could prescribe, the visits I could make, seemed pointless and ridiculous, reduced to childish games in the face of the rural poverty which was closing in on me from all sides" (Dmitrieva 1994, 158). Dmitrieva died in Sochi on February 18, 1947.

References: Buck, Claire, ed., *Bloomsbury Guide to Women's Literature*, London: Bloomsbury (1992); Davies, Mildred, "Valentina Dmitrieva," *Russian Women Writers*, vol. 2, New York: Garland (1999); Dmitrieva, Valentina, "After the Great Hunger," in Catriona Kelly, ed., *An Anthology of Russian Women's Writing, 1777–1992*, Oxford: Oxford University Press (1994); Engel, Barbara Alpern, *Mothers and Daughters: Women of the Intelligentsia in Nineteenth Century Russia*, Cambridge: Cambridge University Press (1983).

Dock, Lavinia Lloyd
1858–1956

Lavinia Dock was an early nursing leader and educator who worked with Isabel Hampton Robb at Johns Hopkins and was inspired by the work of Lillian D. Wald, which enhanced her vision of what the nursing profession should be. She was instrumental in the early years of her career in promoting a professional identity for nurses and in establishing high standards in the nursing profession. Born on February 26, 1858, to Gilliard and Lavinia Loyd Bombaugh Dock, she was raised in Harrisburg, Pennsylvania, and enrolled in the Training School for Nurses in New York at Bellevue Hospital. She graduated in 1886 and a few years later assisted Clara Barton following the devastating Johnstown, Pennsylvania, flood of 1889. She made a lasting contribution to nursing with her publication the following year of the *Textbook for Materia Medica for Nurses*, a guide for nurses on the use of drugs. It served as a textbook for many years and went through several editions.

Isabel Hampton Robb appointed Dock the assistant superintendent of nurses at Johns Hopkins Hospital. She became very involved in the profession, realizing nurses needed an organized voice. In 1893 she organized the American Society of Superintendents of Training Schools and a few years later joined the community of women living in the Settlement House on Henry Street in New York City. Lillian Wald, who had started the house, was a tremendous influence on Dock.

Her work there for the next twenty years formed a foundation for nurses having a huge role in public health care. She was very vocal about problems that others did not want to think about or discuss; she was one of the first nurses to talk about the problem of prostitution and the need for treating venereal disease.

> Elizabeth Blackwell early declared, in a letter to her sister, her determination not to be intimidated or discouraged in the difficult task of attacking the social evil by methods of education, and her books and addresses on this subject are classics in their dignity and nobility of position. . . . From that time on women physicians as an entire body have stood united for a single standard of morals and for the education of the public. In their ranks there can be found no division or opposing opinions on this subject. They are active in the warfare against vice, in every country where medicine has opened its door to women, and in our own country they have been publicly called upon by their colleagues in the medical profession to carry the teachings of hygiene to the women of the land" (Dock 1910, 80–81).

Hygiene and Morality (1910) speaks strongly against prostitution and addresses other public health concerns. She later moved away from nursing and became more involved in the women's suffragist movement and equality for women.

Dock died in Chambersburg, Pennsylvania, on April 17, 1956.

See also: Barton, Clara; Robb, Isabel Hampton; Wald, Lillian D.
References: Dock, Lavinia L. *Hygiene and Morality: A Manual for Nurses and Others, Giving an Outline of the Medical, Social, and Legal Aspects of the Venereal Diseases*, New York: G. P. Putnam's Sons (1910); Sklar, Kathryn Kish, "Dock, Lavinia Lloyd," *American National Biography*, vol. 6, New York: Oxford University Press (1999).

Dolley, Sarah Read Adamson
1829–1909

One of the early women physicians in the United States, Dolley provided leadership for women wanting a career in medicine. When hospitals wouldn't allow women to practice, she assisted and was elected as the first president of the Provident Dispensary Association. The dispensary provided help for the needy women and children of Rochester until 1894.

Born in Chester County, Pennsylvania, on March 11, 1829, Dolley was the third of five children. Her parents were Charles Adamson and Mary Corson Adamson, of Quaker descent. She was educated at the Friends' School in Philadelphia and later became interested in medicine. She was denied admission to many schools until Central Medical College accepted her. She graduated in 1851.

Following an internship at Blockley Hospital, she married Dr. Lester Clinton Dolley, an anatomy professor. They had two children, Loilyn in 1854 and Charles Sumner in 1856. Loilyn died in 1858 of typhoid pneumonia.

Dolley remained in Rochester for life, continuing to be active in her medical practice, which she devoted to women and children, and continuing her education by going to Paris, Prague, and Vienna to learn from their physicians. She became very involved in organizing professional women's associations. Her husband's career at Central Medical College didn't last because the college closed, but he also had a private practice.

She had an unusually good reputation for a woman physician of the time due to her training after her education in college. Even male colleagues had respect for her talents. Dolley died in Rochester, New York, on December 27, 1909.

References: Miller, Genevieve, "Dolley, Sarah Read Adamson," in *Notable American Women 1607–1950,* Cambridge, MA: Belknap Press (1971); More, Ellen Singer, *Restoring the Balance: Women Physicians and the Profession of Medicine, 1850–1995,* Cambridge, MA: Harvard University Press (1999).

du Coudray, Angelique Marguerite
1714/5–1794

Angelique du Coudray was a midwife in eighteenth-century France. Because many newborns died from the brutal practices of women not properly trained or licensed to practice midwifery, King Louis XV appointed her to go on an urgent mission across all of France to train women as well as men to deliver babies. He invested her with broad authority.

Through all her correspondence, which is plentiful, du Coudray does not reveal much about her personal life. She may have been orphaned or abandoned; one can only speculate. She trained with the able midwife Anne Bairsin, passed her examinations, and went to Paris to earn her living. Records show she was a registered midwife in Paris in 1740 at the age of twenty-five. On record also is a petition from 1745 that she and forty other midwives signed, asking the faculty of medicine at the University of Paris to give them lessons. Since 1733 the midwives had been attending sessions conducted by the school of surgery, but the surgeons had stopped these lessons, and the midwives were left with no one to give them ongoing training and instruction. The faculty of medicine, who had a higher status than the surgeons did and who were their old rivals, immediately obliged the midwives.

The midwives complained that many women were practicing without licenses and doing harm. These women, who didn't have the knowledge to deliver babies when complications existed, were competing with the midwives for business and damaging the profession. Louis XV was also concerned about women practicing without a license, but his greater priority was dealing with depopulation. France was losing many soldiers in its battles of the Seven Years War, and newborns were dying. It was at this time, in 1759, that he commissioned du Coudray with training midwives across the country.

Du Coudray realized that she needed training tools and that same year wrote an obstetrical text, *Abrégé de l'art des accouchements* (Summary of the Art of Delivery), which has many illustrations. The book was helpful, but after her trip to Auvergne, where she heard numerous stories of malpractice by midwives, she felt she needed more effective training materials. Illiteracy was very high in the rural areas of France, and the midwives needed hands-on experience as well as the illustrations from her text. She then invented a mechanized anatomical model of a pregnant woman along with a child. The anatomical model aided a great deal, as students could practice turning models of babies into the correct position before birth. Hundreds of these models were made and sent to others to use in training.

Du Coudray never got lost in the mechanics of training, always reminding her students that they would be dealing with human beings and precious new lives. She gave very practical advice as well. In regard to twins, she told her students that if a midwife saw a left foot and a right foot protruding, "before pulling them out she must check that they both belong to one baby. If instead she is holding one foot of each twin, it would be futile and fatal to pull. She will need to push them back in and search around until she is confident that she has found two feet of the same child" (Gelbart 1998, 70).

Many babies died who could have been saved had someone given them the proper attention: "A weak, motionless baby mistaken for dead will be wrapped up and put away in a corner to spare the mother such a sad sight. Some are buried alive, and without baptism" (Gelbart 1998, 137). Du Coudray went on to explain to her students how she had brought four such infants back to life, one having had his toe eaten by a dog. She constantly told midwives in training to pay attention to the baby.

Du Coudray trained 10,000 midwives in

about forty different cities. She earned a reputation that preceded her wherever she went. Not all people were happy with her; she had to deal with jealous women, surgeons who saw her as unwanted competition, and the politics of the day. However, she was able to deal with these problems with equanimity and work within the system. Her letters are very professional. She seems to have derived the motivation for her work from her patriotism.

Du Coudray did not even protest in later years when Louis XVI became king in 1774 and wanted her to train men as veterinarians, because in many rural situations when a woman giving birth was having trouble, people called on the nearest shepherd to help.

Du Coudray was found dead by authorities on April 17, 1794, during the Reign of Terror. She had wisely trained her niece, another able midwife, to take her place, but soon after her niece died in 1825, no one seemed to take the mission as seriously as they had.

References: Gelbart, Nina Rattner, *The King's Midwife: A History and Mystery of Madame du Coudray,* Berkeley: University of California Press (1998); Snodgrass, Mary Ellen, *Historical Encyclopedia of Nursing,* Santa Barbara, CA: ABC-CLIO (1999).

Dufferin Fund

The Dufferin Fund was established in 1885 to fund medical training for nurses, midwives, physicians, and hospital assistants as well as provide for small hospitals and the care of women and children in India. Queen Victoria was convinced there was a great need for medical women in India, and Lady Dufferin, wife of the viceroy to India, initiated the fund. It was the first organized effort to help the women and children of India with a strong argument for its support being that women of the Hindu and Muslim faiths would not see male physicians.

When Lady Dufferin surveyed the conditions in India, she saw firsthand the needs that existed. She worked very hard at promoting the fund's success, and it helped numerous women and children over the years.

While she and her husband were in India, the colonial government was very supportive of the effort, and support also grew in England. When she left India in 1888, however, no one was as enthusiastic in maintaining the same level of assistance that she had achieved.

References: Lal, Maneesha, "The Politics of Gender and Medicine in Colonial India: The Countess of Dufferin's Fund, 1885–1888," *Bulletin of the History of Medicine* 68, no. 1 (Spring 1994): 29–66.

Dunn, Thelma Brumfield
1900–

Thelma Dunn became a leading authority on the tumors in mice and directed the Cancer Induction and Pathogenesis Section of the Pathology Laboratory at the National Cancer Institute.

Born in Pittsylvania County, Virginia, on February 6, 1900, she attended Cornell University and graduated with a bachelor's degree in 1922. She proceeded to the University of Virginia and earned her medical degree in 1926. She interned at Bellevue Hospital in New York and later worked in pathology at the University of Virginia and George Washington University, eventually taking a position at the National Cancer Institute researching cancer.

She wrote a book on cancer in 1975 on the importance of research. Her knowledge of mouse tumors greatly aided in the research she did at the National Cancer Institute. She is a realist about the disease and its consequences but not pessimistic—"a cure may come unexpectedly as insulin did for diabetes, as liver did for pernicious anemia, or as the antibiotics did for bacterial diseases. In the meantime we can continue to fight a limited war, a war of containment where cancer deaths are reduced and life prolonged. We have not yet applied all we know about preventing cancer" (Dunn 1975, 191). She married in 1929 and had three children. She currently lives in Charlottesville, Virginia.

References: *American Men and Women of Science*, 14th ed., New York: Bowker (1979); Dunn, Thelma Brumfield, *The Unseen Fight against Cancer: Experimental Cancer Research—Its Importance to Human Cancer*, Charlottesville, VA: Batt Bates (1975); Kass-Simon, Gabriele, *Women of Science: Righting the Record*, Bloomington: Indiana University Press (1990).

Durocher, Marie Josefina Mathilde
1809–1893

One of the first woman doctors in Latin America, Marie Durocher became a famous Brazilian obstetrician and was awarded the first medical degree of the newly reorganized Medical School at Rio de Janeiro in 1834.

Durocher was born in Paris but moved to Brazil with her family at the age of eight. She married early and had two children. Her husband died young and thus she had to seek a profession. Durocher was active for sixty years, usually dressing in men's clothes because she felt they were more practical than dresses for her work.

References: Lovejoy, Esther Pohl, *Women Doctors of the World*, New York: Macmillan (1957); Ogilvie, Marilyn, and Joy Harvey, eds., *The Biographical Dictionary of Women in Science: Pioneering Lives from Ancient Times to the Mid-20th Century*, New York: Routledge (2000).

Dyer, Helen Marie
1895–1998

Helen Dyer's development of the index of tumor chemotherapy in 1949 was requisite for the National Cancer Institute to develop a chemotherapy program. The index is a compilation of data she had gathered on earlier chemical treatments of tumors and their evolution. She was a gifted biochemist who contributed to the understanding of cancer and its treatment. She was also a proponent of more women going into science disciplines.

Born on May 26, 1895, in Washington, D.C., she was the daughter of Joseph E. Dyer and Florence Robertson Dyer, who had four children. She graduated from Western High School in 1913. She went on to Goucher College in Baltimore to study biology and physiology and graduated in 1917.

She worked for the Civil Service Commission and the Red Cross during World War I. Afterward, she wanted to advance her education in order to teach. She took courses at Mount Holyoke, then went back to Washington, D.C., to take a position at the Hygienic Laboratory, which was part of the Public Health Service. She worked there for seven years, researching the effects of chemotherapeutic drugs on animals. She also studied tumor growth rates.

In order to gain more education, she went to George Washington University to do graduate work. She earned a master's degree and stayed on to teach biochemistry while working on a doctorate degree, which she received in 1935. She continued to teach and had a very good reputation with the students.

She went to the National Cancer Institute in 1942 and stayed for twenty-three years. She was invaluable in creating the index of tumor chemotherapy and published numerous articles on the topic. She also did research on amino acids.

Dyer was active in the Washington Chemical Society and in 1962 was selected as a delegate to the International Cancer Congress in Moscow due to her international reputation. She earned numerous awards and honors over the years, including the Garvan Medal in 1962 for her work in biochemical research.

Dyer never married or had children. She retired in 1965 but continued to do research for several years. She died September 20, 1998, at her home in Washington, D.C., at the age of 103.

References: "Helen Dyer, 103, Cancer Researcher," *Washington Times* (22 September 22, 1998): C6; Ogilvie, Marilyn, and Joy Harvey, eds., *The Biographical Dictionary of Women in Science: Pioneering Lives from Ancient Times to the Mid-20th Century*, New York: Routledge (2000).

E

Edinburgh School of Medicine
1887–1898

Founded in Edinburgh by Sophia Jex-Blake, it was an early medical school for women in Europe. Jex-Blake had very high standards and was considered by many to be too strict. The school closed in 1898 because of competition from other medical schools, particularly the Medical College for Women, which had lower tuition and access to clinical facilities at the Edinburgh Royal Infirmary beginning in 1892.

See also: Jex-Blake, Sophia Louisa
References: Todd, Margaret G., *The Life of Sophia Jex-Blake,* London: Macmillan (1918).

Elders, Minnie Joycelyn
1933–

Joycelyn Elders became the first African American to hold the position of surgeon general in the United States. She was outspoken in her commitment to health reform, health education, and particularly sex education in schools.

Born in Schaal, Arkansas, on August 13, 1933, Elders was the oldest of eight children of Haller and Curtis Jones, who were loving parents. They were sharecroppers with no running water or electricity, and Elders, along with her brothers and sisters, worked in the cotton fields. She was very good in school, earning a scholarship to attend college. She received a B.A. in biology from Philander Smith College in Little Rock,

Arkansas. She then worked as a nurse's aide in the Veterans' Administration in Milwaukee before joining the U.S. Army in 1953. She trained as a physical therapist. Once out of the army, she went to medical school and received her M.D. degree from the University of Arkansas Medical School in 1960.

Elders interned at the University of Minnesota Hospital and did a residency in pediatrics at the University of Arkansas Medical Center. While in Arkansas she also earned an advanced degree in biochemistry. She was an assistant professor in pediatrics there after receiving a National Institutes of Health Career Development Award. In her research, she focused on endocrinology and pediatrics and by 1976 was a full professor.

Governor Bill Clinton of Arkansas appointed her director of the Arkansas Department of Health in 1987. They had met at the funeral for one of her brothers, who had been murdered. While in that office, she increased immunization rates, made it more possible for poor women to get mammograms, and increased early preventive-medicine screenings for children.

Elders could see what early pregnancy and sexually transmitted diseases were doing to young people and the health of the country, and she worked hard on educating the young. She was a strong advocate of sex education and contraception, opposed by many conservative politicians and religious leaders.

President Clinton nominated her in 1993 for the surgeon general position. She faced a battle during her confirmation hearings with many opponents in Congress feeling that she was too liberal. She was eventually confirmed and took office. She is a proponent of plain talk about sex, condoms, and masturbation, which she sees as part of human sexuality. Young people seemed to embrace her frankness, but some of their parents, and some government officials, did not. She served as surgeon general for only fifteen months because of controversy over some of her remarks. She has no regrets and still feels "committed to the issues I have always been about: comprehensive health education, prevention of teenage pregnancy, early-childhood education, school-based clinics to make health care available for all children, a preventive approach to health care for everyone" (Elders and Chanoff 1996, 336).

She married Oliver Elders in 1960 and had two sons, Eric and Kevin. After serving as surgeon general, Elders returned to the University of Arkansas as a pediatric endocrinologist.

References: Elders, M. Joycelyn, and David Chanoff, *Joycelyn Elders, M.D.: From Sharecropper's Daughter to Surgeon General of the United States of America*, New York: Morrow (1996); *Notable Black American Scientists*, Detroit: Gale Research (1998).

Elion, Gertrude Belle
1918–1999

Gertrude Elion received the Nobel Prize in physiology or medicine in 1988 "for demonstrating the differences in nucleic acid metabolism between normal cells and disease-causing cancer cells, protozoa, bacteria, and viruses" (McGrayne 1998, 302). She shared the award with George Hitchings and Sir James Black. It was the first time in thirty-one years that an award was given for drug research, and Elion was one of the few to receive a Nobel Prize without having a doctorate.

Elion developed many new drugs for cancer treatment. Before her research, most children with leukemia were not expected to survive; because of her contributions, a larger percentage of them now survive (Elion 1988, 449). She also laid the foundation for azidothymidine (AZT), the first

drug approved by the FDA for AIDS patients, and made organ transplants possible with the development of a drug to inhibit organ rejection.

Born on January 23, 1918, in New York City, Elion was the daughter of two immigrants. She had one younger brother. Her father, Robert, had come from Lithuania and descended from a long line of rabbis. He aspired to be a dentist and in 1914 graduated from the New York University School of Dentistry. Her mother, Bertha Cohen, had come from Poland. Elion was educated early in the public schools and proved an excellent student, graduating from high school at the age of twelve. She wanted to attend college but was unsure of what to major in. Her father had lost a lot of money in the stock market crash of 1929, but she was able to attend Hunter College for free because of her grades. She felt that the professors at Hunter, an all-female college, didn't expect students to set out on a career, but Elion planned to do so from the beginning.

She majored in science and chemistry, wanting, in emulation of her beloved grandfather, to help others. He had died of cancer when she was fifteen.

She graduated from Hunter with an A.B. degree in 1937. Like many others during the Great Depression, she struggled to find work. For three months, she taught biochemistry at the New York Hospital School of Nursing. Then she found a low-paid position as a laboratory assistant for a chemist. She stayed with the chemist for a year and a half and saved her money. With her savings and some help from her parents, she was able to enter graduate school at New York University in 1939.

She received an M.S. in chemistry in 1941. World War II was just beginning, and there was a shortage of chemists. Wanting to do research, she could find only laboratory jobs, which bored her. Eventually she took a job as an assistant to George Hitchings at Burroughs Wellcome, a pharmaceutical company. "I never felt constrained to remain strictly in chemistry, but was able to broaden my horizons into biochemistry, pharmacology, immunology, and eventually virology" (Elion 1988).

Elion also became interested in getting a doctorate, but because she loved her job and could not keep it and pursue further education, she chose to stay at Burroughs Wellcome. Hitchings was very supportive and encouraged her work on purines and the enzymes involved, letting her make compounds and then experiment to find out how they worked. She began to publish her findings. In 1950, Elion synthesized two cancer-treatment drugs. A purine compound called diaminopurine could interfere with leukemia cells, but the side effects were very strong, and eventually patients relapsed. Elion continued her studies. Later she developed a new compound called mercaptopurine (6-MP), which was also effective; but again, patients with leukemia relapsed after a time. She was committed to making 6-MP better.

Another drug she synthesized was thioguanine, a close relative of 6-MP. When physicians began treating leukemia patients with thioguanine or 6-MP combined with other drugs, they were successful. Still Elion continued to try to make the effects of 6-MP last longer. She also became interested in immune-system suppressants, and research led her to the development of Imuran, a more sophisticated version of 6-MP. It wasn't long before it proved useful in organ transplants, which had usually failed prior to Imuran because recipients' bodies rejected the new organ. By 1961 it had become possible to successfully transplant organs.

Hitchings retired in 1967, and Elion could admit that they'd had their differences and that he never gave her proper credit for her work. She was glad to be on her own to choose her projects without reporting to him.

Antivirals were of interest because scientists felt that any drug developed to kill a virus would also harm the DNA of a healthy cell. Elion returned to the aminopurine, which had been observed to have antiviral properties back in 1948 but was also too toxic. She developed a related compound that was successful against herpes.

Later, in the mid-1970s, her team tested acyclovir, which was successful against viruses but not at all toxic. This develop-ment convinced scientists that enzymes could be specific to viruses. Acyclovir was marketed as Zovirax in 1991.

In 1970, Elion moved with the company to North Carolina. She retired in 1983 and served as a consultant to Burroughs Wellcome. Within one year her division had developed AZT, the first drug approved by the FDA to treat AIDS patients.

In October 1988, a reporter called to tell her she'd won the Nobel Prize. She was surprised until she heard that the other two winners were Hitchings and Sir James W. Black. She was thrilled but stressed that the biggest reward in her career was knowing she had helped develop tools to cure diseases.

She continued to work, teaching Duke University students research methods, consulting at Burroughs Wellcome, and serving on national and international committees.

Elion died February 21, 1999, in Chapel Hill, North Carolina.

References: Elion, Gertrude B., "The Purine Path to Chemotherapy," "Elion, Gertrude B.," Official Web Site of the Nobel Foundation, http://www.nobel.se/medicine/laureates1988/elion-autobio.html; McGrayne, Sharon Bertsch, *Nobel Prize Women in Science*, New York: Carol (1998).

Emerson, Gladys Anderson
1903–1984

Gladys Emerson isolated vitamin E for the first time in 1936 after her husband, Oliver Emerson, discovered it. She contributed much to the understanding of the importance of vitamins and minerals in daily nutrition and aided the government in establishing dietary guidelines. She also contributed a great deal of research on vitamin B deficiencies.

Born July 1, 1903, in Caldwell, Kansas, she and her parents, Otis and Louise Anderson, moved to Fort Worth, Texas. She attended public schools there and eventually graduated from high school in El Reno, Oklahoma. She went on to higher education at the Oklahoma College for Women, graduat-

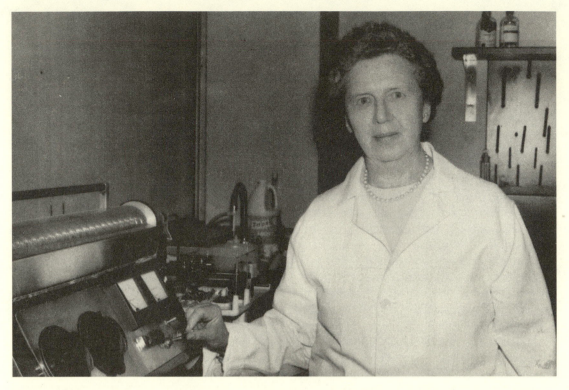

Gladys Anderson Emerson (UCLA School of Public Health/U.S. National Library of Medicine)

ing with A.B. and B.S. degrees in 1925. She attended Stanford and received an M.A. in 1926, followed by a Ph.D. in nutrition and biochemistry from the University of California, Berkeley, in 1932.

She and Oliver traveled to work in Germany for a brief time before beginning work at the University of California, Berkeley. She worked as a research associate there for the Institute of Experimental Biology from 1933 to 1942. She then went to the Merck Institute in New Jersey to head its department of nutrition. During her stay there she did a great deal of work on the vitamins E and B. She did experiments on both rats and monkeys to determine the effects of various vitamin deficiencies.

She next took a position as head of the Department of Nutrition and Home Economics at the University of California in Los Angeles. She was an enthusiastic teacher and lecturer on nutrition. By this time she was known as an expert in the field and had frequent requests for lectures around the country.

She and her husband divorced in 1940, and she never remarried or had children. One of the highest honors she received was the Garvan Medal, in 1952. It is given in the field of chemistry to a woman who has made significant accomplishments.

Emerson died of cancer on January 18, 1984, at her home in Santa Monica, California. She was buried on January 24, 1984, next to her parents in El Reno, Oklahoma.

References: Folkers, Karl, "Gladys Anderson Emerson (1903–1984): A Biographical Sketch," *Journal of Nutrition* 115, no. 7 (July 1985): 837–841; *Notable Twentieth-Century Scientists Supplement*, Detroit: Gale Research (1998).

Erxleben, Dorothea Christiana
1715–1762

Germany's first woman doctor, Dorothea Erxleben, was fortunate enough to practice publicly as a physician by being bold enough to petition King Frederick II for consent to attend the University of Halle with her brother. She was born in Quedlinburg in 1715 to Christian Polycarpus Leporin and Anna Sophia Meinecken. She felt early on that she benefited from reading and aspired to learn all she could. By the time her brother entered the University of Halle, she had prepared herself for further study and was interested in medicine. She had learned a great deal from her father, a physician who supported her goal.

With King Frederick II's approval, she and her brother went to the University together. Many opposed her attendance, feeling that females were far too fragile to ever be well educated, much less become physicians.

When Austria and Germany went to war and her brother was called into military service, she left school because she was not comfortable attending classes without him. She married Johann Erxleben, a deacon, and assumed responsibility for his five children, adding four of her own. While raising her family, she did practice medicine even though she did not have a university degree.

In 1753 she was accused of not treating patients correctly after one of her patients died. She addressed the charges and was allowed to defend her dissertation and take the exams to prove her knowledge. She did an excellent job on the exams, receiving her degree on June 12, 1754. She continued her medical practice until her death in 1762.

References: Schiebinger, Londa L., *The Mind Has No Sex? Women in the Origins of Modern Science*, Cambridge, MA: Harvard University Press (1989).

Eskelin, Karolina
1867–1938

Karolina Eskelin was the first woman to receive a doctorate (1895) in medicine in Finland and the first woman to be a surgeon in Finland. She was allowed to practice medicine as a physician at the Surgical Hospital in Helsinki prior to founding another hospital in Tampere. She also founded a second private hospital in Helsinki. She briefly vis-

ited the United States and practiced medicine in Oregon and Massachusetts.

References: Lovejoy, Esther Pohl, *Woman Doctors of the World*, New York: Macmillan (1957); Olkkonen, Tuomo, "Suomen Ensimmainen Naistohtori," *Opusculum* 5, no. 3 (1985): 122–128; Riska, Elainne, "Women's Careers in Medicine: Developments in the United States and Finland," *Scandinavian Studies* 61 (Spring–Summer 1989): 185–198.

Evans, Alice Catherine
1881–1975

Alice Evans's pioneering work in milk bacteria led to the acceptance of pasteurization. She was the first woman to serve as a bacteriologist for the U.S. Department of Agriculture (USDA).

Born in Neath, Pennsylvania, on January 29, 1881, she was the daughter of Anne B. Evans and William Howell Evans and had one brother, Morgan. Both her parents were teachers, and her father was also a farmer. She became a teacher as well and, after four years, enrolled in a program for rural teach-

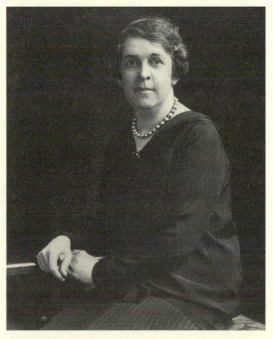

Alice Catherine Evans (Underwood & Underwood/ U.S. National Library of Medicine)

ers at Cornell that her brother had told her about.

There Evans became interested in science and completed a degree in bacteriology in 1909. She went on to the University of Wisconsin for a master's degree. Upon graduation, she worked for the government, investigating the microbes in cow's milk. After obtaining a position with the USDA in its dairy division, Evans discovered, in 1917, that bacillus abortus, which causes Bang's disease in cows and was thought to be a harmless germ to humans, was very similar to the bacteria known as *Micrococus melitensis*, which was from raw goat's milk and made people sick with what was called undulant fever. Undulant fever had been a problem since the nineteenth century. Evans concluded that the disease that became known as brucellosis could be contracted by humans from drinking both cow's and goat's milk.

Later scientific investigations led to the realization that many people who had brucellosis were at times misdiagnosed as having influenza or tuberculosis.

Evans published her findings but was ignored because she held no doctorate degree. She moved on to work for the U.S. Public Health Service but continued to argue about the importance of pasteurizing milk. No one listened until two other researchers, Dr. Charles M. Carpenter of Cornell University and Dr. Karl F. Meyer of the University of California, confirmed her findings. Carpenter found that the same germ that led to undulant fever in humans caused Bang's disease (brucellosis) in animals. Meyer suggested a new genus be named *Brucella* to incorporate both organisms. By the 1930s, the dairy industry was pasteurizing all milk in the United States.

During her own research, Evans contracted brucellosis in 1922 and suffered with it for twenty years. Nonetheless, she continued her bacteria research, which included looking for the cause of meningitis and streptococcus infections. In 1928 she became the first woman to become president of the Society of American Bacteriologists. She retired in 1945 but stayed active in microbiology research until her death from a stroke on September 5, 1975, in Alexandria, Virginia.

References: Ogilvie, Marilyn, and Joy Harvey, eds., *The Biographical Dictionary of Women in Science: Pioneering Lives from Ancient Times to the Mid-20th Century*, New York: Routledge (2000); Stevens, Marianne Fedunkiw, *American National Biography*, vol. 7, New York: Oxford University Press (1999).

F

Fabiola, Saint
d. ca. 399

Saint Fabiola founded a public hospital in Rome that was the first such hospital in western Europe. She was also responsible for establishing a hospice in Porto, Italy, with the help of St. Pammachius. A Christian noblewoman, Fabiola dedicated her life to helping the poor and needy after converting to Christianity and following the teachings of St. Jerome. She studied the scriptures, as she knew Latin, Hebrew, and Greek.

Fabiola came from a wealthy family descended from Julius Maximus. She married very young and then separated from the church because she married a second time before her first, abusive, husband died. Upon the death of her second husband and her public penitence, she sold her possessions and worked for the good of the poor. At the hospital she founded, she attended to the patients herself regardless of their disease or condition.

She followed Jerome to Bethlehem in 395 and stayed with her relative, Oceanus. She returned to Rome following the Huns' threat to invade Palestine in 396. She contemplated a long journey due to her restlessness but died before she could commence. All of Rome admired her greatly. December 27 is her feast day.

References: Carter, E. D., "Fabiola, St." *New Catholic Encyclopedia*, New York: McGraw-Hill (1967); "Fabiola, Saint," *Encyclopedia Britannica*, vol. 4, Chicago: Encyclopedia Britannica (1997).

Farquhar, Marilyn Gist
1928–

A cell biologist, Marilyn Farquhar has contributed a significant amount of research on renal disease and more recently on the characteristics of G proteins.

Born on July 11, 1928, in Tulare, California, to Brooks Dewitt Gist and Alta Green Gist, Farquhar had one older sister. She was educated in the public schools and then attended the University of California at Berkeley. She majored in zoology as a premed student. She graduated in 1949 and was one of only three women admitted to medical school at the University of California in San Francisco.

After two years, she became interested in the study of diseases. She changed her course of study and received a Ph.D. in pathology in 1955 at the University of California, Berkeley. She went with her husband, John Farquhar, to the University of Minnesota and studied kidney disease. Cell biology was a new field, and electron microscopy made it possible for scientists to see much more detail.

Farquhar returned to the University of California at San Francisco in 1962 and eventually became a full professor of pathology. Her first marriage ended in divorce, and in 1970 she married George Palade, a future Nobel Prize winner.

Farquhar has published hundreds of articles and papers on cell biology, renal disease, kidney problems, and G proteins. In 1988 she was elected to the National Academy of Sciences. Currently she serves as professor of pathology and is the chair of cellular and molecular medicine at the University of California, San Diego. She has two sons, Bruce and Douglas, by her first marriage.

References: *Notable Twentieth-Century Scientists,* Detroit: Gale Research (1995); Shearer, Benjamin F., and Barbara S. Shearer, *Notable Women in the Life Sciences: A Biographical Dictionary,* Westport, CT: Greenwood Press (1996).

Felicie, Jacoba
1280–?

Jacoba Felicie was a very learned healer in the thirteenth century in Paris. She was possibly as skilled as male physicians of the time were.

Most women then could not obtain licenses to practice medicine and were not admitted to universities, with the exception of Italian universities, and thus they had limited training. Skilled physicians sometimes taught women. Felicie, an empiric, was prosecuted several times for practicing medicine without a license.

References: Hughes, Muriel Joy, *Women Healers in Medieval Life and Literature,* New York, King's Crown Press (1943); Ogilvie, Marilyn, and Joy Harvey, eds., *The Biographical Dictionary of Women in Science: Pioneering Lives from Ancient Times to the Mid-20th Century,* New York: Routledge (2000).

Female Genital Mutilation

Many cultures use female genital mutilation (FGM) to circumcise young girls. Many of these girls die from the procedure or develop physical and emotional problems.

Over the past two centuries, women who were subjected to this procedure have sought the help of female physicians and medical missionaries. Many have also tried to escape those societies that practice this procedure, which is often bound up in cultural and religious beliefs. FGM is now against the law in many countries due to better awareness of the damage it can do.

With so many undesirable effects of excision and infibulation it might appear most extraordinary that such practices survive. But the practices themselves have been kept so secret and there are indeed many who have not suffered the after-effects described, themselves, and are therefore quite unaware of the medical hazards. Moreover many rural dwellers still do not associate certain medical conditions with the excision operation. The lack of communication sometimes between the educated urban population and unschooled rural people encourages the continued belief in traditional mythological rationalizations for the customs, and ideological arguments remain unchallenged. (Sanderson 1981, 44)

See also: Ramsey, Mimi; el Saadawi, Nawal
References: Sanderson, Lilian Passmore, *Against the Mutilation of Women: The Struggle to End Unnecessary Suffering,* London: Ithaca Press (1981); Toubia, Nahid, and Susan Izett, *Female Genital Mutilation: An Overview,* Geneva: World Health Organization (1998).

Fenselau, Catherine Clarke
1939–

Catherine Fenselau contributed to the development of mass spectrometry and its use in analyzing chemical compounds to determine molecular mass, structure, and composition. Researchers use the method extensively today to determine the benefits of many drugs in treating diseases.

Born in York, Nebraska, on April 15, 1939, Fenselau became interested in science in high school. She was encouraged to go to college at Bryn Mawr and graduated with an A.B. in chemistry in 1961. She chose Stanford for graduate study and received her Ph.D. in 1965. By this time she was married to Allan H. Fenselau. At Stanford she began working in the new field of mass spectrometry.

Her first teaching job was at Johns Hopkins School of Medicine, where she rose from instructor to professor. She worked there from 1967 to 1987. In 1985 she won the Garvan Medal from the American Chemical Society for her outstanding contributions to chemistry.

She left Johns Hopkins for a position at the University of Maryland, Baltimore County, as professor and chair of the Department of Chemistry. Her interests in mass spectrometry led to studies of laetrile, an anticancer drug. The World Health Organization also asked her to study the metabolism of clofazamine, a drug used to treat leprosy.

In 1992 Fenselau received a Merit Award for her work from the National Institutes of Health. Currently she is a professor in the Department of Chemistry and Biochemistry at the University of Maryland, College Park. She has two sons.

References: Roscher, Nina Matheny, "Catherine Clarke Fenselau," in Benjamin F. Shearer and Barbara S. Shearer, eds., *Notable Women in the Physical Sciences: A Biographical Dictionary,* Westport, CT: Greenwood Press (1997).

Ferguson, Angela Dorothea
1925–

Angela Ferguson did pioneering research in the diagnosis and treatment of sickle cell anemia. She also made it clear that more research was needed on African American children so that black pediatricians like herself would know what norms to expect in their clients and what advice to give mothers.

She was born in Washington, D.C., on February 15, 1925, to a poor family. Her father taught at a segregated high school and also served in the U.S. Army Reserves, but he did not earn enough during the depression to support a family of eight. Angela worked in the school cafeteria in exchange for meals, and many times at home dinner consisted of only potatoes or cocoa and water.

Never intending to go to college, Angela attended Cardoza High School. It was here that she discovered her love of and gift for science, particularly chemistry and mathematics. She took summer-school courses to catch up with some of the other students and graduated in 1941.

She decided to seek a career in science and was accepted at Howard University. Her parents could afford her first year there, since she lived at home. After that she obtained scholarships for tuition and fees and covered other expenses by working in the laboratories at Freedmen's Hospital, the teaching hospital at Howard University and the predecessor of Howard University Hospital. She graduated from Howard in 1945.

Her interests changed to biology and medicine with a desire to help children, and she pursued pediatrics training in medical school at Howard University. She graduated with her medical degree in 1949 and interned in all departments of Freedmen's Hospital. After passing her final examinations, she went into private practice. During this time, she realized that research focused primarily on children of European descent, and she did not have sufficient information to treat her black patients.

Howard University School of Medicine hired her to begin to rectify this lack, and during her research, she discovered that many black children suffered from sickle cell anemia. It was a very hard disease to diagnose, as its symptoms vary by age and are common to other ailments. She studied hundreds of cases in order to determine the most obvious signs and shared her findings with colleagues. One of her greatest contributions was promoting the use of a blood test at birth to determine if African American babies had the disease. She also developed helpful treatments for sickle cell anemia, among them increasing fluid intake to help the flow of blood.

In 1965 her work changed dramatically when she became involved in building a new teaching hospital at Howard University. From the beginning of the project, she advised government officials and others on what was needed in a teaching hospital. The new Freedmen's Hospital opened ten years later, and Ferguson held the position of associate vice-president for health affairs for over twenty years, until she retired in 1990. She is married to Dr. Charles M. Cabaniss and has two daughters.

References: Kessler, James H., *Distinguished African American Scientists of the 20th Century*, Phoenix: Oryx Press (1996); "Scientist," *Ebony* (August 1960): 44.

Flexner Report
1910

The Flexner Report came about as a result of concerns over educational standards. In the late nineteenth century and the early twentieth century, large numbers of proprietary colleges and universities were starting up without sufficient standards and governing boards in place. The Carnegie Foundation, charged with the evaluation of education in the country because of these developments, appointed Abraham Flexner to investigate the problem. His 1910 Flexner Report drastically changed medical education in the United States and Canada in the following decades. Flexner was very critical of proprietary medical schools, reinforcing the importance of scientific education and clinical experience. His report encouraged standardization in medical school curriculums and resulted in massive reforms and the closing of many schools over the next several years.

Unfortunately for women, the report resulted in the closing of some of the schools that allowed them to enter, and some of the schools that survived continued to refuse admittance to women for quite some time. Thus despite its positive ramifications for medical education as a whole, the report resulted in a decline in women physicians during the early part of the twentieth century.

References: Flexner, Abraham, *Medical Education in the United States and Canada: A Report to the Carnegie Foundation for the Advancement of Teaching*, New York: Carnegie Foundation for the Advancement of Teaching (1910); King, L. S., "Medicine in the USA: Historical Vignettes, XX. The Flexner Report of 1910." *JAMA* 251, no. 8 (February 24, 1984): 1079–1086.

Footbinding

For over a century, it was the custom in China for women to bind their feet in order to make them tiny. According to Pruitt, "A girl's beauty and desirability were counted more by the size of her feet than by the beauty of her face" (1945, 22). Also, Hong says, "Bound feet were associated with security, mobility and status" (1997, 25).

Western medical missionaries were among the first to help the women who suffered from the practice. Footbinding emotionally affected the women physicians more than men in the field because the custom was associated with male dominance and kept Chinese women and girls in despair. It was the female missionaries, stirred by their own reform movements at home in Western Europe, Canada, and the United States, who fueled the antifootbinding movement of the late nineteenth and early twentieth centuries.

In the missionaries' eyes tiny-footed girls usually looked as if they were in pain, for instead of jumping about happily they needed help in walking, as if they were wounded. Footbinding was consequently denounced as an evil which crippled approximately half the population, added to the misery of the poverty stricken, increased child deaths, prevented women from supporting themselves and from caring adequately for their children, inhibited 'the cheer and cleanliness' of their homes, and confined women and their thoughts to the narrowest of spheres" (Hong 1997, 55).

Girls with bound feet could not attend school or engage in any physical activity; many suffered infections, broken bones, intense pain, and sometimes death. "My grandmother had wanted me to have bound feet. She told me that big feet were not beautiful. I thought that was fine, so I had my feet bound, but it was very painful. When you bind your feet, you have to wear at least two pairs of cloth shoes, plus several layers of cloth strips binding your feet tightly inside the shoes" (Young 1995–1996, 535). The Chinese outlawed the custom in 1902.

References: Hong, Fan, *Footbinding, Feminism, and Freedom: The Liberation of Women's Bodies in Modern China,* London: F. Cass (1997); Pruitt, Ida, *A Daughter of Han,* New Haven, CT: Yale University Press (1945); Wang, Ping, *Aching for Beauty: Footbinding in China,* Minneapolis: University of Minnesota Press (2000); Young, Helen Praeger, "From Soldier to Doctor: A Chinese Woman's Story of the Long March," *Science and Society* 59, no. 4 (Winter 1995–1996): 531–547.

Fowler, Lydia Folger
1822–1879

Lydia Fowler became the second female physician in the United States in 1850 and was the first woman to become a professor at a U.S. medical school. She lectured frequently and argued for the need of women in the medical profession.

Fowler was born May 5, 1822, in Nantucket, Massachusetts, to Gideon and Eunice Macy Folger. She had a good basic education, including math and science, and left school in 1838 to teach in Norton at the Wheaton Seminary. She married Lorenzo Niles Fowler in 1844 and had a daughter, Jessie Allen, in 1856.

Lorenzo Fowler was a phrenologist who lectured extensively on this new science. Lydia accompanied him and eventually began speaking on physiology and hygiene. She decided to enroll at Central Medical College in New York, which was one of the first medical schools to accept women on a regular basis. She learned a great deal about anatomy and became a lecturer at the college. Later on she was promoted to professor in order to teach in the area of midwifery and the diseases of women and children. Her post was short-lived because the school merged with a competitor in New York. Fowler left to begin private practice. She also taught and gave periodic lectures to women.

Eventually the women's rights movement and the temperance drive took more of her time. She and her husband moved to London

in 1863, where she continued to be involved in the temperance movement. She died of pleuropneumonia on January 26, 1879.

References: Ford, Bonnie, "Lydia Folger Fowler," in Frank N. Magill, ed., *Great Lives from History, American Women Series,* vol. 2, Pasadena, CA: Salem Press (1995).

Franklin, Martha Minerva
1870–1968

Martha Franklin was a leader and organizer of black nurses in the United States at the end of the nineteenth century and beginning of the twentieth century. She founded the National Association of Colored Graduate Nurses (NACGN) in 1908 with support from other black nurses, notably Mary Eliza Mahoney and Adah Belle Samuels Thoms. She also had support from the National Medical Association (NMA), the major black physicians' association of the time.

Born in New Milford, Connecticut, to Henry J. Franklin and Mary E. Gauson on October 29, 1870, Franklin had a sister, Florence, and a brother, William. Her father had been a soldier in the Civil War. She attended public school in Meriden, Connecticut, where there were few blacks. She chose a nursing career and went to Philadelphia, where she became the sole black graduate of the December 1897 class of the Women's Hospital Training School for Nurses.

Like most black nurses, Franklin experienced discrimination. The American Nurses Association did not allow blacks to join, and she felt that having no voice was a major obstacle to progress. She conducted a survey of 1,500 black nurses and urged a meeting.

In 1908 a meeting finally took place, and the NACGN was officially founded with Franklin as president. There were fifty-two nurses at the first meeting in New York City. By 1940 there were over 12,000 members.

Franklin worked very hard within the association and with other groups who were supportive. She became a registered nurse in New York after completing a postgraduate course at Lincoln Hospital. She worked as a nurse in the public schools and continued to obtain more education as needed. Franklin died on September 26, 1968. In 1976 she was posthumously inducted into the Nursing Hall of Fame.

See also: Mahoney, Mary Eliza
References: Davis, Althea T., *Early Black American Leaders in Nursing: Architects for Integration and Equality*, Boston: Jones and Bartlett (1999); Davis, Althea T., "Franklin, Martha Minerva," *American National Biography*, vol. 8, New York: Oxford University Press (1999).

Franklin, Rosalind Elsie
1920–1958

Rosalind Franklin contributed an enormous amount of information toward the understanding of DNA's structure. Her work was vital to the discovery of nucleic acids and their molecular structure.

Born in London on July 25, 1920, to Ellis and Muriel Waley Franklin, she grew up with three brothers until a sister came along when she was eight. She received a good education at St. Paul's Girls' School, where she became very interested in science. Her parents were devoted to public service and were philanthropists. Her father helped numerous Jews escape from Nazi Germany. Many in her family were socialists, as was she. Relatives were oftentimes involved in women's causes, and their work had an impact on her.

Her father did not encourage her interest in science because he wanted her to go into social work. After he refused to pay for her education at Cambridge, an angry Aunt Alice and her mother agreed to finance her schooling. Later her father relented and was supportive. She attended Newnham College at Cambridge University in London and received a degree in chemistry in 1941. She stayed at Cambridge and studied gas-phase chromatography while on a research scholarship. She earned her Ph.D. in 1945 while studying the structure of coal and carbons to help in the war effort. She contributed a great deal to the industry by helping to find high-strength fibers in carbon.

Once the war ended she turned her attention to X-ray crystallography and diffraction in order to find out more about how molecules form. In 1947 she went to France and began work at the Laboratoire Centrale des Services Chimiques de l'Etat. There during the next three years, she furthered her work on carbon fibers. She then returned to England and in 1950, Sir John Randall at King's College asked her to join Maurice Wilkins and Raymond Gosling, who were already working at King's on DNA; Randall wanted someone to study the photos Gosling had already taken.

Franklin preferred to work independently and from the beginning did not get along with Wilkins. There were further problems regarding the roles each would play, and the partnership did not last. Franklin and Gosling did work well together and published five papers.

Franklin found King's College very formal. The segregation of men and women there was a hindrance to cooperative research efforts. She led a social life outside of the college, keeping busy also with social reforms. She continued to work on DNA and its structure, making a lot of headway and producing some of the best existing photos of DNA. Working with coal had helped her to work with structures that were not totally crystalline. She was able to show that the DNA molecule could exist in either a more crystalline A form or a B form.

Wilkins eventually showed James D. Watson one of Franklin's photos without her knowledge or permission. The photo gave Watson a piece to the puzzle that he and Francis Crick had been looking for, and they were able to publish an article on the structure of DNA. They would win the Nobel Prize in medicine in 1962 along with Wilkins, four years after Franklin's death to ovarian cancer.

Franklin went on to Birkbeck College in 1953 and studied virus structures. Her work there helped lay the foundation for biomolecular science. She died on March 20, 1958, after having been diagnosed with cancer in 1956. Franklin continued to work despite being gravely ill.

Franklin was very dedicated to her work

and was not good at small talk. Although most admired her, some colleagues found her difficult. In *The Double Helix*, James Watson's account of the discovery of the structure of DNA, Franklin is portrayed in a very negative way. Some critics have called the book very cruel, and some scientists feel Watson should have given a good deal of credit to Franklin for her work on DNA. Franklin did not appear as an entry in the *Dictionary of National Biography* until the 1993 *Missing Persons* volume was published.

References: Klug, Aaron, "Franklin, Rosalind Elsie," *Dictionary of National Biography: Missing Persons*, Oxford: Oxford University Press (1993); McGrayne, Sharon Bertsch, *Nobel Prize Women in Science: Their Lives, Struggles, and Momentous Discoveries*, Secaucus, NJ: Carol (1998); Sayre, Anne, *Rosalind Franklin and DNA*, New York: Norton (1975).

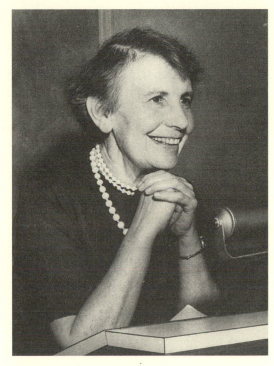

Anna Freud (U.S. National Library of Medicine)

Freud, Anna
1895–1982

Anna Freud was a pioneer in psychoanalysis. She carried on after her father and established her own theories in child therapy.

Born in Vienna, Austria, on December 3, 1895, the last of six children, she was the daughter of the founder of psychoanalysis, Sigmund Freud, and his wife, Martha Bernays. She was educated as a teacher, but her father had a profound impact on the direction her work would take.

She worked closely with her father in Vienna until the Nazi invasion, at which time she and her family escaped to England. She continued her work there and with Dorothy T. Burlingham established a nursery and later a clinic in Hampstead in order for children to receive medical and educational services following World War II.

Freud's work focused on child therapy and human defense mechanisms. She built on her father's work but also contributed much to our understanding of children and how their environments affect them. She had tremendous energy and was an excellent public speaker, appealing to audiences of diverse backgrounds. She also was a clear writer who published a number of papers and books during her lifetime.

Psychoanalysts are still developing many of her ideas, and she is widely read. "She has gone forward where he left off, giving her life to children from unhappy homes, to children in the midst of the terrors of war, to normal children in their puzzling, inspiring variety" (Coles 1992, 198). Freud died October 9, 1982, in London.

References: Coles, Robert, *Anna Freud: The Dream of Psychoanalysis*, Reading, MA: Addison-Wesley (1992); Jahoda, Marie, "Freud, Anna," *Dictionary of National Biography: 1981–1985*, London: Oxford University Press (1990); Limentani, Adam, *Between Freud and Klein: The Psychoanalytic Quest for Knowledge and Truth*, London: Free Association Books (1989); Sheehy, Noel, Antony J. Chapman, and Wendy A. Conroy, *Biographical Dictionary of Psychology*, London: Routledge (1997).

Friend, Charlotte
1921–1987

Charlotte Friend was the first scientist to discover that a virus could cause cancer. Many were skeptical about this at the time, but her hard data, published in 1957, were convincing. Friend was also an activist for women's rights and a leader among women in science. She was elected to the National Academy of Sciences in 1976 and became the first woman president of the New York Academy of Sciences and later, president of the American Association for Cancer Research.

Born March 11, 1921, during the depression, Friend grew up in New York City along with her two older sisters and a younger brother. Her parents, Morris Friend and Cecelia Wolpin, had emigrated to the United States from Russia as young adults. Her father died when she was three years old, and her mother moved the family to the Bronx to be closer to her own extended family there.

Friend was educated at Hunter High School and later Hunter College. She worked at a doctor's office at night while going to college. She loved New York City and took advantage of the many free cultural and educational opportunities as she was growing up. She developed a love of art, music, and science.

Upon graduation in 1944 she enlisted in the navy and worked in Shoemaker, California, at the naval hospital's hematology laboratory. After World War II ended, she used the GI Bill to go to graduate school at Yale. She earned a Ph.D. in 1950 in bacteriology.

Friend's first job after graduation was working at the Sloan Kettering Institute for Cancer Research in New York City. She was free to do research that interested her, and it was here that she was able to isolate what became known as the Friend leukemia virus (FLV), which caused leukemia in rats. She published her findings in 1957 in the *Journal of Experimental Medicine.* Many researchers asked for samples of the virus from her, and numerous research projects followed.

In 1966 she moved on to Mount Sinai Hospital to work in its new medical school's Center for Experimental Cell Biology. She was both a professor and the director. She continued her research there, and her cell cultures, which were used all over the world, made a significant impact on cell and molecular biology. She received many awards during her lifetime.

Friend, who never married, developed lymphoma when she was sixty and suffered with it for six years. She died in New York City on January 13, 1987.

References: Diamond, Leila, "Charlotte Friend (1921–1987)," *Nature* (23 April 1987): 748; Diamond, Leila, "Friend, Charlotte," *American National Biography*, vol. 8, New York: Oxford University Press (1999); Diamond, Leila, and Sandra R. Wolman, *Viral Oncogenesis and Cell Differentiation: The Contributions of Charlotte Friend*, New York: New York Academy of Sciences (1989).

Fulton, Mary Hannah
1854–1927

Mary Fulton founded the Hackett Medical College for Women, the first women's medical college in China. A physician and medical missionary, she was bold enough to take on the responsibility of educating Chinese women medical students when the college that originally admitted them, Canton Medical Missionary Hospital, decided not to continue to educate women. Had it not been for Fulton, the female medical students would have had to discontinue their education.

Born May 31, 1854, in Ashland, Ohio, she received a good education at Lawrence University and received her B.S. from Hillsdale College in 1874.

She taught in public school in Indianapolis, Indiana, before entering the Women's Medical College of Pennsylvania, from which she received her medical degree in 1884. She took a great interest in doing medical missionary work in China, and that same year, the Presbyterian Board of Foreign Missions appointed her and her brother, Albert, a Presbyterian minister, to serve in South China.

They initially settled in Canton, and following a brief stay in Kwangsi, which proved to be too violent, returned to Canton. Fulton was very successful in setting up dispensaries and worked at the Canton Medical Missionary Hospital. When there was a fallout between two of the male leaders of the hospital, one physician left and took all his male students with him. The female medical students were left with no teachers or support. Fulton took it upon herself to set up a women's and children's medical hospital and later the Hackett Medical College for Women.

Throughout the late nineteenth century she treated bubonic plague, endured the opium wars, and treated women slaves in China. "I often returned from attending those ill at home, sick at heart. In every house I found either bound feet, those afflicted with tuberculosis or those addicted to the use of opium; sometimes all three" (Fulton 1915, 106). The bubonic plague was devastating to the Canton population: "John Kerr, the director of the Canton Missionary Hospital, lamented that in 'the great city of Canton, . . . there was no Sanitary Board, the government adopted no sanitary or preventive measures, there was no isolation of cases, no removal of filth or rubbish, no water supply, no system of drainage, and . . . Chinese medicine and Chinese superstitions had full and unrestricted sway'" (Benedict 1996, 135).

Despite these overwhelming problems, Fulton persevered in establishing the medical school, and also a school for nurses. She retired to Pasadena, California, after poor health forced her to leave China. She wrote of her missionary work and died on January 7, 1927.

See also: Guangzhou, China

References: Balmer, Randall, and John R. Fitzmier, *The Presbyterians*, Westport, CT: Greenwood Press (1993); Benedict, Carol, *Bubonic Plague in Nineteenth-century China*, Stanford, CA: Stanford University Press (1996); Cadbury, William Warder, and Mary Hoxie Jones, *At the Point of a Lancet: One Hundred Years of the Canton Hospital, 1835–1935*, Shanghai: Kelly and Walsh (1935); Fulton, Mary H., *"Inasmuch": Extracts from Letters, Journals, Papers, etc.*, West Medford, MA: Central Committee on the United Study of Foreign Missions (1915); Tucker, Sara W., "Opportunities for Women: The Development of Professional Women's Medicine at Canton, China, 1879–1901," *Women's Studies International Forum* 13, no. 4 (1990): 357–368.

G

Geneva Medical College
1835–1872

Geneva Medical College was the first institution of higher education in the United States to confer a medical degree upon a woman, Elizabeth Blackwell, the first female physician in the United States.

Geneva College wanted a medical school in order to bring in more money. This move was very problematic, as the College of Physicians and Surgeons in New York (later part of Columbia University) was against it. College officials and others persisted until the college's doors opened in 1835.

At the time Elizabeth Blackwell attended, the college had a two-year program. The school had a faculty of physicians who also engaged in private practice when the college was not in session. The school did quite well until the 1850s and 1860s brought much new competition from other medical schools; some of these, unlike Geneva College, were near hospitals.

In 1872, Geneva Medical College conferred its last medical degree. Most of the medical school faculty then moved to Syracuse University, which had better facilities.

Geneva Medical College had been a small part of Geneva College, which was started in 1796 as Geneva Academy, gaining a charter to become a college for men in 1825 with the help of John Henry Hobart. It was known as Geneva College until 1852, when it became Hobart College, named after its founder. It is known as Hobart and William Smith Colleges today.

References: Smith, Warren Hunting, *Hobart and William Smith: The History of Two Colleges*, Geneva, NY: Hobart and William Smith Colleges (1972).

Giliani, Alessandra
1307–1326

Alessandra Giliana was the first female prosector. She studied with and was an assistant to Mondino dei Luzzi, considered a great anatomy teacher of the time, at the University of Bologna in Italy.

She was skilled at dissecting cadavers and used a colored dye that dried quickly to show the smallest of blood vessels to students. This demonstration was an indispensable learning aid for medical students of the time. She died very young on March 26, 1326.

References: Hughes, Muriel Joy, *Women Healers in Medieval Life and Literature*, New York: King's Crown Press (1943); Shearer, Benjamin F., and Barbara S. Shearer, *Notable Women in the Life Sciences: A Biographical Dictionary*, Westport, CT: Greenwood Press (1996).

Goodrich, Annie Warburton
1866–1954

Annie Goodrich implemented new standards for nurses that became nationally accepted and directly improved patient care in the United States. In Washington, D.C., in 1918, Goodrich also established the first U.S. Army School of Nursing and served as the first dean.

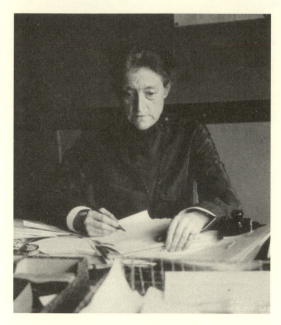

Annie Warburton Goodrich (U.S. National Library of Medicine)

Born in Brunswick, New Jersey, on February 6, 1866, she was the second child of Annie Williams Butler and Samuel Griswold Goodrich. She and her older sister, Grace, had five more siblings: John, Samuel, Chauncey, Catherine, and Sophie. The family moved to New York City when she was still very young. She was tutored at home and then in 1877 went to Berlin, Connecticut, to attend Miss Churchill's Private School. The family then moved to England, where her father's job selling insurance took them, and she finished her secondary education at private schools abroad.

They returned to Hartford, Connecticut, in 1885 because of her father's failing health. Goodrich later moved to Boston and earned a living by being a companion to socialite Miss A.S.C. Blake. In 1890, Goodrich entered the New York Hospital Training School for Nurses, prompted by her feeling that she could earn a living being a better nurse than the woman who aided her aging grandparents could.

Upon graduation she stayed and worked at the hospital for a few months, then was highly recommended to take the position as superintendent of nurses at the New York Post-Graduate Hospital. She helped improve the nursing-education standards and stayed for seven years before moving on to work at St. Luke's Hospital for two years. In 1902 she took a position as the superintendent of nursing at New York Hospital.

She was there until 1907, when she resigned to take work at Bellevue and Allied Hospitals as the general superintendent. The state of New York also hired her to oversee its licensing and registration of nurses; many training schools were in need of educational standardization.

She worked as an assistant professor at Columbia in 1917 in nursing administration until she was needed in World War I. For the U.S. Army hospitals during the war she became the chief nursing inspector to the hospitals in the United States and France. She organized the U.S. Army School of Nursing in Washington, D.C., in order to meet the demands of nurses training for work in the military.

She later became the first dean of Yale's School of Nursing, which had high standards for entrance and graduation. The first woman to get a degree at Yale graduated in the field of nursing. Goodrich also assisted in starting Yale's master's degree program. From the beginning she realized that "tragedy can result from placing responsibility in hands that lack the intelligent skill which results from mastery of both the science and the art of nursing" (Werminghaus 1950, 75).

Goodrich retired from Yale in 1934 and served as a consultant to a number of organizations. Later, when World War II was under way, she helped the U.S. Public Health Service organize the Cadet Nurse Corps. She died in Cobalt, Connecticut, on December 31, 1954.

Because of her high expectations and perseverance, the nursing profession made great progress. She wrote, served on many organizational committees, and worked tirelessly to care for the sick and to educate those who would take up the job that she would leave behind. She stated, "Knowledge is more than power; it is a definite responsibility" (Koch 1951, 148).

References: Carey, Charles W., Jr., "Goodrich, Annie Warburton," *American National Biography*, vol. 9, New York: Oxford University Press (1999); Koch, Harriett Rose Berger, *Militant Angel*, New York: Macmillan (1951); Werminghaus, Esther A., *Annie W. Goodrich: Her Journey to Yale*, New York: Macmillan (1950).

Gordon, Doris Clifton Jolly
1890–1956

Doris Gordon was the second woman to become a physician in New Zealand and the first woman in Australasia to be recognized by a fellowship (granted in 1925) to the Royal College of Surgeons of Edinburgh.

Born in Melbourne on July 10, 1890, she was the daughter of Lucy Clifton Crouch and Alfred Jolly. They emigrated in 1894 to New Zealand and lived first in Wellington, then later, in 1905, in Tapanui, Otago.

Doris did not attend school until she became interested in becoming a medical missionary. She graduated from the Tapanui District High School and went on to the University of Otago Medical School, graduating in 1916. She became a house surgeon at Dunedin Hospital that same year.

She married William Patteson Pollock Gordon, a physician, in 1917. Following World War I she and her husband set up practice in Stratford on the North Island. She spent much of her career dealing with childbirth matters, particularly pain medications for women going through childbirth, and other obstetric and gynecologic concerns of the times. She helped establish a chair in obstetrics at Otago Medical School and founded the New Zealand Obstetrical Society. High standards were very important to her.

"We are young enough not to be encouraged by antiquity. Comparatively speaking we have no shortage of money. Certainly skyscraper hospital buildings are not popular because of our earthquake menace, and amazing population spurts in northern areas leave many hospitals in the predicament of the small boy who habitually outgrows his pants. But we can be proud of our compulsory standard of floor space per bed, our spacious theatre suites, our general standard of surgery, and very proud of our unified nursing stand" (Gordon 1958, 55–56).

She had four children, three sons and a daughter. She felt being a mother was extremely fulfilling. She was strong-minded and determined and did not hesitate to get involved in political matters. She strongly opposed government control of medicine, feeling doctors could make better decisions in health matters. She remained active with public health concerns all her life. Doris Gordon died on July 9, 1956, at the Marire Hospital.

References: Bryer, Linda, "Gordon, Doris Clifton," *Dictionary of New Zealand Biography*, vol. 4, *1921–1940*, Wellington: Bridget Williams Books and the Department of Internal Affairs (1998); Gordon, Doris Jolly, *Doctor Down Under*, London: Faber and Faber (1958).

Guangzhou, China

Guangzhou, China, became the center for Protestant missionary work in the nineteenth century, welcoming female medical missionaries and also serving as an educational center for women physicians in China, first through the Canton Medical Missionary Hospital and then through the Hackett Medical College for Women.

Guangzhou is in the province of Guangdong, but Westerners had also come to know the city as Guangdong—Canton—by late in the sixteenth century. The first women's medical college in China was founded there by Mary Hannah Fulton in 1902 and thrived until the late 1920s, when political changes forced its closure.

See also: Fulton, Mary Hannah
References: Cohen, Saul B., *The Columbia Gazetteer of the World*, New York: Columbia University Press (1998); Rubinstein, Murray A., *The Origins of the Anglo-American Missionary Enterprise in China, 1807–1840*, Lanham, MD: Scarecrow Press (1996).

H

Hamilton, Alice
1869–1970

Alice Hamilton was a physician who progressively advocated occupational health among workers in the industrial trades; she also served as the first female faculty member at Harvard Medical School in 1919. As a pioneer in occupational medicine, she became the foremost authority in the new field during her lifetime. Without her perseverance, occupational health hazards would have gone undetected in many industries in the United States.

Born in New York City on February 27, 1869, to Montgomery Hamilton and Gertrude Pond, she grew up in Fort Wayne, Indiana, in a fourth-generation home. She and her siblings, Edith, Margaret, and Norah, were all very close in age, and their parents taught them at home. A brother, Arthur, whom everyone called Quint, was born when she was seventeen.

Hamilton felt her home education was not very sound. Her lessons had included reading, languages, history, and literature but very little math or science. Also, her mother had instilled in her a deep social consciousness. Gertrude Pond Hamilton felt very strongly about the shortcomings of society that allowed cruelty to prisoners, blacks, child laborers, and the poor. She admired those who did something about a problem as opposed to only talking about it.

As was the family tradition, when Alice was seventeen she attended a school in Farmington, Connecticut, for two years. The school was inadequate in some ways, but there Alice began lifelong friendships.

When she returned home, she and her sister Edith determined to prepare for a career, as the family's finances were dwindling.

Alice chose medicine, the only other choices for women at the time being teaching and nursing, neither of which appealed to her. She also felt she could do the most good as a physician. She was not well educated in the sciences, however, so she got some tutoring in physics and chemistry and then attended a small medical school in Fort Wayne for a year to study anatomy.

Once her father was convinced she was serious about a medical career, she enrolled at the Medical School at the University of Michigan in Ann Arbor. There she loved the atmosphere and the depth of courses offered. She also did not have to fight the sexism that existed in so many other schools. "The school was coeducational and had been for about twenty years, so we women were taken for granted and there was none of the sex antagonism which I saw later in Eastern schools. A man student would step aside and let the woman pass through the door first, the women had the chairs if there were not enough to go round, but when it came to microscopes or laboratory apparatus it was first come, first served" (Hamilton 1943, 40).

Graduating in 1893 from medical school at the University of Michigan, Hamilton wanted to pursue bacteriology and pathology, but she was urged to take on some hospital work for the added experience. She held two internships, two months in the Hospital for Women and Children in Minneapolis and nine months in Boston at the New England Hospital for Women and

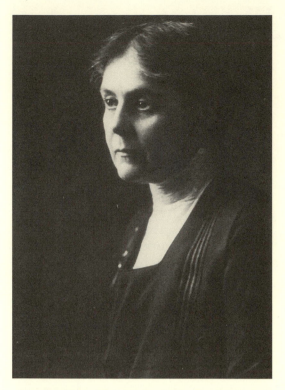

Alice Hamilton (U.S. National Library of Medicine)

Children. In this work, she became aware of a wide variety of problems in public health.

Hamilton's professors told her that to specialize in bacteriology and pathology, she would need some education in Germany, so she and Edith traveled to Leipzig in 1895. She worked in Leipzig and Munich, returning to study at Johns Hopkins Medical School in Baltimore.

The Women's Medical School of Northwestern University was where Hamilton first began teaching. It was her desire to go to a settlement house, Hull House in Chicago, and work, but it was hard to get in because many new students were interested in working there. She was able to gain a room at Hull House in 1897 and lived there while teaching at Northwestern. At Hull House, Hamilton realized she needed more education on industrial diseases. She saw many working-class people suffering from lead and carbon monoxide gas poisoning and pneumonia.

In 1910, Hamilton headed a commission

in Illinois to study industrial diseases. At this time, awareness of occupational hazards was growing, and Hamilton's work would focus on many of these specific health hazards.

The commission's report in 1911 led Illinois and six other states to pass occupational disease laws. The laws required employers to provide periodic medical exams for workers and incorporate safety measures. Violators could be prosecuted.

Following her work with the Illinois commission, Hamilton worked for the federal government in various capacities from 1911 to 1920, studying the deleterious effects of working with lead, rubber, munitions, and rayon. In 1915, U.S. munitions factories were busy making explosives for France to use in World War I. Hamilton realized that no one knew much about the health effects of munitions production, and doctors knew very little, if anything, about nitrous fumes. On one of her first trips to New Jersey, she witnessed two workers involved in making picric (an explosive) for the French. The two men, one black and one white, had orange stains on their skin and yellow in their hair and eyebrows.

I edged nearer and being greeted with a friendly grin by the Negro, ventured a question: "Dyeing cotton goods?" "No, Miss, we're working over to the Canary Islands, making picric for the French." "Is it dangerous?" I asked. "Not this yellow stuff ain't, but there's a red smoke comes off when the yellow stuff is making and it like to knocks you out and if you don't run it gets you. You don't suspicion nothing much, you goes home and eats your supper and goes to bed, and then in the night you starts to choke up and by morning you're dead. . . . Sure it's true, Miss. The man who had the bunk under me, he died that way. I ain't going to stay myself after next pay day." (Hamilton 1943, 185)

She saw this dangerous munitions work everywhere; nitrous fume poisoning was very frequent and the cause of many deaths in workers making explosives for the war effort.

Hamilton was a pacifist during the war, but she did not make her views public because she felt she was doing important work and did not want to jeopardize her job. She was on good terms with most of the government officials she worked with.

After the war ended, her reputation as an authority in the field of public health gained her an appointment to the Harvard Medical School in 1919, a time when the school still did not admit women as students. She stayed there and taught until retiring in 1935, never attaining a position higher than assistant professor.

She served on many state, national, and international committees working for public health and social reform. She supported and spoke for women in industry and for the protection of their health in legislation and regulations. Her major contribution was the work *Industrial Toxicology* in 1934 and its subsequent revised edition in 1949, which was the first work of its kind to enlighten professionals on dangerous industrial practices.

In her autobiography, which she wrote during World War II, she notes that the progress between the two wars was very evident. Even though the same kinds of dangerous materials were used for making weapons, more safety regulations were in place, and engineers and doctors knew much more about protecting workers. Even employers found that a high turnover of workers in these industries was not a profitable answer to the problems. "Industrial medicine had at last become respectable" (Hamilton 1943, 198).

Hamilton suffered from increasingly poor health during her nineties; deafness and a series of strokes hampered her. She died on September 22, 1970, in Hadlyme, Connecticut, at the age of 101. It seemed appropriate that the Occupational Safety and Health Act was passed a few months later. President Nixon signed it on December 29, 1970. The act serves to ensure safety and health in the workplace.

References: Corn, Jacqueline Karnell,

"Hamilton, Alice," *American National Biography* vol. 9, New York: Oxford University Press (1999); Hamilton, Alice, *Exploring the Dangerous Trades: The Autobiography of Alice Hamilton, M.D.*, Boston: Little, Brown (1943); Sicherman, Barbara, *Alice Hamilton: A Life in Letters*, Cambridge, MA: Harvard University Press (1984).

Han Suyin
1917–

An early physician in Asia, Han Suyin is best known for writing fiction, particularly *A Many Splendored Thing*, which was made into a movie in 1955. Her writings include autobiographical stories, historical and political accounts of revolutionary China, and romances.

Born in Sinyang, China, as Elizabeth Chou on September 12, 1917, she served as a physician after receiving an education at the University of London and the University of Brussels. She worked at the Queen Mary Hospital in Hong Kong from 1948 to 1952 and then went to the Johore Bahru

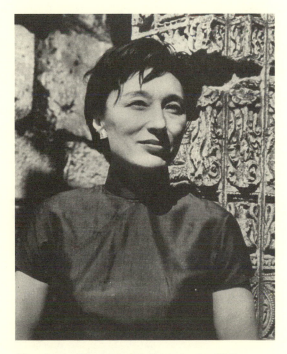

Han Suyin (World Health Organization/U.S. National Library of Medicine)

Hospital in Malaya. She maintained a private practice for about ten years.

Her later years have been substantially filled with political and literary endeavors; in her early life she showed perseverance in pursuing a medical education when few women sought such a profession. She was one of the first Chinese women physicians in Asia.

References: *International Who's Who of Women,* London: Europa (1997).

Hautval, Adelaide
1906–1988

Adelaide Hautval was a French physician and psychiatrist who aided women in the German concentration camps during World War II. She later testified about the medical experiments on Jewish women in the camps of Auschwitz. She was recognized in 1965 by Yad Vashem as one of the Righteous Among the Nations, an honor bestowed on the courageous men and women who risked their lives to help the Jews under persecution in Nazi Germany.

Born in France to a Protestant family, Hautval studied medicine in Strasbourg and then worked in many psychiatric clinics there and in Switzerland. She encountered resistance from the Nazis upon trying to cross occupied France in 1942 in order to attend her mother's funeral. She was arrested and imprisoned and witnessed the inhumane treatment of the Jewish prisoners by the Gestapo. She protested continually and was eventually sent to Auschwitz to work as a doctor treating sick Jewish women.

During her time there she was asked to practice gynecology and agreed until she discovered that inhumane medical experiments were being performed on Jewish women. They were sterilized by means of X rays or ovariectomies, sterilization being part of the grand plan for all Jewish women after the awaited Nazi victory. Hautval refused to participate and instead gave medical aid as best she could to women who had typhus. Had the Nazis known any of the women had typhus, they would have killed

them immediately because of its infectious nature. Hautval hid some of the women on top of the bunks in her block.

She was later sent to Birkenau and gave medical aid as best she could under the circumstances. She then worked at Ravensbruck until liberation. She testified in 1964 in a libel trial in England involving the actions of Wladyslaw Dering, a physician who had participated in the medical experiments at Auschwitz. "Justice Frederick Horace Lawton, in his summation to the jury called Hautval 'perhaps one of the most impressive and courageous women who have ever given evidence in the courts of this country'" (Gutman 1990, 650).

Hautval died in 1988. A book of her writing about her experiences and the inhumanity of the Nazi medical experiments was published in 1991.

References: Epstein, Eric Joseph, and Philip Rosen, *Dictionary of the Holocaust: Biography, Geography, and Terminology,* Westport, CT: Greenwood Press (1997); Gutman, Israel, *The Encyclopedia of the Holocaust,* New York: Macmillan (1990); Hautval, Adelaide, *Médecine et Crimes Contre l'Humanité,* Le Mejan, Arles: Actes Sud (1991); Rozett, Robert, and Shmuel Spector, *Encyclopedia of the Holocaust,* New York: Facts on File (2000).

Hazen, Elizabeth Lee
1885–1975

Along with Rachel Fuller Brown, Elizabeth Hazen was responsible for discovering the first antifungal antibiotic that could be used safely on humans. Most scientists considered this biomedical discovery to be the most important since Sir Alexander Fleming discovered penicillin in 1928. She and Brown subsequently donated all their royalties from the patent to scientific research.

Hazen was born in Rich, Mississippi, on August 24, 1885. Her parents were William Edgar Hazen and Maggie Harper Hazen. Both died when she was a child, and an aunt and uncle adopted her. She attended college at Mississippi Industrial Institute and College. After receiving her B.S., she taught school in order to earn money for graduate study at Columbia University.

Hazen earned her master's degree in 1917 and worked at the West Virginia Hospital's bacteriological laboratory while pursuing her Ph.D. at Columbia. She earned it in 1927 and went to work for the New York State Department of Health. Her work in analyzing bacteria and possible vaccines led to her interest in finding an antifungal antibiotic. She eventually worked with Rachel Fuller Brown, and they developed Nystatin. Hazen and Brown patented their discovery in 1950, and E.R. Squibb and Sons developed a method for mass production. Nystatin became available to the public in 1954.

Nystatin proved to have many uses. It is a treatment for Dutch elm disease, fights molds in foods, and saved priceless artworks that had developed fungus after a flood in Italy.

Hazen and Brown were both interested in furthering women's education in science. Their donation of all income from the Nystatin patent benefited numerous students and researchers. Hazen became a professor at Albany Medical College in 1958. She died on June 24, 1975, in Seattle, Washington.

See also: Brown, Rachel Fuller
References: Baldwin, Richard S., *The Fungus Fighters: Two Women Scientists and Their Discovery*, Ithaca, NY: Cornell University Press (1981); Ogilvie, Marilyn, and Joy Harvey, eds., *The Biographical Dictionary of Women in Science: Pioneering Lives from Ancient Times to the Mid-20th Century*, New York: Routledge (2000); Vare, Ethlie Ann, and Greg Ptacek, *Mothers of Invention: From the Bra to the Bomb: Forgotten Women and Their Unforgettable Ideas*, New York: Morrow (1988).

He Manqiu
1920?–

He Manqiu became one of the first Chinese female doctors by training during the Long March in harsh and primitive conditions.

Born to a liberal father, she had one brother and was close to her grandmother. Her father was supportive of her early education at a missionary school in Chengdu, and she "wanted to participate in the revolution and help liberate women for a long time. A lot of students in Chengdu were organized to cut off pigtails and unbind feet, to propagate the spirit of the May 4th movement against feudal ideas. Although I was young, I accepted the idea of women being liberated" (Young 1996, 536).

He Manqiu joined the Red Army when she discovered women could become soldiers. It was during a stay at a short-staffed hospital that she developed a desire to learn about medicine. She became a nurse and after that had an opportunity to take an exam and become a medical student in the Chinese army. During the long march, she and the other students learned medicine under primitive conditions as they had no paper and pencils (only sticks for writing in the dirt), and had to memorize everything the teachers taught. For cadavers they had to use what they found.

On our way back we just happened to find an intact, fresh corpse in a cave. We felt sure that this person had had no family to prepare him for death and that no one would try to find the body because this corpse had had no funeral or burial. We had seen several funerals in this Tibetan area. The family always claimed the dead body and disposed of it in one of several ways. One funeral practice was to flay the skin and expose the body to the vultures. Another was cremation, and the third was to put the body in a river or stream. Sometimes when a person died, the body was tied to a tree and stones were piled up around until it was completely covered. That's why it wasn't easy to find a cadaver in such a place. Of course, we couldn't use our own soldiers or prisoners of war. Usually when our soldiers died we claimed the bodies and then buried them, because the Communist Party was humane. If we hadn't found that person's body in the cave, we would have had to wait for the body of a criminal who had been sentenced to death. (Young 1996, 545)

He Manqiu continued to work as a physician for many years in the Chinese military and retired to Beijing.

References: Young, Helen Praeger, "From Soldier to Doctor: A Chinese Woman's Story of the Long March," *Science & Society* 59, no. 4 (Winter 1996): 531–547.

Healy, Bernadine
1944–

Bernadine Healy has the distinction of being the first woman appointed to head the National Institutes of Health (NIH), in 1991–1993 under George Bush. She was also the first woman to hold the position of dean of the College of Medicine and Public Health at Ohio State University before assuming her duties as president of the American Red Cross, the first physician to hold that title. She was also CEO of the organization until her resignation in 2001.

Healy was born on August 2, 1944, in New York City. She is the second of four daughters of Michael J. and Violet McGrath Healy. Her parents operated a perfume business at home while she was growing up in Queens. She graduated from Hunter College High School and went on to Vassar, where she majored in chemistry, graduating in 1965. She received her M.D. from Harvard Medical School in 1970 along with 9 other women in a class of 120.

She did her internal medicine and cardiology postgraduate work at Johns Hopkins University School of Medicine and Hospital, where she later served as full professor and directed the coronary care unit.

Healy has done extensive research as well as worked with patients of all ages and backgrounds. Her excellent management skills have proved an asset wherever she has worked within the medical community. While she served the Research Institute of the Cleveland Clinic Foundation as director, funding rose from $8 million to $36 million in only five years. She is one of the few med-

ical professionals who don't see management duties as detracting from research and patient care. Her leadership has influenced thousands of physicians, politicians, and patients. "As a doctor and researcher, I have dedicated my life to alleviating human suffering," Healy says. She was pressured to resign her position at the Red Cross following controversial remarks after the terrorist attacks on September 11, 2001 (she had asked U.S. Muslims to support Israel's inclusion in the International Red Cross). She is married to Dr. Floyd Hoop and has two daughters.

References: *Encyclopedia of World Biography,* vol. 7, Detroit: Gale (1998); Stapleton, Stephanie, "Former NIH Chief to Lead Red Cross," *American Medical News* (2 August 1999): 241; www.redcross.org/healyart.html.

Heikel, Rosina
1842–1929

Rosina Heikel was the first female physician in Finland, receiving her medical degree from the University of Helsinki in 1878. Her parents were Carl Johan Heikel and Kristina Elisabet Dobbin. She did well in school and, like her brothers before her, wanted to study medicine.

When she was ready for university study, no medical schools in Finland were open to her. She went to Stockholm and took a physiotherapy course, studied midwifery back in Helsinki, and then went back to Stockholm to learn more about physiology and anatomy. She was eventually allowed to study medicine by special permission of the emperor.

After completing her degree, she was restricted to practicing medicine on women and children. She worked as a pediatrician and gynecologist in Helsinki most of her life. Outside of her medical career she was very involved in the women's rights movement in Finland (Naisasialiitto Unioni) and was a proponent of women's education.

References: Forsius, Arno, "Emma Rosina Heikel (1842–1929)—Suomen ja Pohjoismaiden ensimmainen naislaakari," http://www.saunalahti.fi/arnoldus/heikel.html;

Lovejoy, Esther Pohl, *Women Doctors of the World*, New York: Macmillan (1957); "Rosina Heikel: First Woman Doctor in Finland, 1842–1929," *Women of Learning*, http://www.helsinki.fi/akka-info/tiedenaiset/english/heikel.html; Seppanen, Anni, "Medical Women in Finland," *Journal of the American Medical Women's Association* 5, no. 7 (1950): 291.

Hemenway, Ruth V.
1894–1974

A pioneering medical missionary in China prior to World War II, Ruth Hemenway grew to embrace practical medical science to meet the needs of the Chinese in the early decades of the twentieth century and to introduce some measure of health care in rural areas. She placed health care above her Christian missionary goals in order to better serve the people she saw in need.

Born in Williamsburg, Massachusetts, in 1894, she grew up on her father's farm and had an early desire to become a physician. She graduated from Northampton High School in 1910 and then taught school in order to save money for medical school.

She continued to work odd jobs while attending Tufts Medical School. China was in great need of physicians, and Hemenway was motivated by her religious convictions to serve others; she also wanted to learn about other cultures and religions. Having grown away from traditional religions, she nevertheless realized that she would require support from an organized religious group in order to serve as a missionary. She accepted support from the Methodist Women's Board of Foreign Missions in 1924 and was destined for Mintsing, Fukien.

She arrived, began working in primitive conditions, and realized a great need for sanitary practices, health clinics, and basic education. Early on she conducted a clinic in a village church:

> Hordes of people of all ages and both sexes began to push up to the table. We made them walk single file past the opposite side of the table. But with each patient came children and babies, sisters-in-law, mothers-in-law, and a few neighbors. Many men were present and they all shoved themselves into the front row so that they could hear all the histories and symptoms. No privacy was possible. A sick person at each end of the table shouted her symptoms to one of us doctors. She had to yell louder than all the screaming babies and shrieking relatives as well as shouting men who attempted to help her out in her narration. One baby's ears were packed with dirt. When I asked why, the young mother told me that her baby was only two years old, and she was afraid he was too young to bathe. (Hemenway 1977, 44–45)

Hemenway was in China from 1924 until 1941 during very turbulent political times. Although the villages she worked in were generally far removed from the revolution, sometimes it came very close. She continued to focus on proper health care service to the people who needed it most. During this period she occasionally spent brief periods in the United States and elsewhere. On one sojourn in the United States to recover from an illness, she realized she had developed an appreciation of China's "long history of philosophy and high ethical teachings, her love of beauty in nature, in literature, in music and all arts. I thought of China's young people with their great artistic ability, their high intelligence, their reverence for learning, their respect for the aged, and their passionate patriotism. I remembered Chinese ways of courtesy and gentleness; their fine sensitivity and intuition were characteristics in even the illiterate mountain people. Even the poorest people possessed a wonderful graciousness and dignity. Confucius and sons had given their people a great deal" (Hemenway 1977, 92).

Hemenway died in 1974.

References: Hemenway, Ruth V., *Ruth V. Hemenway, M.D.: A Memoir of Revolutionary China, 1924–1941*, Amherst: University of Massachusetts Press (1977).

Hildegard of Bingen
1098–1179

Hildegard's writings include a great deal of information on the medicinal properties of plants, minerals, and animals. This information came to her in visions that both she and her parents believed were a gift from God. The use of the spiritual to explain the physical world was acceptable during her time; science was considered a bridge between the physical and spiritual worlds. Hildegard used her knowledge to treat the sick. She was well respected during and after her time, and many health practitioners sought out her writings.

She was born in summer 1098 in Bermersheim, south of Mainz, Germany, the tenth child of Hildebert and Mechthilde. Her parents were wealthy and belonged to the nobility. Hildegard began having her visions at a very early age. Apparently they were so strong that she was ill much of the time. Her parents sent her to Disibodenberg, where her Aunt Jutta and others at the Benedictine monastery educated her. When her aunt died she became abbess of the convent. In 1147 she founded her own convent at Rupertsberg. She died at Rupertsberg, near Bingen, in 1179.

References: Flanagan, Sabina, *Hildegard of Bingen, 1098–1179: A Visionary Life*, London: Routledge (1998); Pagel, Walter, "Hildegard of Bingen," *Dictionary of Scientific Biography*, vol. 6, New York: Charles Scribner's Sons (1970–1980); Shearer, Benjamin F., and Barbara S. Shearer, *Notable Women in the Life Sciences: A Biographical Dictionary*, Westport, CT: Greenwood Press (1996); Snodgrass, Mary Ellen, *Historical Dictionary of Nursing*, Santa Barbara, CA: ABC-CLIO (1999).

Hoby, Lady Margaret
1571–1633

Throughout her life, Lady Margaret Hoby played the role of a physician in taking care of neighbors and family. Her diary is the earliest that shows the deep influence of Puritanism on the lives of Elizabethan women.

The daughter of Arthur Dakins and Thomasine Genevieve, Hoby married three times. Her last husband was Sir Thomas Hoby. She was educated in the household of Henry Hastings and became the caregiver for workers of her husband's estate. It is not clear how vast her medical knowledge was, but it is clear that she believed that God was the great healer: "I may truly conclude it is the Lord, and not the phisision, who both ordaines the medesine for our health and orderethe the ministring of it for the good of his children" (ca. 1599; Hoby 1998, 13).

She witnessed much death due to disease and plagues, which reinforced her faith in God. "This day I hard the plague was so great at whitbie that those wch were cleare shutt themselues vp, and the infected that escaped did goe abroad: Likewise it was reported that, at London, the number was taken of the Liuinge and not of the deed: Lord graunt that these Iudgementes may Cause England wt speed to tourne to the Lord" (ca. 1603; Hoby 1998, 195). In her day, the faithful saw disease as a punishment from God. She had no children and died in 1633. She was buried in the chancel of Hackness Church on September 6, 1633.

References: Hoby, Lady Margaret, *The Private Life of an Elizabethan Lady: The Diary of Lady Margaret Hoby, 1599–1605*, ed. Joanna Moody, Stroud, Gloucestershire: Sutton (1998); Slack, Paul, "Hoby, Margaret, Lady," *Dictionary of National Biography: Missing Persons*, Oxford: Oxford University Press (1993).

Hodgkin, Dorothy Mary Crowfoot
1910–1994

Dorothy Hodgkin received the Nobel Prize in chemistry in 1964 for her use of crystallography as an exceptional analytical tool in shedding new light on the structure of molecules. She identified the structure of over 100 molecules, including vitamins D and

B-12, insulin, and penicillin. She was the second woman after Florence Nightingale to be a recipient of Britain's Order of Merit and also received the Royal Medal, the Royal Society's highest honor, in 1965. She was the first woman to receive this honor.

She was born in Cairo, Egypt, then a British colony, on May 12, 1910. Her father, John Crowfoot, worked for the British government in the education department, and her mother, Grace Mary Hood Crowfoot, enjoyed weaving in the ancient methods and botanical studies. After the outbreak of World War I, the family was dispersed. When Dorothy was four, the Crowfoots sent her and her three younger sisters to England for safety; there, they stayed with a nursemaid and had their grandmother nearby. They saw their mother only once during the four years of the war, but Dorothy felt the separation made her more independent.

After the war, her mother taught the girls at home for a time. Dorothy attended the Sir John Leman School from 1921 to 1927. She was interested early on in chemistry and biochemistry, and also in crystals.

She graduated from Somerville College at Oxford University in 1931. She then took an opportunity to work with John D. Bernal at Cambridge University. He was working on sterol crystals and had a well-financed laboratory. She continued her exploration of X-ray crystallography on protein crystals.

In 1934 she was diagnosed with severe rheumatoid arthritis. Hodgkin complained little during her life about the pain she endured from this crippling disease, and it did not slow her work or determination.

She accepted a job at Somerville College even though she would miss Bernal and his well-equipped lab. At Somerville she had to work in antiquated laboratories, and there was a shortage of equipment. She also did not enjoy the isolated life of a woman scientist at Oxford. Many clubs excluded women, which she felt was a huge problem. She did work off and on at Cambridge when she could while teaching chemistry at Somerville.

While at Somerville, she and her research student, C. H. Carlisle, determined the structure of cholesterol iodide. "For the first time,

X-rays had revealed the structure of a molecule that synthetic and organic chemists could not decipher" (McGrayne 1998, 237).

This success encouraged Hodgkin to study as many crystals as she could. Before long, other scientists learned of her work and began sending samples for her examination.

In 1937, she married Thomas L. Hodgkin; they would have three children, Luke, Elizabeth, and Toby. Thomas was involved in politics and was a member of the Communist Party; Dorothy was interested in the world peace movement. Having lost four of her brothers in World War I, Dorothy would be involved in controversies throughout her life because she campaigned for peace during the post–World War II and Cold War years.

She had obtained her Ph.D. in 1937 from Oxford and soon thereafter became interested in cracking the code for insulin and penicillin. With the outbreak of World War II, she focused on penicillin. At that time many chemists thought this work could not succeed because penicillin was far too complex. Dorothy was determined to find its chemical structure using X-ray crystallography. "Due to the increasing number of casualties in World War II, soldiers were in dire need of the medicinal properties of penicillin, as the number of bacterial infections contracted during the war was increasing at a rapid rate. The world, however, was at a standstill in terms of mass-producing penicillin because its chemical structure was still unknown" (Van der Does 1999, 170).

By 1944, Hodgkin had determined the structure of penicillin. She was promoted from fellow to university lecturer at Oxford in 1946 and received international recognition. She aided in founding the International Union of Crystallography, a political worry to some Western governments because the union welcomed members from any country and did not exclude those who belonged to the Communist Party. This inclusiveness suited Hodgkin's goal of unity in the world of science.

Her next success was with B-12, a much larger molecule than penicillin and key in curing anemia. John White worked with her on this mystery. She was finally promoted to full professor at Oxford in 1958 and had a new laboratory. In 1964 she received the Nobel Prize in chemistry. She kept on the trail of insulin, which had interested her thirty years before, and determined its structure in 1969. "She had the imagination to insist that the problem she chose could be solved, even though she had to wait for many years for the answer. In fact Dorothy pioneered many of the methods of macromolecular structure determination that we now take for granted" (Glusker 1994, 2469). Hodgkins died on July 29, 1994.

References: Glusker, Jenny P., "Dorothy Crowfoot Hodgkin," *Protein Science* 3, no. 12 (December 1994): 2465–2469; McGrayne, Sharon Bertsch, *Nobel Prize Women in Science*, Secaucus, NJ: Carol (1998); *Nobel Lectures: Chemistry 1963–1970*, River Edge, NJ: World Scientific (1999); Van der Does, Louise Q., and Rita J. Simon, *Renaissance Women in Science*, Lanham, MD: University Press of America (1999).

Honzakova, Anna
1875–1940

Anna Honzakova was the first Czech woman to graduate from a Czechoslovakian university and become a physician. After graduating from Minerva high school in Austria, she attended medical school at the University of Czechoslovakia in Prague. She obtained her physician credentials in 1902. She went on to serve as a school physician at a girls' grammar school and later specialized in gynecology and midwifery. She authored a book on protecting children against tuberculosis and also wrote a book about Anna Bayerova.

She was born in Kopidlno on November 16, 1875. She served as the first president of the Women's Medical Association of Czechoslovakia. She died on October 13, 1940.

See also: Bayerova, Anna
References: *Ceskoslovensky Biograficky Slovnik*, Prague: Academia (1992); Lovejoy, Esther P., *Women Doctors of the World*, New York: Macmillan (1957).

Hoobler, Icie Gertrude Macy
1892–1984

Icie Hoobler made important contributions to the field of nutrition, particularly the nutrition of nursing mothers and their infants, by studying nutrient values of vitamins and analyzing milk. She also discovered that cottonseed products varied in toxicity. This finding later resulted in better manufacturing methods that "greatly reduced or removed the toxicity and made the cotton seed products safer to use in animal foods" (Hoobler 1982, 56).

Born in Gallatin, Missouri, on July 23, 1892, Hoobler had two brothers and a sister. Their parents, Perry Macy and Ollevia Elvaree Critten Macy, managed a farm. Hoobler received her early education in a one-room schoolhouse and later attended Central College for Women, as did her sister.

In the beginning she wanted to please her father, who wanted a musician in the family. She spent three years of intense practice on the piano only to discover music was not for her. She did enjoy her classes with Lily G. Egbert, an enthusiastic female biology teacher, and thought about a career in science. She received an A.B. degree in English in 1914.

She wanted to attend the University of Chicago, but her parents were concerned that she was too young and inexperienced for a big-city university. Instead she attended Randolph-Macon College for Women for a year to prepare. She was further encouraged in her endeavor to study science and went to the University of Chicago in 1915 to earn enough credits to obtain a B.S. After receiving that degree, she taught chemistry at the University of Colorado and at the same time earned her M.S. degree.

She entered Yale University Graduate School in 1918 and received her Ph.D. in 1920 in physiological chemistry. It was at Yale that she did her study on cottonseeds and their toxicity. She was at the same time aware of new developments in the sciences. "What intrigued me most was the fact that chemistry and physics were becoming increasingly relevant in the study of biology and physiology. Body and mind processes were being recognized as physiological in nature and the basis of mental activity. The interlinking of the human body and mind chemically and physiologically had a profound effect on my desire to ultimately be involved in these areas of study and research" (Hoobler 1982, 69).

Her first position was as an assistant chemist at Western Pennsylvania Hospital. She had to work many hours in the laboratory and faced much discrimination, such as not being allowed to eat in the doctors' dining room and not having a women's restroom nearby. The lack of a convenient restroom led to a serious bout of nephritis, a kidney infection; it was only after a year's leave that she was well enough to return to work. After complaining to no avail, she submitted her resignation. However, once the president of the board of trustees found out what was happening, facilities were improved after she left.

She moved on to become director of the Nutrition Research Laboratories at the Merrill-Palmer School and Children's Hospital in Detroit. There, she demonstrated good organizational skills and became an expert on nutrition. She studied metabolism, the chemical characteristics of growth in children and how nutrition affects growth, human milk composition, and the chemistry of red blood cells. On June 11, 1938, she married Dr. Raymond Hoobler, who encouraged her to pursue her professional goals. He died after only five years. Hoobler continued her work and eventually retired in Gallatin, Missouri. She died on January 6, 1984.

Hoobler wrote her autobiography in part "because of my hope that young women students of like desires and intellectual interest as my own, may find some optimistic guidance and encouragement to enter the science arena where their participation and full life commitment are needed and their unique talents and skills may be given full expression, in a worthy, womanly, and satisfying manner" (Hoobler 1982, 3).

References: Hoobler, Icie Gertrude Macy, *Boundless Horizons: Portrait of a Pioneer Woman Scientist*, Smithtown, NY: Exposition Press (1982); Shearer, Benjamin F., and Barbara S. Shearer, *Notable Women in the Physical Sciences: A Biographical Dictionary*, Westport, CT: Greenwood Press (1997).

Horney, Karen Theodora Clementina Danielsen
1885–1952

Karen Horney was a physician and world-renowned psychoanalyst who challenged Freud's theories. She received a great deal of respect within the psychiatric community in the early twentieth century and is still respected today.

Born September 16, 1885, in Blankense, Germany, Horney was the daughter of Clotilde Marie Van Ronzelen Danielsen and Berndt Henrik Wackels Danielsen. She received her medical education at the University of Freiburg and received her medical degree in 1915 from the University of Berlin. She specialized in psychiatry and was deeply involved in psychoanalysis, which Karl Abraham had brought to Berlin.

She had married Oskar Horney, a doctoral student, in Freiburg. She became unhappy and asked Abraham, a follower of Freud, to psychoanalyze her. She began lecturing and teaching on the techniques of psychoanalysis. In the 1920s her marriage ended in separation and later divorce. She had three daughters.

She differed very much with Freud's view of "penis envy" and also was the first to argue that "womb envy" existed. She believed cultural factors had a greater influence on women's subordination to men. She wrote persuasively and challenged some of Freud's other views as well, such as his view that biological development is a primary force in personality development. She gained many followers over the years.

Fascism was rising in Germany, and in 1932 she moved to Chicago to work at the Institute for Psychoanalysis. She stayed two years before leaving for New York City. Her lectures there at the New School for Social Research at the New York Psychoanalytic

Institute were very popular and caused much friction between the Chicago and the New York psychoanalytic institutes. There seemed to be two growing schools of thought, one espousing Freud's theories and the other, Horney's.

The New York Psychoanalytic Institute eventually demoted Horney, and she resigned. She founded the Association for the Advancement of Psychoanalysis, where she worked for the last nine years of her life.

Horney had a very good understanding of the relationship between physical ailments and psychological illness. "It is impossible to tell from a cough alone whether the patient has a cold or tuberculosis. The same is true of functional female disorders, especially in borderline cases. The physician must determine whether they require physical or psychological treatment, or some combination of the two. As I have suggested, this can be a very difficult diagnosis. If the patient's problems are psychological, in whole or in part, the physician must further decide whether his help will suffice or whether psychoanalytic therapy is called for" (Horney 2000, 116).

She died in New York City on December 4, 1952.

References: Horney, Karen, *The Unknown Karen Horney, Essays on Gender, Culture, and Psychoanalysis*, New Haven, CT: Yale University Press (2000); Paris, Bernard J., *Karen Horney: A Psychoanalyst's Search for Self-Understanding*, New Haven, CT: Yale University Press (1994); Quinn, Susan, *A Mind of Her Own: The Life of Karen Horney*, New York: Summit Books (1987); Sokal, M. M., "Horney, Karen (Danielsen)," in Martin Kaufman, Stuart Galishoff, and Todd L. Savitt, eds., *Dictionary of American Medical Biography*, Westport, CT: Greenwood Press (1984).

Hubbard, Ruth
1924–

Ruth Hubbard was the first tenured female professor at Harvard. She is a prominent biologist who has worked to educate scien-

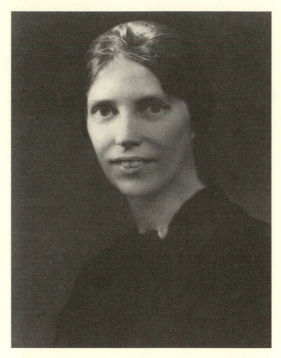

Ruth Hubbard (Bachrach/U.S. National Library of Medicine)

tists in the applications of genetics research, encourage women in the sciences, and climb the ladder of academia at Harvard.

Born March 3, 1924, in Vienna, Austria, Hubbard grew up making rounds with her physician father, Richard Hoffman. Her mother, Helene, was also a physician. At an early age, Ruth assumed she would be a doctor. Her family moved to the United States in 1938 following Hitler's annexation of Austria. She attended school in Brookline, Massachusetts, and then entered Radcliffe College for premedical studies. She later saw that a traditional medical career was unusual for a woman and turned her attention to biochemistry: "The fact that women were more successful in gaining access to biochemistry than to anatomy and physiology has its parallel in the fact that biochemistry was also more accessible to Jews than were anatomy and physiology. It may be that the young, aspiring science of biochemistry was simply more open than the old, established medical sciences" (Hubbard 1990, 44).

She earned her Ph.D. in 1950. She enjoyed research more than teaching, a preference that presented problems for many women. Either universities hiring research scientists were not hiring women or institutions that were hiring women had small or inadequate research facilities. Hubbard, however, had the good fortune of working at George Wald's laboratory at Harvard and eventually worked her way up, combining teaching and research. Her early interests lay in photochemistry and vision, retinal pigments, and photoisomerization. She later became concerned about the emphasis on genetics as the sole basis for explaining people's characteristics. She is also very concerned about ethical standards in genetic research.

Beyond asking what genetic research should be done and how it should be applied, we need to question the current emphasis on genes as determining our development, health, and behavior. Focusing on genes leads almost inevitably to an assignment of values: these genes are good, those genes are bad. We may start with relatively clear-cut cases like Tay-Sachs disease, which is invariably fatal in early childhood, but we almost immediately get into gray areas where people leading quite ordinary lives can suddenly find themselves stigmatized as defective.

Scientists and physicians should not be given the right to assign such labels, but the problem is greater than that. The labels themselves are inherently wrong, no matter who is doing the labeling. There is no way to say which lives are or are not valuable. I am glad Woody Guthrie was born, though he developed Huntington Disease. I am glad for all the blind poets and musicians, from Homer to Stevie Wonder. Who knows, maybe Helen Keller would have led a completely undistinguished life instead of becoming a famous writer and political activist had her immune system not failed her as a child. (Hubbard and Wald 1997, 161)

As a feminist and scientist, Hubbard has written for both scholarly and popular publications. She writes clearly about her concerns within the scientific community. Aware of the advances in medical science over the years, she is also aware of and outspoken about the dangers of proceeding without a conscientious effort to maintain proper policies and procedures for the good of humanity.

Hubbard is professor emerita at Harvard. She married Frank Hubbard in 1942, but they later divorced. She married George Wald in 1958, and they had two children, Elijah and Deborah Hannah.

References: Hubbard, Ruth, *The Politics of Women's Biology*, New Brunswick, NJ: Rutgers University Press (1990); Hubbard, Ruth, and Elijah Wald, *Exploding the Gene Myth: How Genetic Information Is Produced and Manipulated by Scientists, Physicians, Employers, Insurance Companies, Educators, and Law Enforcers*, Boston: Beacon Press (1997); Kropf, Allen, and Ruth Hubbard, "The Photoisomerization of Retinal," *Photochemistry and Photobiology* 12, no. 4 (October 1970): 249–260.

Hugonay, Countess Vilma
1847–1922

Countess Vilma Hugonay was the first female physician to graduate at a medical school in Hungary. She was motivated to receive medical training after her first child died. She received her M.D. in 1879 at the University of Zurich but for many years was allowed to practice only midwifery. In 1897, she was finally allowed by the Hungarian Ministry of Culture to practice as a physician.

References: Lovejoy, Esther Pohl, *Women Doctors of the World*, New York: Macmillan (1957); Ogilvie, Marilyn, and Joy Harvey, eds., *The Biographical Dictionary of Women in Science: Pioneering Lives from Ancient Times to the Mid-20th Century*, New York: Routledge (2000).

Hyde, Ida Henrietta
1857–1945

Ida Hyde broke down the barriers in Germany to advanced education for women and was the first women to work in the medical school at the University of Heidelberg. She did research on a variety of physiological aspects of health and wrote two textbooks as well as numerous papers on physiology, all of which were well received.

She was born in Davenport, Iowa, on September 8, 1857, to Babette Loewenthal and Meyer H. Hyde. Her father left the family, and her mother, her brother, and she moved to Chicago, where Hyde attended public schools. She eventually taught in the public schools and introduced science courses. In 1891 she received an A.B. degree from Cornell with a major in the biological sciences.

She continued her studies that year at Bryn Mawr College, but after a professor at the University of Strassburg heard about her research project on jellyfish, he invited her to Germany on a fellowship in 1893. At that time there were no German universities that allowed women students, but she was allowed use of the laboratory. When she could not gain entrance at Strassburg, she persisted with the University of Heidelberg, which accepted her as a Ph.D. candidate. She graduated with honors in 1896.

Hyde worked at the Naples Zoological Station, doing research on octopus salivary glands, then came back to the United States to work at Harvard Medical School. She studied the heart's blood flow and also taught at some preparatory schools. In 1898 she moved to the University of Kansas, becoming professor of physiology in the medical school.

Hyde was active in community health and lectured on numerous public health concerns while at Kansas. She also began a program to examine children with communicable diseases. Her research included many aspects of physiology. "She studied the effects of the environment and nutrition on the nervous system, the reactions of various animals to drugs, alcohol, and stress, and the effects of caffeine on humans. She also developed a microelectrode that enabled her to stimulate and study a single cell" (Shor 1999, 613). From 1922 to 1923 she went to the University of Heidelberg and did research on radium and its biological effects.

Hyde worked hard to ensure equal educational opportunities for women in the sciences. She was the first woman to become a member of the American Physiological Society (1902). She died in California on August 22, 1945.

References: Shor, Elizabeth Noble, "Hyde, Ida Henrietta," *American National Biography*, vol. 11, New York: Oxford University Press (1999).

I

Inglis, Elsie Maude
1864–1917

Elsie Inglis was a pioneer and leader of women physicians in Scotland, founded the Elsie Inglis Hospital for Women and Children, and for the cause of World War I founded the Scottish Women's Hospitals. She proposed, and had accepted by some of the Allies, women medical units in the field to treat wounded soldiers.

Born in Naini Tal, India, at a Himalayan hill station where her father worked in the civil service, she had seven siblings and was encouraged at an early age to gain a good education. Her father was very supportive of her decision to go into medicine.

She first attended the Edinburgh School of Medicine for Women, which had been founded and was run by Sophia Jex-Blake. She later went to Glasgow to attend the Medical College for Women because she was interested in surgery and the college had better facilities for those interested in clinical practice. She passed her Triple Qualification in 1892 and went to work in the Hospital for Women in London as a house surgeon.

During these early years she worked with Elizabeth Garrett Anderson and other pioneers in England. She went to Dublin and took a three-month course in midwifery in the Rotunda. There were more mixed classes there (both men and women), and she felt the teaching was exceptional. She later opened a practice in Edinburgh with Dr. Jessie MacGregor.

Inglis's father died in 1894. The loss of the man who had always supported her career and with whom she had corresponded almost daily was a severe blow to her. In 1899 the University of Edinburgh admitted women to the medical examinations; Inglis passed and became an official physician with a medical degree. From then on her practice grew, and she responded to the needs she saw in the community. She opened a clinic, called a hospice, that was staffed by women and included a maternity ward. As the hospice grew, it was clear that her idea of locating it on High Street, near her patients' homes, had been a good one. Eventually, "she had a small ward of five beds for malnutrition cases, a baby clinic, a milk depot, health centres, and the knowledge that the Hospice has the distinction of being the only maternity centre run by women in Scotland. This affords women students opportunities denied to them in other maternity hospitals" (Balfour 1919, 133).

Inglis never denied treatment to those who could not afford it. According to one of her patients, "'That woman has done more for the folk living between Morrison Street and the High Street than all the ministers in Edinburgh and Scotland itself ever did for any one. She would never give in to difficulties. She gave her house, her property, her practice, her money to help others'" (Balfour 1919, 136).

Over the next decade, Inglis continued her work as a physician in London and Dublin. She also continued to work for women's suffrage and to promote equality in education for women, involvements she had taken up while still in medical school. Her organizational skills were well honed when World War I broke out. She decided to form a unit of women to help with caring for the wounded in the field. Suddenly the Edinburgh Suffrage offices became the Scottish Women's Hospitals. Inglis had an enormous circle of friends in the medical community as well as the suffrage movement, and all were willing to help her.

Britain did not accept the women's medical units, but the French and others were glad to have them. The Scottish Women's Hospitals went to France, Belgium, Corsica, Serbia, and Russia. Inglis and her unit did much work in Serbia even after being taken prisoner. She and her colleagues worked under horrendous conditions with inadequate facilities and medical supplies. She returned to England briefly after being released, only to take a medical team to Russia, where help was badly needed. She stayed with her units until the Bolshevik Revolution was inevitable and they had to pull out. She returned to England and died the day after she arrived, on November 25, 1917.

See also: Anderson, Elizabeth Garrett; Edinburgh School of Medicine; Jex-Blake, Sophia Louisa; Scottish Women's Hospitals

References: Balfour, Lady Frances, *Dr. Elsie Inglis*, New York: George H. Doran (1919); Leneman, Leah, *In the Service of Life: The Story of Elsie Inglis and the Scottish Women's Hospitals*, Edinburgh: Mercat Press (1994); Ogilvie, Marilyn, and Joy Harvey, eds., *The Biographical Dictionary of Women in Science: Pioneering Lives from Ancient Times to the Mid-20th Century*, New York: Routledge (2000).

J

Jacobi, Mary Corinna Putnam
1842–1906

One of the most prominent women physicians and educators of the late nineteenth century, Mary Jacobi was the first woman to teach at the all-male New York Postgraduate Medical School. She was also a gifted writer, a leader in promoting equal education and training for women in medical schools when few were allowed entrance, and a vocal activist in the women's suffrage movement of the late nineteenth century.

Born in London, England, on August 31, 1842, Jacobi was the daughter of George Palmer Putnam, a New York publisher who had taken his family to London to open an office there, and Victorine Haven. Mary was the oldest of eleven children and was determined early in life to be a physician. Her father returned with his family to New York in 1847. She graduated from school in 1859, although much of her education had taken place at home.

She first studied at the College of Pharmacy in New York and was the first female graduate in 1863. She spent some time in New Orleans during the Civil War, tending to an injured brother and writing both nonfiction and fiction. Upon leaving New Orleans, she enrolled in the Female Medical College of Pennsylvania and graduated in 1864. Some faculty members there felt she had not had enough education to graduate, particularly the dean, Edwin Fussell. However, Ann Preston, a professor at the college, strongly supported Jacobi and felt she should be allowed to take graduation examinations: "[Fussell] contends that she has not

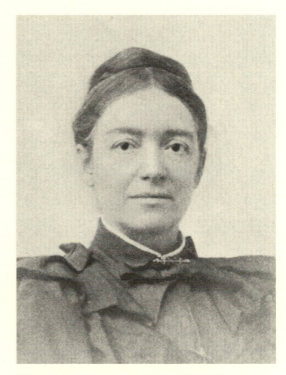

Mary Corinna Putnam Jacobi (MCP Hahnemann University)

fulfilled the requirements, then that she is incompetent, and intermittently that her credentials were not sufficient for advanced placement. He then escalates the charges to misrepresentation and a possibility of deliberate fraud. When he calls her 'unworthy,' it is not clear whether his objections are technical, relating to formal requirements; principled, relating to competence and knowledge; or moral, relating to deceptions" (Gartner 1996, 474). Fussell resigned following this incident, and Ann Preston became the dean.

Following her internship at the New England Hospital for Women and Children, Jacobi was convinced that she still did not have enough knowledge to practice medicine, a concern of most women physicians of the time. The schools that were started just for women did not have access to the kinds of medical laboratories or teaching hospitals that would have allowed them to better train their students.

Jacobi sought admission to the University of Paris and was denied numerous times. She studied on her own, was taught by observing physicians working in hospitals, and eventually obtained admission to the university. She graduated with honors in 1871. During this time she lived on her writing and on what her family could send her.

Following her final examinations, she still felt challenged. "I was prepared for a much more difficult examination, and internally I don't consider the passing this one even well (that other youth was accepted in spite of the most innumerable and awful blunders, so you see the mere fact of passing does not count for much), to be any great shakes; still as it is almost the first school in the world, and as the examination is really much more minute and extensive than at home, I suppose it counts for something" (Putnam 1925, 183).

She began working at the Women's Medical College of the New York Infirmary, which had been founded by Elizabeth Blackwell. She taught pharmacology and therapeutics. She strived to strengthen the curriculum and in 1874 became head of pediatric outpatients at Mount Sinai Hospital. She served as a professor of children's diseases at New York Postgraduate Medical School in 1882.

Her views on some aspects of medicine and medical education differed in some respects from Elizabeth Blackwell's. She felt women should not specialize in women's and children's diseases but instead should be well rounded. She also did not oppose experimentation on animals (Blackwell was an antivivisectionist).

She viewed a male physician as an equal. "Perhaps Jacobi's successes in the male pro-

fessional world were due at least in part to her willingness to accept men as equals. Certainly Jacobi did not share Blackwell's ambivalence toward romantic attachments to men, and her private correspondence never reveals the suspicion of marriage characteristic of many accomplished women of her generation" (Morantz-Sanchez 1985, 194).

She married a well-known pediatrician pioneer, Abraham Jacobi, in 1873. They had three children, only one who survived to adulthood. She also maintained a close relationship with many of her siblings.

Much of her medical writing focused on pathology and neurology. She did not set limits for herself as to what she would write about. "If Ann Preston and Hannah Longshore ventured into territories of language closed to women, Mary Putnam Jacobi laid claim to vast tracts of forbidden ground: menstruation, hysteria, nervous disease, the interior of the uterus. Other nineteenth-century women physicians were active scientists or prolific popular writers; few combined both genres, and none as productively as Mary Putnam Jacobi" (Wells 2000, 147).

Before her death from a brain tumor, she published the article "Description of Early Symptoms of the Meningeal Tumor Compressing the Cerebellum. From Which the Writer Died. Written by Herself," which was reprinted in *Mary Putnam Jacobi, M.D.: A Pathfinder in Medicine* (1925). She circulated the report to her physician friends. She died on June 10, 1906.

See also: Blackwell, Elizabeth; Medical College of Pennsylvania; Preston, Ann
References: Gartner, C. B., "Fussell's Folly: Academic Standards and the Case of Mary Putnam Jacobi," *Academic Medicine* 71, no. 5 (May 1996): 470–477; Gartner, Carol B., "Jacobi, Mary Corinna Putnam," *American National Biography,* vol. 11, New York: Oxford University Press (1999); Morantz-Sanchez, Regina Markell, *Sympathy and Science: Women Physicians in American Medicine,* New York: Oxford University Press (1985); Putnam, Ruth, *Life and Letters of Mary Putnam Jacobi,* New York: G. P. Putnam's Sons (1925); Wells, Susan, *Out of the Dead House: Nineteenth-Century Women Physicians and the*

Writing of Medicine, Madison: University of Wisconsin Press (2000).

Jacobs, Aletta Henriette
1854–1929

Aletta Jacobs was the first Dutch female medical doctor in the Netherlands. She obtained a license to practice medicine in 1878. She led the way for more women entering universities in the Netherlands and was an activist for social reforms and women's suffrage.

Born on February 9, 1854, Jacobs was the youngest of eight children of Abraham and Anna de Jongh Jacobs. She was born and raised in Sappemeer, a small village in Groningen. She had six brothers and four sisters. Her father was a country doctor who made rounds, and her mother kept house. Jacobs received a good education, as her father and mother felt education was important.

She enjoyed the outdoors and was quite a tomboy. She was a good student, at times being assisted by her father and older brothers. She wanted to be a doctor like her father and easily passed the exam to become a pharmacist's assistant. The local boys' high school allowed her to sit in on classes, and the University of Groningen permitted her to attend classes for one year. She realized later that "ultimately, the opening of the Dutch universities to women depended on my progress during this first year" (Jacobs 1996, 13).

She did very well even though she was often ill in her student days and received her medical credentials after defending her doctoral thesis on March 10, 1879. She became the first female doctor in the Netherlands. She wanted to continue her studies and did travel to London to visit the New Hospital for Women opened by Elizabeth Garrett Anderson. Jacobs and Anderson were both interested in many social issues of the times, and they got along well together.

In September 1879, Jacobs went to Amsterdam to attend a medical conference and was encouraged to get further training in London. This was her intent, but "during the conference, I received so many requests from Amsterdam families asking me to replace their regular doctor and I was approached by so many mothers wanting me to supervise the health of their children that it seemed to me wiser not to return abroad" (Jacobs 1996, 35).

She set up a practice in Amsterdam and offered free clinics to the poor, treating women from many different backgrounds for many years. Many of them had too many children and were relieved when Jacobs advocated birth control, a subject little discussed at the time.

This approach led to much controversy, with some accusing Jacobs of promoting abortion and some fearing that her views would lead to underpopulation. This opposition did not deter her either from promoting birth control or from speaking out about venereal diseases.

She treated many prostitutes at her clinics. "I have seen much misery caused by marriages involving young men who did not realize that they were still suffering from a venereal disease when they wed the woman of their dreams. In addition, as the only woman doctor in the Netherlands, I was consulted by prostitutes about diseases that I never even knew existed" (Jacobs 1996, 102).

Despite criticism, Jacobs continued to consult with young people who came to her for advice. During the early days of her practice, she had met another social reformer and activist, Carel Victor Gerritsen. They worked together for many years and shared similar interests in public welfare. They married in 1892, and in September 1893, Jacobs realized she was expecting their first child. The baby died following a mistake by the midwife. "I simply cannot describe how devastated we felt. It took me years to recover from my grief. But looking back, despite all the sorrow I still count myself lucky that I know how it feels to be a mother, that I have held my child in my arms, even though it was for but one day" (Jacobs 1996, 120).

Gerritsen suffered much with poor health, although he was continually involved in politics and spoke on social concerns, as did Jacobs. He died of liver and stomach cancer on July 5, 1905. Following his death, Jacobs turned her attention to women's suffrage work until World War I. During the war she was a committed pacifist, believing that women's presence as nurses during the war seemed to condone violence if they did not actively protest against it. "It was our duty to protest against the mindless destruction of art treasures, the breaking up of families, the barbaric sacrificing of young lives" (Jacobs 1996, 167).

She traveled to North America and visited many public health institutions and women's rights groups, even gaining an audience with President Woodrow Wilson. Once the war was over she worked hard for various peace initiatives and women's rights.

Jacobs died on August 10, 1929.

See also: Anderson, Elizabeth Garrett
References: Jacobs, Aletta, *Memories: My Life as an International Leader in Health, Suffrage, and Peace*, New York: Feminist Press (1996); Ogilvie, Marilyn, and Joy Harney, eds., *Biographical Dictionary of Women in Science*, New York: Routledge (2000).

Jalas, Rakel
fl. 1930s

Rakel Jalas was a leading psychiatrist in Finland prior to 1948. She was a consultant to the Ministry of Social Affairs and was elected to the Finnish parliament in 1948.

References: Lovejoy, Esther Pohl, *Women Doctors of the World*, New York: Macmillan (1957); Seppanen, Anni, "Medical Women in Finland," *Journal of the American Medical Women's Association* 5 (1950): 291.

Jemison, Mae Carol
1956–

Better known as the first female African American astronaut, Mae Jemison is first a physician who has been able to apply her medical skills in space experiments. She has contributed to medicine, engineering, and space science.

Born on October 17, 1956, in Decatur, Alabama, she grew up in Chicago with a brother and a sister. She is the daughter of Charles Jemison, a carpenter, and Dorothy Jemison, a schoolteacher. She had an early interest in space flight and was not deterred by the fact that at the time, no blacks or women were part of the space program.

She attended Morgan Park High School in Chicago, where she was interested in astronomy as well as space flight and in dance and art. Upon graduation she entered Stanford University with an interest in biomedical engineering and graduated in 1977 with a degree in chemical engineering.

After graduation she applied to NASA's astronaut-training program and to the medical school at Cornell, graduating in 1981. She worked for the Peace Corps and helped administer the medical programs in Sierra Leone and Liberia, where she learned to work with people of various backgrounds. When she returned to the United States, she worked for a health maintenance organization as a physician before finally being accepted into the space program in 1987. She worked for NASA for the typical five years before being eligible to serve on a shuttle mission. On September 12, 1992, she and six others traveled into space on the *Endeavor* to conduct numerous experiments. She studied weightlessness, motion sickness, tissue growth, and the loss of calcium in bones.

Jemison's background in both engineering and medicine allows her to make unique contributions; she was recently involved in coordinating a space-based communications system to support health care delivery in the developing world. She feels very strongly that people of all backgrounds and races have a right to have input on the direction of the space program. Jemison currently lives in Houston.

References: Bailey, Martha J., *American Women in Science, 1950 to the Present: A Biographical Dictionary*, Santa Barbara, CA: ABC-CLIO (1998); "Jemison, Mae C.," *Current Biography Yearbook*, New York: H. W.

Wilson (1993); Welch, Rosanne, *Women in Aviation and Space*, Santa Barbara, CA: ABC-CLIO (1998).

Jex-Blake, Sophia Louisa
1840–1912

Sophia Jex-Blake was the leader of the movement in Great Britain to open medical schools to women. Along with Elizabeth Garrett Anderson, she founded the London School of Medicine for Women. Jex-Blake was born in Sussex, Hastings, on January 21, 1840, to Thomas and Maria Emily Jex-Blake. Three years before Sophia was born, her grandfather had the family name of Blake officially changed to Jex-Blake in honor of his grandmother, Elizabeth Jex. Sophia was the youngest of three children; she had a brother, Thomas, and a sister, Caroline. Three other children had died in infancy. Her father was the proctor of Doctors Commons.

Sophia's parents educated her at home until she was eight. The various boarding schools she attended after that found the energetic and bored Sophia hard to handle. As a late teen, she began thinking about a vocation; she did not want to marry, the goal of most girls her age.

She considered teaching but was very disappointed in the education she had received in girls' schools with teachers she felt should have been better educated. She persuaded her parents to allow her to attend Queen's College for Women. She thrived at college, hungry for knowledge and taking a full load of courses in many areas: math, philosophy, English, French, religion, astronomy, and history. Because of her proficiency in math, she was asked to be a tutor. By her second year she was teaching women for the Society for Promoting the Employment of Women, founded in 1858 to help women learn simple skills so that they could acquire work as clerks and in shops. This work brought her into contact with women who had fallen on hard times, and she sent some of these people to her parents for assistance. Active members of the Anglican Church, they were quick to help the needy.

Sophia completed her studies in 1861 and then felt a need to go abroad. She visited various countries, teaching on occasion and learning as much as she could about different cultures. She visited the United States in 1865 and worked under Dr. Lucy Sewall at the New England Hospital for Women and Children. In 1868 she began her own medical study in New York under Elizabeth Blackwell.

Returning to England upon the death of her father, Sophia looked to her own country for the remainder of her medical education. The Medical Act of 1858 seemed to have closed all roads to women seeking an education in medicine, but she persevered and was finally accepted by the medical school at Edinburgh.

Thus began a long battle for her and the four other women undertaking medical studies at Edinburgh. Although at first the women were only occasionally subjected to heckling and rude behavior, more and more male professors and students came to resent their presence. In November 1870, a mob of protestors, some drunk and not even students, gathered at Surgeon's Hall to prevent the women from attending class. Several hecklers, mudslingers, and trash throwers showed up to perform. Supportive male classmates helped them get through the entrance and into the buildings. In the same year, college officials denied the women entrance to the Edinburgh Royal Infirmary, where medical students were required to obtain clinical training. The women challenged this decision.

In January 1871, Mr. Craig, the student Jex-Blake had indicated as the instigator of the riot at Surgeon's Hall, filed a defamation writ against her. Mr. Craig worked for Professor Christison, who was adamantly against having females educated in medicine. Sophia defended herself in court four months later. The jury found in favor of the claimant but awarded him one farthing instead of the 1,000 pounds he wanted. Sophia and her female colleagues, who had served as her witnesses, were seen as the victors.

The women also had to fight to take the professional examinations; the faculty did not support giving them to women. The university court had ruled the women would have to accept certificates of proficiency instead of medical degrees, or leave. The women students sued the university and won the right to stay in medical school in 1872, but that judgment was reversed in 1873. They were not allowed to take the degree examinations until the Russell Gurney Enabling Act of 1876.

Helping the women's cause during these years was public opinion. A wave of public sympathy and support countered every setback the women experienced. Why admit the women and then prevent them from completing their education? Jex-Blake's mother and brother were also very encouraging.

In 1874, Jex-Blake founded the London School of Medicine for Women. Clinical work had to wait until 1877, when the Royal Free Hospital opened its doors to women. In the meantime, Sophia had obtained her M.D. in Berne. She returned to qualify in Great Britain by taking the license of midwifery at the College of Surgeons. This plan was foiled when the examiners resigned en masse. In response, Parliament passed the Russell Gurney Enabling Act of 1876, which obligated all medical examining bodies to examine women (except in the field of surgery) and stipulated that women had the same rights as men to enter the medical profession. That same year Sophia Jex-Blake gained license to practice medicine through the Irish College of Physicians. She was finally able to start a private practice in Edinburgh and begin her career.

In her busy practice, she was especially popular with working-class women. Within months of opening her practice, she established an outpatient clinic where poor women could receive care for a few pence. She saw patients at her dispensary, traveled to their homes, or received them in her home. During these years she was attentive to political developments regarding medical education for women. She was deeply concerned about a bill in 1878 that would have required medical practitioners to obtain qualifications in both internal medicine and surgery. At the time, no examining body that qualified surgeons examined

women. She gathered some opponents of the bill, but eventually it was deferred and then dropped. However, it wasn't until 1885 that women could qualify to practice surgery.

In 1894, Edinburgh University finally allowed women to graduate from the medical program. Jex-Blake's mother, who had suffered from a long illness, died in 1881. Afterward, an assistant at the dispensary died suddenly, and Sophia blamed herself for not noticing that the assistant had been working too hard. Suffering from depression over these losses as well as exhaustion, she didn't practice medicine for almost two years.

There are no letters or diaries from this period. Margaret Todd, a friend of Sophia's later in life, received all her personal papers, but many assume that she destroyed all the documents prior to committing suicide.

In 1883, Jex-Blake returned to her work. Her practice thrived once again, and she also was pleased to see the Edinburgh Hospital and Dispensary become Scotland's first hospital staffed by women for the treatment and care of women.

In 1887, Sophia and friends opened the Edinburgh School of Medicine for Women. It wasn't long, however, before the school was competing with the second women's medical college, the Medical College for Women. It had been founded in part by women younger than she who had left her school because they disagreed with her ideas and strict standards.

The new college had a lower tuition and obtained access to the Edinburgh Royal Infirmary for clinical practice in 1892. Sophia's Edinburgh School of Medicine for Women was forced to close in 1898, and Sophia retired to Sussex the following year.

Once in Sussex, she continued to follow the progress of women medical students. Her home was always a haven for students, friends, and colleagues. She continued to suffer from heart problems off and on, having had a heart attack before leaving Edinburgh. In her later years, the problem worsened, and she died on January 7, 1912. Margaret Todd, a very close friend and a writer who became a physician, wrote a biography of Sophia in 1918.

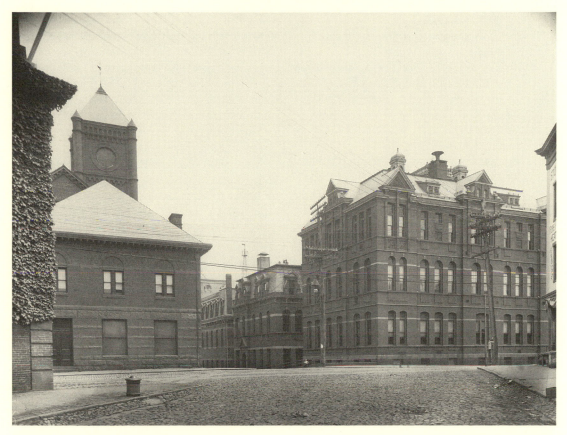

Johns Hopkins University (Library of Congress)

See also: Anderson, Elizabeth Garrett; Blackwell, Elizabeth; Edinburgh School of Medicine; Medical Act of 1858; Russell Gurney Enabling Act of 1876; Sewall, Lucy Ellen
References: Jex-Blake, K., "Jex-Blake, Sophia Louisa," *Dictionary of National Biography 1912–1921: Supplement 3*, London: Oxford University Press (1927); Roberts, Shirley, *Sophia Jex-Blake: A Woman Pioneer in Nineteenth-Century Medical Reform*, London: Routledge (1993); Todd, Margaret G., *The Life of Sophia Jex-Blake*, London: Macmillan (1918).

Johns Hopkins University

Johns Hopkins University was among the first major medical schools in the United States to admit women. The university would not have been able to open its medical school in 1893 had it not been for the fundraising abilities of four women: Miss M. Carey Thomas, Miss Mary Elizabeth Garrett, Miss Mary Gwynn, and Miss Elizabeth King. They were daughters of the trustees of Johns Hopkins and proponents of the women's rights movement.

When the women proposed raising the funds needed to open the medical school, $500,000, they made sure the university would admit women and hold to very high standards for all students. The requirements for admittance included a bachelor's degree; language skills in Latin, German, and French; and a background in biology, chemistry, and physics. Most of the faculty were taken aback at such high standards. As Dr. William Osler reportedly said to Dr. William Welch, it was lucky they got in as professors because they could not have made it as students (Bernheim 1948, 31).

The medical school opened with four renowned physicians as the founding medical educators: William H. Welch, William S.

Halsted, William Osler, and Howard Kelly. The school was a huge attraction for women medical students, who wanted to attend the traditionally male schools because of their better facilities and their hospital affiliations. Here, women could gain practical experience as well as a good academic education.

References: Bernheim, Bertram Moses, *The Story of Johns Hopkins: Four Great Doctors and the Medical School They Created*, New York: Whittlesey House (1948); "Women (or the Female Factor)," http://www.hopkinsmedicine.org/history.html#women.

Joliet-Curie, Irene
1897–1956

Irene Joliet-Curie was a Nobel Prize–winning chemist and physicist who, along with her husband, Frederic, discovered artificial radioactivity. Like her mother, she studied the medical possibilities radioactivity offered. She also contributed much toward the understanding of the neutron.

Born to the famous couple Pierre and Marie Curie on September 12, 1897, in Paris, Irene was the older of two daughters. Her sister, Eve, was born in 1904. They were both educated at home. Her grandfather, Eugene Curie, who came to live with the family when she was very young, had a great influence on her. She was taught by a group of elite scientists who were friends of the Curies. For a time her mother taught her physics, Paul Langevin taught her mathematics, and Jean Perrin taught her physics.

Her mother sent her to the College Sevigne, where she graduated before the outbreak of World War I. She also studied math and physics at the Sorbonne. She eventually gained licenses in physics and math while also working as a nurse during the war. She helped her mother set up the equipment for taking X rays of the wounded soldiers.

It was during the war that Irene became much closer to her mother. They shared a similar mission in helping wounded soldiers. "An intimate and charming comrade-ship linked Mme Curie and this young girl. The Polish woman was solitary no longer. She was able to talk of her work or of her personal worries now with a collaborator and friend" (Curie 1937, 301). Marie Curie had complete confidence in Irene's ability to help even though she was very young.

After the war Irene completed her doctoral degree in physics and began working for her mother at the Radium Institute of the Sorbonne. There she met Frederic Joliot, who had been hired as a laboratory assistant. Since he had no experience working with radioactive materials, Marie Curie turned his training over to Irene. They eventually found they had similar interests, and in 1926 they married.

They began collaborating and studied polonium, which Irene's parents had discovered to be radioactive. They found that when polonium was placed next to aluminum, positrons and neutrons poured out of the aluminum. When they announced their finding at the Solvay Conference in Belgium in 1933, many scientists were skeptical, and they were discouraged. However, a few scientists, including Wolfgang Pauli, encouraged them.

They returned to Paris to continue their experiments and soon saw that they had been correct; further experiments with aluminum in close proximity to polonium produced radioactivity. This discovery of artificial radiation would have a huge impact on chemistry, biology, and medicine. They received the Nobel Prize in chemistry in 1935.

In 1937 Irene began working at the Radium Institute as a professor and became interested in the results of assailing uranium with neutrons. She did much of the original research that Otto Hahn was able to build on in order to discover atomic fission. He would win a Nobel Prize in chemistry in 1944.

She and Frederic had two children, Helene in 1927 and Pierre in 1932. She enjoyed motherhood immensely and also thrived working in the laboratory even though she suffered for many years with tuberculosis. As World War II approached, Frederic began to work more on nuclear fission. He and Irene did not think an atomic bomb could be produced by the end of the war; moreover, they were more interested in nuclear energy because at the time France was very reliant on other countries for fuel.

During the war the Joliots, particularly Frederic, had less time for their research and spent more time on politics. Frederic eventually headed the most organized of the French Resistance groups. When the Germans occupied Paris and were a threat to the lab where he and Irene did their research, he worked on protecting it. He also had to arrange for Irene and their children to be smuggled out of the country to Switzerland in 1944.

Another important issue was protecting the uranium that France had, along with the "heavy water" (water enriched by deuterium) that was necessary for the atomic generator they wanted to construct. When the Nazis asked Frederic where the heavy water was, they were aware that Frederic had put it on a ship bound for England. However, they did not know which ship. Frederic gave them the name of one of the ships he knew had sunk. He also managed to keep the uranium safe.

Irene was very proud of Frederic. He had worked with the Resistance to get Jewish children out of Germany, giving them non-Jewish names and cards, and to shelter Jewish families until the end of the war. He assisted many who escaped from Germany.

Frederic joined the Communist Party and was against nuclear power for weapons. This position eventually hurt his career. Irene was also a controversial political figure during and after the war. They both eventually lost favor with many people because of their Communist views. However, Irene continued to be more interested in research than in politics and went on with her experiments even as she grew more ill from radiation exposure.

Eventually she went to look for natural sources of uranium in France and its overseas territories. Unlike many physicists, she was very knowledgeable about mineralogy and geology, particularly about minerals that produced natural radioactive substances. This work she did in conjunction with the French Atomic Energy Commission from 1946 to 1950. Frederic, with her help, had been successful in constructing Zoë, France's first nuclear reactor, in 1948. She also continued her research at the Radium Institute and spoke out for women's rights whenever she could.

She knew that the exposure to radiation had taken a toll on her, and she became weaker as time went on. By 1950, many scientists realized the dangers of working with radiation, and new precautions were in place in labs around the world. "To the end, she maintained her faith in science. During the last year of her life, she wrote, 'Science is the foundation of all progress that improves human life and diminishes suffering'" (McGrayne 1998, 142). Like her mother, she suffered from leukemia. She died on March 17, 1956. Both her children became scientists.

References: Curie, Eve, *Madame Curie: A Biography*, New York: Doubleday (1937); McGrayne, Sharon Bertsch, *Nobel Prize Women in Science: Their Lives, Struggles, and Momentous Discoveries*, Secaucus, NJ: Carol (1998); McKown, Robin, *She Lived for Science: Irene Joliot-Curie*, New York: J. Messner (1961); Perrin, Francis, "Joliot-Curie, Irene," *Dictionary of Scientific Biography*, vol. 7, New York: Scribner (1973); Shearer, Benjamin F., and Barbara S. Shearer, *Notable Women in the Physical Sciences: A Biographical Dictionary*, Westport, CT: Greenwood Press (1997).

Jones, Mary Amanda Dixon
1828–1908

Mary Jones was a physician who excelled in gynecological surgery when it was still a new and controversial specialty. In the nineteenth century, Jones was considered just as much an expert in the area as many male surgeons. She is a controversial figure in the history of women in medicine because she defied the norm for women physicians of her day and proceeded on a course that alienated her from many of her female colleagues. The scandal surrounding her surgical ability made the headlines in 1892. Public sentiment, professional opinion, and the social norms of the time all played a part in the trials that followed.

Born February 17, 1828, in Dorchester County, Maryland, she was one of several children of Noah Dixon and Sarah Turner. Her family was Methodist, middle-class, and in the shipbuilding business. She was able to obtain a good education at Wesleyan Female College, graduating in 1845.

She worked upon graduation as an instructor of physiology and literature at Wesleyan, then moved on to teach at the Baltimore Female College. She eventually took a position at a girls' seminary as the principal. All along she studied medicine with some local physicians.

After her marriage in 1854, she moved west. She had three children and eventually the couple moved back to Baltimore so that her husband, John Quincy Adams Jones, could practice law. She then left the family and went to New York City in 1862 and received a degree from the Hygeio-Therapeutic College.

After the Civil War ended, she lived in Brooklyn with her children while her husband stayed in Baltimore. She lectured on health issues for a time and was involved in some of the women's rights events of the day. Her practice was quite successful, but she decided in 1872 to pursue a traditional medical degree from the Women's Medical College of Pennsylvania, graduating after the required three years in 1875.

It is not known why she went on to get a traditional degree, but this course was not uncommon for women at that time. She also would certainly have been presented with patients who had problems she did not have the skill to handle. Upon graduation she opened her private practice again and specialized in surgery and problems of women. She again sought further education in 1881 with Benjamin Franklin Dawson, the founder of the *American Journal of Obstetrics and Diseases of Women and Children*.

Gynecology and surgical procedures in this area were still a relatively new field. "As a surgeon, she was bold, radical, and innovative, quick to criticize the temporizing of more conservative colleagues and anxious to advertise her innovations in technique. In this she mirrored the behavior of many of the leading men she most admired" (Morantz-Sanchez 1999, 79).

Rather than quietly treat patients, Jones wrote extensively and engaged in self-promotion in order to gain a good reputation. Some other women physicians thought she was too forward. Many male physicians found her to be very competent and were impressed with her knowledge not only of surgery but also of pathology. She also worked on keeping a dialogue open between herself and the male professionals she admired, both in the United States and abroad.

Beginning in 1889 the *Brooklyn Eagle* published a series of articles accusing her of various unethical methods, from mismanagement of funds for her hospital to unnecessary surgeries. She was also accused of not educating patients enough before they had surgery. Hysterectomies were quite controversial at the time. Many had the view that a woman's reproductive system belonged to the nation and that it was every woman's duty to have children; by performing hysterectomies on young women, a physician was hurting the country. The fact that Jones performed so many hysterectomies came up in some of the newspaper articles and in a trial when she was accused of manslaughter. She was found to be innocent, but she then sued the *Brooklyn Eagle* to seek restitution. She lost that battle, and her career was irreparably damaged.

After losing the libel suit, she left Brooklyn and went to New York City with her son, Charles, also a physician. She spent the rest of her years publishing articles and died in 1908. Her son continued to practice medicine in Brooklyn and New York City.

References: Morantz-Sanchez, Regina, "Jones, Mary Amanda Dixon," *American National Biography*, vol. 12, New York: Oxford University Press (1999); Morantz-Sanchez, Regina Markell, *Conduct Unbecoming a Woman: Medicine on Trial in Turn-of-the-Century Brooklyn*, New York: Oxford University Press (1999).

Jones, Mary Ellen
1922–1996

Mary Ellen Jones was a prominent researcher who discovered carbamyl phosphate, a compound requisite for the biosynthesis of arginine and urea. She also led her peers in DNA and cancer research and was the first woman to be a department head in the School of Medicine at the University of North Carolina at Chapel Hill.

Born in LaGrange Park, Illinois, on December 25, 1922, Jones was the daughter of Elmer and Laura Klein Jones. She attended the University of Chicago, majoring in biochemistry, and graduated in 1944. She worked for four years to save money for graduate studies at Armour and Company. She worked as a bacteriologist in quality control until 1948, when she went to Yale to study enzymology, completing her dissertation in 1951. She became increasingly interested in enzymes as she studied and worked in Fritz Lipmann's laboratory at Massachusetts General Hospital. He would later win a Nobel Prize for his discovery of coenzyme A and its importance to metabolism.

She wrote well and was able to obtain a position as an assistant professor at Brandeis University in 1957, rising to associate professor in 1960. She built a well-respected laboratory in the Department of Biochemistry. In 1966 she followed her husband, Paul Munson, to the University of North Carolina, where he was chair of the pharmacology department. She again worked in biochemistry, but after her divorce from Munson, she moved in 1971 to the University of Southern California's medical school and remained until 1978. She then returned to the University of North Carolina and worked until she retired in 1995.

Throughout her career, Jones studied proteins, enzymes and their actions, nucleotides, metabolism, and biosynthesis. She was a strong supporter of women and minorities in science and was very encouraging to all her students. She had two children, Ethan and Catherine. Jones died of cancer in Waltham, Massachusetts, on August 23, 1996.

References: Bailey, Martha J., *American Women in Science,* Santa Barbara: ABC-CLIO (1994); Fountain, Henry, "Mary Ellen Jones, 73, Crucial Researcher on DNA," *New York Times* (7 September 1996): 13; Traut, Thomas, "Biographical Memoirs: Mary Ellen Jones," http://www.nap.edu/readingroom/books/biomems/mjones.html.

Jordan, Lynda
1956–

A top researcher in biochemistry, Lynda Jordan has worked to uncover the secrets of phospholipase A2 (or PLA2) and its role in diabetes, arthritis, preterm labor, asthma, and other respiratory problems. Discovering the enzyme code may lead to new treatments, which are desperately needed.

Born in Roxbury, Massachusetts, on September 20, 1956, Jordan had to undergo harsh beginnings as a black woman in her quest to become a scientist. Her mother's second husband, Charles Jordan, had twelve children, and the children grew up in a rough housing project. At Dorchester High School, Jordan frequently got into trouble and didn't think too much about higher education until a speech for the Upward Bound program given by Joseph Warren inspired her. She began to apply herself in math and science and excelled in her studies. She went on to college and graduated from North Carolina A&T in 1974 and later received her master's at Atlanta University and her Ph.D. at MIT in 1985. From 1985 to 1987 she did research at the Pasteur Institute in Paris.

Despite the fact that some opposed her return to North Carolina A&T to teach, she wanted to return to the historical black college and give back to the university and its students. She built a well-equipped laboratory there for top-notch research and also takes every opportunity to encourage those from underrepresented groups to further their education.

Her work has focused on enzymes, particularly A2. She recently served two years as the MLK Visiting Professor at MIT and currently is a professor at North Carolina A&T. She is also a minister.

References: Coleman, Sandy, "At Home in the Lab and Pulpit," *Boston Globe* (18 April 1999): 1ff.; Hawkins, B. Denise, "Sister, Scientist, Mentor: Lynda Jordan," *Black Issues in Higher Education* 11, no. 21 (15 December 1994): 14–17.

Joteyko, Josephine
1866–1929

Josephine Joteyko was one of the first female Polish physicians. She excelled at medical studies and published numerous articles that were well received by both male and female colleagues of her day.

Born in Pocsujki on January 29, 1866, she went to Warsaw with her family when she was very young so that she would be able to obtain a good education. She attended the Varsovie secondary school and then studied science at the University of Geneva. She went to Brussels to study medicine and later to the University of Paris, obtaining her M.D. in 1896.

Her first position was at the Institute Solvay in Brussels as an experimental physiologist. She became interested in psychology, and in 1903 she headed research at the Kasimir Laboratory of Psychology at the Université Libre of Brussels until 1921. She wrote many articles and was the editor of *Revue Psychologique* for a time. She also lectured at several European universities. Her research focused on nutrition, physiology, muscle fatigue, and pain. She received several European awards for her work.

During the last years of her life she returned to Warsaw to teach science. She died in 1929.

References: Lovejoy, Esther Pohl, *Women Doctors of the World*, New York: Macmillan (1957); Ogilvie, Marilyn Bailey, and Joy Harvey, eds., *Biographical Dictionary of Women in Science: Pioneering Lives from Ancient Times to the Mid-20th Century*, New York: Routledge (2000).

K

Kagan, Helena
1889–1978

One of the earliest women physicians in Israel while it was still under Ottoman rule, Helena Kagan gained acceptance as a physician even before women were given licenses to practice medicine. She was the first woman to be awarded the Medal of the Freedom of Jerusalem in 1958.

She was born September 25, 1889, in Tashkent, Uzbekistan. Her father was an engineer. Hard times came when her father refused to convert to Christianity and lost his job. Her parents were still able to pay for her and her older brother to attend school. She graduated in 1905.

She went to Bern University in Switzerland to study medicine, graduating in 1910. She continued to study there, particularly pediatrics, for four more years. She went to Jerusalem in 1914 to practice medicine but was not able to obtain a license. Instead she assisted a physician at Jerusalem Municipal Hospital and trained young Arab and Jewish women as nurses for the typhus epidemic. After the outbreak of World War I, the physician she worked for died, and she had to take over for him. Because of the shortage of doctors, she found herself in charge of the typhus and cholera wards at the hospital as well as overseeing the prison hospital.

She eventually received a work permit and in 1916 founded a small children's hospital, which would eventually become part of the Hadassah Medical Organization. She worked there as head of the pediatrics department until 1925. She founded a homeless shelter for children in 1927 and some nurseries for working mothers. She supervised and trained many of the workers in these nurseries.

She worked for a time at Bikur Cholim Hospital in Jerusalem and was also associated with Hebrew University for many years. She received an honorary doctorate in 1967. She was one of the sole reasons for the expansion of health care in Israel, as she was really on her own for much of her early work. She established the Israel Pediatric Association in 1927 and in 1975 received a special Israel Prize in recognition of all her work. She passed away in 1978.

References: Hellstedt, Leone McGregor, *Women Physicians of the World: Autobiographies of Medical Pioneers*, Washington, DC: Hemisphere (1978); Kagan, Helenah, *Reshit darki bi-Yerushalayim*, Tel-Aviv: Vitso, Histadrut 'olamit le-nashim Tsiyoniyot; Tel-Yitshak ha-midrashah ha-Liberalit 'a. s. Dr. Y. Forder (1980); Lovejoy, Esther Pohl, *Women Doctors of the World*, New York: Macmillan (1957).

Kaufman, Joyce Jacobson
1929–

Joyce Kaufman is a talented scientist whose ability to combine chemistry, physics, pharmacology, computing, and biology has significantly aided in the understanding of how drugs affect the central nervous system.

Born in New York City on June 21, 1929, she attended Johns Hopkins University and received a bachelor's degree in chemistry in

1949, followed by a master's degree in 1959 and a D.E.S. (diplôme d'études supérieures) in theoretical physics from the Sorbonne in 1963.

Kaufman has worked at various companies doing research in many areas, including physiochemical studies and the nervous system. She has worked at Johns Hopkins University in both the chemistry department and the School of Medicine's anesthesiology and surgery departments. She has an unusual gift for understanding many science disciplines and their interrelationships.

She married Stanley Kaufman in 1948 and has one daughter.

References: *American Men and Women of Science,* 20th ed., New York: Bowker (1998); Bailey, Martha J., *American Women in Science: 1950 to the Present,* Santa Barbara, CA: ABC-CLIO (1998).

Kelsey, Frances Oldham
1914–

Frances Kelsey fought to ban thalidomide in the United States and determined to keep a drug company from distributing it in 1962, thus saving thousands of unborn babies from deformities. Her persistent skepticism about the drug and its testing made her a heroine with the public and earned her the President's Award for Distinguished Federal Civilian Service in 1962. She also helped establish the groundwork for tougher drug laws and brought greater awareness to the public as to the dangers of new drugs that do not have proper and thorough testing.

Born in Cobble Hill, British Columbia, she developed an interest in science as she "grew up in the country where she collected everything from bugs to bird eggs" (Bren 2001, 27). She went to McGill University in Montreal and earned a bachelor's degree in 1934. She continued her studies during the depression and obtained her master's in pharmacology the next year. She then accepted a scholarship from the University of Chicago, where E.M.K. Geiling was establishing a new pharmacology department.

While working, she earned her Ph.D. and became a faculty member at the University of Chicago. She married Dr. Fremont Ellis Kelsey in 1943, and they had two daughters. She worked at various jobs as a physician and teacher before being hired by the U.S. Food and Drug Administration in 1960. It was here that she did her important work on studying thalidomide and its effects, studying reports from Europe on its effects on humans, and requiring the drug company that was marketing it to provide more information.

Kelsey continues to work for the FDA.

References: Bren, Linda, "Frances Oldham Kelsey: FDA Medical Reviewer Leaves Her Mark on History," *FDA Consumer* 35, no. 2 (March–April 2001): 24–29; Grigg, William, "The Thalidomide Tragedy—25 Years Ago," *FDA Consumer* 21, no. 1 (February 1987): 14–17; Mintz, Morton, "'Heroine' of FDA Keeps Bad Drug off of Market," *Washington Post* (15 July 1962): A1.

Kenny, Elizabeth
1886–1952

Elizabeth Kenny was an Australian nurse who treated polio victims with methods that went against the medical practices of the time but eventually gained acceptance by the American Medical Association and others interested in treating polio victims before a vaccination was developed. A nurse serving in the backcountry, she treated people with hot packs and stimulation, using her instincts rather than prescribed, traditional methods. "Kenny clinics" were established around the country.

Born in Warialda, New South Wales, on September 20, 1886, she had very little formal training as a nurse. Her parents were Michael and Mary Kenny, and she was one of nine children. Her father was a veterinarian.

She served in the Australian bush from 1911 until World War I. It was during this early period of her career that she came across victims of poliomyelitis. The popular treatment of the day was to splint or cast the affected limbs right away. Having no idea of the accepted treatment in those early years, however, she developed her own technique of physical therapy. She treated her first case with warm, moist packs applied to the affected muscles. She then worked with the muscles to retrain them and make them more flexible. Using the same treatment with several other patients was successful. When she reported her treatments to Dr. Aeneas McDonnell, he was surprised and shocked that the children had survived. He informed her of the accepted method of the day. "Then he fetched from his library some impressive-looking tomes that dealt with this baffling disease. What I discovered in their pages left me speechless with astonishment. It simply could not be that I, in contraposition to wise authorities, had blundered upon a treatment that had met with success!" (Kenny 1943, 29). She told Dr. McDonnell she had treated the symptoms she saw—spasms; this symptom was not even mentioned in the book.

She treated many other types of ailments and delivered numerous babies in less than desirable surroundings. She traveled mainly by horseback, spending many nights under the sky. By 1913 she had a cottage hospital in Clifton not far from her mother's house. When World War I broke out, she volunteered and served at the front in France.

There were many dangers in serving as a nurse at the front as well as aboard the ships going to and from. During one troublesome but ultimately successful trip, her ship was reported as lost off the coast of Africa. Upon going to headquarters the next morning, she "presented my pay book to the pay officer. He looked at the book, took my name, and consulted his records. Then he informed me that I had been lost at sea and was dead. Under the circumstances, he could not possibly give me any money. The announcement gave me pause. It was difficult to believe that a ghost should feel so keenly the need of replenishing her wardrobe. But the paymaster was obdurate. He was very busy at the time, and took no further notice of me. Even the fact that he was dealing with someone who had been dead for several days failed to awaken the slightest interest in his official heart" (Kenny 1943, 42–43).

She eventually straightened out the problem, and later when the other members of her unit came, "I guided them through the intricate process by which they were restored to the land of the living, and we all went out to celebrate our resurrection" (Kenny 1943, 43).

After a shrapnel wound to her leg and knee, she managed to survive the influenza epidemic of 1918 while tending hundreds of patients on a ship bound for Australia. Soon thereafter she suffered a heart attack and was treated in Germany before returning again to her home country.

Kenny recovered and resumed her nursing work when the war was over. She invented a stretcher on wheels, the Sylvia Stretcher, after seeing so many in battle and at home die on the way to medical care via a bumpy road. Traditional stretchers could put the patients in shock, and many did not survive these trips. Her stretcher kept patients off the ground, allowing the tires and not the patients to absorb the bumps and also allowing Kenny to treat the patient for shock while in transit. Kenny named the stretcher after the little girl whose accident inspired it and patented it in 1927 so that it could be made available in more areas.

In the years that followed, Kenny struggled to gain acceptance for her methods of treating infantile paralysis. She tried in Australia and England but was disappointed each time. Kenny felt part of the problem was that officials perceived her as claiming a cure. "In the first place, I did not—and do not—claim a cure for infantile paralysis. I had written a personal letter to each member of the English committee emphasizing this fact. Infantile paralysis, like any other disease, takes its toll in human suffering. . . . Discovery of a cure would be enough to electrify the world. In the meantime, if the toll can be reduced and the legacy made less severe, any treatment accomplishing such results should be worthy of the most careful consideration before it is dismissed as useless" (Kenny 1943, 176–177).

After failing to win support from the established medical communities in Australia and Great Britain, in 1940 she went to the United States and demonstrated her methods of treatment on polio victims. In Minneapolis, she gained some listeners and eventually supporters who helped spread the idea and founded Kenny clinics in numerous places.

She died on November 20, 1952, after having been given diplomatic status by the U.S. Congress, having lunched with President Roosevelt, and most important, having seen her method of treatment accepted and able to help hundreds of polio victims suffering from pain.

References: Cohn, Victor, *Sister Kenny: The Woman Who Challenged the Doctors*, Minneapolis: University of Minnesota Press (1975); Hiestand, Wanda C., "Think Different: Inventions and Innovations by Nurses, 1850 to 1950," *American Journal of Nursing* 100, no. 10 (October 2000): 72; Kaufman, Martin, Stuart Galishoff, and Todd L. Savitt, eds., *Dictionary of American Medical Biography*, Westport, CT: Greenwood Press (1984); Kendall, Florence P., "Sister Elizabeth Kenny Revisited," *Archives of Physical Medicine and Rehabilitation* 79, no. 4 (April 1998): 361–365; Kenny, Elizabeth, *And They Shall Walk*, New York: Dodd, Mead (1943); Snodgrass, Mary Ellen, *Historical Encyclopedia of Nursing*, Santa Barbara, CA: ABC-CLIO (1999).

Kenyon, Josephine Hemenway
1880–1965

Josephine Kenyon was a pediatrician partially responsible, following the lead of Luther Emmett Holt, for fueling the boom in "baby books" during the early twentieth century. Her 1934 publication *Healthy Babies Are Happy Babies: A Complete Handbook for Modern Mothers* was remarkably successful.

She was born to Charles Carroll Hemenway and Ida Eliza Shackelford in Auburn, New York, on May 10, 1880. Her father was a Presbyterian minister. In 1891 the family moved to Glasgow, Missouri, after her father took a job as president of Pritchett College. She attended college there and received her bachelor's and a master's in 1898 and 1899, respectively.

She wanted a career in medicine and went to Bryn Mawr College in Pennsylvania to study biology before entering the School of Medicine at Johns Hopkins University in Baltimore. She had the great fortune to obtain training from some of the most prominent teaching physicians of the day: William Henry Welch, Sir William Osler, William Stewart Halsted, and Howard Kelly, still known as the Big Four at Johns Hopkins.

Following graduation she worked at the Johns Hopkins University Hospital for a year before moving to Babies Hospital in New York City in 1905. She studied childhood diseases and worked with Luther Emmett Holt and Martha Wollstein, pioneers in pediatrics. Following a six-year residency, she opened her own practice and in 1911 married James Henry Kenyon, a neurosurgeon on the staff of Babies Hospital.

Josephine had a great interest in educating the public on childcare and hygiene. She had done some lecturing on the topic before leaving Babies Hospital and was appointed as a lecturer at Columbia University's Teachers College in 1913. It was in this area that she would gain national recognition.

In the early 1920s she began writing advice for mothers in *Good Housekeeping* and contributed popular articles on child and baby care to other lay publications of the day. She appealed to so many women because she was a mother herself (of two daughters) and a physician. Her book *Healthy Babies Are Happy Babies* was so popular that it went through five revised editions and nineteen printings.

Kenyon stressed that a mother's health was as important as the baby's was. Ahead of her day, she also talked about the child's emotional health while maturing. She stressed the importance of children taking responsibility within the family: "We have heard much of the unquestioning obedience of the children of an older generation and the wonderful men and women who resulted from that discipline. In my opinion, the strong men and women developed, not because of this implicit obedience or from fear of the consequences of disobedience, but because these people, when young, had to take definite responsibilities as part of the working unit—the family" (Kenyon 1934, 276).

Kenyon maintained affiliations with many hospitals and universities and was called to speak on childcare innumerable times. She worked for various charitable and religious organizations whose aim was to make babies, mothers, and children safer. She also worked in educating women on proper conduct in the military while around soldiers and worked with various social leaders of the day. She closed her private practice in 1950 and moved to Colorado to be near family. Kenyon died on January 10, 1965, in Boulder, Colorado.

References: Kenyon, Josephine Hemenway, *Healthy Babies Are Happy Babies: A Complete Handbook for Modern Mothers,* Boston: Little, Brown (1934); "Kenyon, Josephine Hemenway," [obit] *JAMA* 192, no. 1 (5 April 1965): 75; Opitz, Donald L., "Kenyon, Josephine Hemenway," *American National Biography,* vol. 12, New York: Oxford University Press (1999).

Klein, Melanie
1882–1960

Melanie Klein was one of the most influential psychoanalysts in Great Britain. Her work has had a lasting impact on psychoanalysts and physicians. She built on the ideas of Freud and extended them. Her innovative method of analyzing child's play helped her later with adult psychoanalysis. Today many child clinics still employ her methods.

Born in Vienna, Austria, on March 30, 1882, she had three siblings. Her father, Moritz Reizes, was a physician and Jewish scholar, and her mother was Libusa Deutsch from Hungary, who for a time ran a store selling exotic plants. Her childhood was marred by the early deaths of her sister, Sidonie, and her brother, Emmanuel. Her father died when she was eighteen.

She received a good education and had a desire to become a physician like her father. However, her financial situation and early marriage to a second cousin, Arthur Stephan Klein, changed her course. They moved to Budapest and were there until 1919, then went to Switzerland for a time. The marriage ended in divorce in 1923 after they had had three children, Melitta, Hans, and Eric.

It was in Budapest that Klein began reading Sigmund Freud's work and became very interested in psychoanalysis. She was encouraged by Sandor Ferenczi and later by Karl Abraham, who recognized her gift at analyzing children. She presented a paper in 1921 on the development of children and received full membership in the Hungarian Psycho-Analytical Society.

She continued her studies in Berlin. There had been no work on the analysis of children under the age of five or six, and she developed a method for understanding very young children who could not yet talk by analyzing the way they played with toys. She felt she could interpret much about a child by the associations observed during free play.

She was asked to speak in England a number of times and moved there permanently in 1926. Her methods and results caused conflict in the field of psychoanalysis. She had traced Freud's views further back to the infant child, and many Freudian thinkers believed she did not have sufficient proof of the capability she attributed to infants. Many colleagues, however, embraced her methods. There was not a distinct division in the British Psychoanalytical Society between the Klein and Freud theories until a series of controversial discussions took place. Then it was clear there were two schools of thought (each of which has survived).

She contributed a great deal to psychoanalytic theory by studying infants and children the first ten years she was in London. After her oldest son was killed in 1933 in a mountaineering accident, she began to look at depression, sorrow, and emotion. She used her own dreams in writing about sorrow and mourning.

Her research involved studying many children with problems and analyzing their behavior. One of the more controversial aspects of Klein's work is that she analyzed her own children. Many analysts today find that disturbing. She had a very troubled relationship with her psychoanalyst daughter, Melitta Schmideberg, who openly argued with and lashed out at her mother in professional meetings.

Klein's pioneering work in child psychoanalysis has endured and helped numerous children and adults around the world. She passed away on September 22, 1960.

See also: Freud, Anna

References: Grosskurth, Phyllis, *Melanie Klein: Her World and Her Work,* New York: Knopf (1986); MacGibbon, Jean, "Klein, Melanie," *Dictionary of National Biography, 1951–1960,* London: Oxford University Press (1971); Segal, Hanna, *Melanie Klein,* New York: Viking Press (1980); Sheehy, Noel, Antony J. Chapman, and Wendy A. Conroy, *Biographical Dictionary of Psychology,* London: Routledge (1997).

Krajewska, Teodora
1854–1935

Teodora Krajewska was a Polish physician who was one of the first female physicians to serve in Bosnia and Herzegovina. She faced cultural barriers but succeeded in helping Muslim women as a social worker, healer, and educator.

She was born in Warsaw in 1854. Her father, Ignacego Kosmowskiego, was a teacher. She had several sisters and was educated in Warsaw. She obtained her medical degree around 1892.

She traveled to Bosnia along with Anna Bayerova of Czechoslovakia to help women in the Muslim faith receive proper health care, many for the first time. She helped with the establishment of better local health services and lived and worked in Dolnja Tuzla and Sarajevo for almost thirty years, from 1893 to 1922.

Krajewska died in 1935.

See also: Bayerova, Anna

References: Krajewska, Teodora Kosmowska, *Pamietnik,* Krakow: Krajowa Agencja Wydawnicza (1989); Necas, Ctibor, "Dr. Med. Teodora Krajewska, Lekarka Urzedowa W Dol. Tuzle I Sarajewie," *Archiwum Historii i Filozofii Medycyny* (Poland) 50, no. 1 (1987): 75–98.

Kubler-Ross, Elisabeth
1926–

Elisabeth Kubler-Ross revolutionized the way physicians, psychiatrists, and other health care providers view death and gave them a tremendous amount of information in order to better understand the stages of death, the acceptance of death as a part of life, and most important, the tools needed to counsel the terminally ill and their families. Medical and counseling centers around the world continue to use her ideas and findings.

Born in Zurich, Switzerland, on July 8, 1926, Kubler-Ross was one of triplet girls. Her parents, Emmy Villiger Kubler and Ernst Kubler, were strict at home but spent a lot of recreational time with their three daughters and an older son. She enjoyed her family but had a hard time finding her own identity, as so many persons of multiple births do. She had the same kinds of clothes and toys as the other girls and in her early days wanted to be different from them.

When Kubler-Ross was very young she had a serious bout with pneumonia and developed a bond with her roommate in the hospital.

> That evening she stirred more than normal. As I tried to get her attention, she kept looking past me, or through me. 'It's important that you keep fighting,' she explained. 'You're going to make it. You're going to return home with your family.' I was so happy, but then my mood changed abruptly. 'What about you?' I asked. She said that her real family was 'on the other side' and assured me that there was no need to worry. We traded smiles before drifting back to sleep. I had no fear of the journey my new friend was embarking on. Nor did she. It seemed as natural as the sun going down every night and the moon taking its place" (Kubler-Ross 1997, 29).

Her friend died peacefully that night. From this experience, she learned that dying can be a relief from pain and thus a positive event.

She did well in school, especially in science. In 1942 she set her sights on medical school, but her parents didn't see that she needed higher education. After a maid position away from home did not work out, she found a job as a lab assistant, thinking the experience would help her get into medical school. In her work in the lab, she took blood from people with late-stage venereal disease. She felt she was "called" to help those who were ill. "In those days, before penicillin, VD sufferers were treated like AIDS patients would be in the 1980s—they were feared, abandoned, shunned, locked away" (Kubler-Ross 1997, 55). She found she could help them physically and emotionally by just listening to them and responding sympathetically.

The hospital where she worked was overwhelmed with refugees from all over Europe after the Normandy invasion in 1944. She later became a member of the International Voluntary Service for Peace and traveled about helping all she could, finally reaching Poland in 1948. She had promised a doctor at the hospital where she worked in Switzerland that she would help the Polish people recover from the aftermath of the war.

The devastation was overwhelming. She helped to rebuild schools and nurse the ill in a small farming town called Lucima. A trip to one of Hitler's death camps, Maidanek, forever etched the horror of hatred in her mind as she visited those who had lost their entire families. She also experienced discrimination when people who thought she was Polish refused to help her when she became seriously ill on the trip home. She would see such discrimination again in the treatment of AIDS patients.

Returning home, she was still determined to become a physician and went back to lab work at the hospital. She talked with patients, taking an interest in their problems and fears, and was able to handle more responsibility. She had seen that healing involved more than physical care, and she was interested in mental as well as physical health.

In 1951 she began medical school at the University of Zurich, intending to follow the Swiss model of a physician—a country doctor who served the community. She passed her Matura, excelling in all sections except Latin.

Numerous times while at the University of Zurich she saw C. G. Jung but avoided meeting him. She didn't want to become a psychiatrist, just a physician.

She met her future husband, Emmanuel Robert Ross (Manny), in medical school, but at the time she was not impressed with any of the American medical students: "My first impression of them as a group, based on how they handled the corpse, was not a good one. They made jokes about the dead man's body, jumped rope with his intestines and teased me about the size of his testicles. It wasn't funny. I thought they were disrespectful, insensitive cowboys" (Kubler-Ross 1997, 94).

Despite that, she and Manny dated through medical school, and they married in 1958, a year after graduating. They went to the United States and both worked as interns at Glen Cove Community Hospital on Long Island, New York. She then took a resident position in psychiatry at Manhattan State Hospital because she needed a job.

The situation at Manhattan State Hospital was appalling to her. Mentally ill patients were used for experiments with psychotic drugs, beaten and punished, or totally ignored. She began listening to the patients and responding to their needs, and in turn they responded with better behavior. Mental patients had to learn to do chores like making their beds and they would be rewarded with such incentives as going outside for a walk. She had another job offer after her first year at the hospital but decided to stay. She obtained releases for many functional patients and helped others finds jobs outside the hospital.

She started an open-house program, finding families in the neighborhood who would visit the patients and develop relationships with them. Patients began to look forward to these visits, and a large percentage of them got well and were released.

Such numbers of recoveries were unprecedented at the hospital.

After two miscarriages in as many years, Kubler-Ross gave birth, in 1960, to her first child, Kenneth Lawrence. She had only one more year of residency, and it was too late to change her acquired psychiatry specialty. Montefiore Hospital accepted her, and not content to be only a wife and mother, she went back to work. At Montefiore, she worked with many terminally ill patients, talking frankly to them about death.

Kubler-Ross lost her own father during this time. He was very ill in Switzerland, and the doctors would not grant his request to die at home. Kubler-Ross arrived and signed papers releasing the hospital from responsibility. She and her mother then took her father home, where he died peacefully in 1960.

After she finished her residency in 1962, she and her husband obtained jobs in Denver at the Colorado School of Medicine. It was here that she gave her first lecture on death.

In 1963 she had a second, premature, child, Barbara Lee. After the birth, Manny took a job in Chicago and she underwent psychoanalysis for three years as a requirement of her training at the Psychoanalytic Institute. She worked at Billings Hospital, which is affiliated with the University of Chicago, as a physician and assistant professor of psychiatry from 1965 to 1970. She disagreed with the traditional practices of the psychiatrists in her department at Billings, whose treatments relied mainly on drugs. She felt that psychiatrists should focus more on the individual patient's personality and family life.

She began regular lecturing on death in 1967; at each lecture, she was accompanied by a terminally ill patient who was willing to talk to the audience about his or her feelings. Priests, nurses, rabbis, counselors, social workers, and students crowded in to find out about a subject no one else wanted to deal with. Physicians did not often attend because as a group, they looked upon death as failure to cure the patient. In 1969, a copy of an article she had written for the Chicago Theological Seminary on the purpose of her death-and-dying seminars found its way to an editor at Macmillan in New York. In response to a call from Macmillan, she wrote her *On Death and Dying* in a little over three months. In the book, Kubler-Ross describes the five stages of dying: denial, anger, bargaining, depression, and acceptance. Macmillan published the book that same year. It continues to be popular today and is required reading for numerous college and university courses. It is also useful for therapists, clergy, social workers, and families dealing with death issues.

Soon after the publication of *On Death and Dying, Life* magazine highlighted one of her seminars. The *Life* article featured a young girl named Eva who was dying of leukemia. In response to the piece, hundreds of people and organizations asked Kubler-Ross to give lectures. She was suddenly famous, the world's expert on death and dying.

Over the next few years, Kubler-Ross had some paranormal experiences that alienated some of her followers. "She had been commissioned, she felt, to use her renown to declare to anyone who would listen that man indeed possessed a spirit and that his spirit survived death—which she now refers to as the 'transition'" (Gill 1980, 313). She continued to write about death and life after death. In 1983 she was asked to help with AIDS, an endeavor that totally absorbed her. Again, she felt that caring and unconditional love would be more helpful than science. She conducted thousands of AIDS workshops all over the world.

Kubler-Ross currently lives in Arizona. Some critics argue she has no scientific proof or clinical trials to support her claims of success with psychotic patients and the terminally ill. As a result of her work, however, there is more awareness today of the right of the dying to determine their own destiny and a hospice movement to support this right. Many physicians now also support patients' rights to not avail themselves of life-sustaining medical equipment.

References: Gill, Derek L. T., *Quest: The Life of Elisabeth Kubler-Ross*, New York: Harper & Row (1980); Kubler-Ross, Elisabeth, *On Death and Dying*, New York: Macmillan (1969); Kubler-Ross, Elisabeth, *The Wheel of Life: A Memoir of Living and Dying*, New York: Scribner (1997).

L

Lachapelle, Marie-Louise Duges
1769–1821

Marie-Louise Lachapelle became the chief midwife at the Hotel Dieu in Paris. She was instrumental in training many midwives.

Born in Paris on January 1, 1769, she was the daughter of Louis Duges and Marie Jonet Duges. Her mother was a midwife and her father, a health officer. Lachapelle began assisting her mother, who was the head midwife at the Hotel Dieu, at an early age.

She married in 1792 and had a daughter; her husband died a few years later. She began working with her mother at the Hotel Dieu to support herself, becoming head of the maternity department after her mother died in 1795.

She developed excellent techniques in delivering babies even in difficult circumstances, techniques that she later recorded in a published work. Some of her training came from Franz Carl Naegele at the University of Heidelberg in Germany. He was a famous obstetrician of his day and respected her talent a great deal.

Lachapelle did much to raise the standards and proficiencies of midwives in the nineteenth century. She died on October 4, 1821.

References: Lovejoy, Esther Pohl, *Women Doctors of the World*, New York: Macmillan (1957); Shearer, Benjamin F., and Barbara S. Shearer, *Notable Women in the Life Sciences*, Westport, CT: Greenwood Press (1996); Uglow, Jennifer S., *International Dictionary of Women's Biography*, New York: Continuum; Macmillan (1982).

LaFlesche Picotte, Susan
1865–1915

Susan LaFlesche Picotte was the first Native American woman to earn a medical degree. She returned to her reservation to serve the needs of the Indians she identified with, as well as others who were in need of medical attention. Speaking both her native tongue and English, she was able to bridge some of the cultural differences between her people and those in surrounding communities. Born on June 17, 1865, on the Omaha Reservation in Nebraska, she was the youngest of five children of Chief Joseph LaFlesche and his wife, Mary. She received much encouragement from her family to advance her education as a representative of the Omahas. Chief LaFlesche had already learned that to progress, the Indians had to adapt to a changing world that was more and more populated by whites. He realized that education was the key and would enable Indians to contribute to the changing society.

Susan did well in school. Her oldest sister, Susette, was a teacher, and she made all her sisters speak English when they were together. She attended both the Elizabeth Institute for Young Ladies (New Jersey) and the Hampton Institute in Virginia, where she graduated with honors in 1886. With financial assistance from the Women's National Indian Association, she entered the

Medical College of Pennsylvania and graduated in 1889.

She served an internship at the Women's Hospital in Philadelphia, affiliated with the Women's Medical College of Pennsylvania, treating outpatients, observing surgery, and preparing medications. She also went on rounds with the resident physician to some very poor neighborhoods. This was valuable experience, since she had had little clinical training while in medical school.

In order to serve the Indians of her tribe, she applied for a physician position with the Omaha Agency Indian School. The commissioner of Indian Affairs believed in Indians becoming educated and serving their people, and she got the job. She quickly returned to the Omahas, becoming a medical leader and organizer. She served members of the Omaha tribe for over four years regardless of the problems with getting supplies, low pay, difficult physical conditions, and the obstacles of travel.

"Making home visits was no easy task. Omahas were scattered over an undeveloped, undulating terrain that was thirty miles long by fifteen miles wide. Most of the so-called roads were little more than poor dirt tracks, which were so bad that a single horse could not pull a wagon on them" (Tong 1999, 94). During this time, she spoke whenever she could to groups off the reservation about the Omahas and her work with them. She was a good speaker who did not alienate whites, and she knew she had to work with them in order to improve conditions for Native Americans.

In the 1890s, La Flesche worked unceasingly to end drinking among the Indians. It had led to illness and death and was destructive to family and community relationships. Her efforts were fruitless, and she became quite frustrated. She blamed the whites for making alcohol available, and although some religious groups supported her efforts to enforce the law against providing alcohol to Indians, cooperation from law enforcement was not forthcoming. She continued to fight against drinking, as her father before her had done.

She married Henry Picotte, half Sioux and half French, and had two sons, Caryl and Pierre, who both were able to attend college. After her husband's death in 1905, she settled in Walthill in the year of its founding, 1906, and continued to speak for the betterment of Indians everywhere. She helped organize the County Medical Society, served on the local health board, and stood firm on eradicating alcohol on reservations and instilling good sanitation and nutrition practices.

Her final efforts were toward getting a local hospital. She helped raise funds, a long and hard task. "A few years before her death, Susan asserted that she believed 'in prevention of diseases and hygienic care' more than she did 'in giving or prescribing medicine.' She said her 'constant aim' was 'to teach these two things, particularly to young mothers,' and her 'greatest desire in having the hospital built was to save the little children'" (Tong 1999, 177).

This goal may well have arisen because she had seen many infants and children die from disease while she was waiting for medical supplies.

In 1913 she attended the opening of the hospital at Walthill, which remained a vital part of health care in the area until 1947. On September 18, 1915, La Flesche succumbed to a long bout with a cancerous bone infection. In that year, hospital officials gave the hospital her name. She was buried in the nearby Bancroft cemetery next to her husband, Henry.

References: Tong, Benson, *Susan LaFlesche Picotte, M.D.: Omaha Indian Leader and Reformer*, Norman: University of Oklahoma Press (1999).

Lancefield, Rebecca Craighill
1895–1981

Rebecca Lancefield was a bacteriologist and researcher. She was a pioneer in classifying and identifying the various strains of streptococci.

Born in Ft. Wadsworth, New York, on January 5, 1895, she was the daughter of Colonel William E. Craighill and Mary Wortley Byram Craighill and had five sisters. She attended Wellesley College, graduating in 1916 with a degree in zoology. After her father died, she taught for a year to help support her sisters. Seemingly headed for a teaching career at Teachers College in New York, she persuaded the administrators to let her pursue a master's in bacteriology.

She excelled and took a part-time position with the Rockefeller Institute, working with Oswald Theodore Avery and Alphonse Raymond Dochez, who were studying streptococcal bronchopneumonia for the surgeon general of the United States. She left to finish her master's and married Donald Lancefield. Her husband finished his Ph.D. in 1921, and they both went to Oregon for a few years to work. Later they returned to New York, and Lancefield went back to work for the Rockefeller Institute, where she would stay for the rest of her career.

While she was there, her laboratory grew in reputation, becoming the world leader in identifying different strains of strep. She developed a unique classification system that is still used today.

Lancefield had one daughter, Jane. She died on March 3, 1981.

References: Elliott, S. D., "Obituary: Rebecca Craighill Lancefield, 1895–1981," *Journal of General Microbiology* 126, pt. 1 (September 1981): 1–4; McCarty, Maclyn, "Rebecca Craighill Lancefield," *Biographical Memoirs*, vol. 57, Washington, DC: National Academy of Sciences (1987); Shearer, Benjamin, and Barbara S. Shearer, *Notable Women in the Life Sciences: A Biographical Dictionary*, Westport, CT: Greenwood Press (1996).

Lazarus, Hilda
1890–198?

Hilda Lazarus was an Indian physician who served for many years as the director of the Vellore Christian Medical College when it became coeducational in 1947 and set a new precedent for Indian medical education. She was instrumental in making the transition to coeducation acceptable.

Born January 23, 1890, in India, Lazarus was one of twelve children, nine of which survived to adulthood. Her grandfather was one of the earliest Brahmins to convert to Christianity. Her parents were well educated, and her father served as principal of the London Mission High School, Visakhapatnam. Despite frequent illnesses as a child, Lazarus was a good student who studied physiology at a local college in order to prepare for medical school. She had decided early on that she wanted to be a physician and obtained her M.D. from the University of Madras in 1917.

She began her career with the Women's Medical Service and served briefly at the Lady Hardinge Medical College Hospital in New Delhi. After a few months she was transferred to the Dufferin Hospital in Calcutta and had to deal with multiple languages in treating patients as well as a tremendous workload.

> There I had to attend to all emergencies, all special paying patients, outpatients, and a ward of twenty beds, as well as being responsible for all statistics. The only languages I was acquainted with were English, Telugu, and Tamil, but here I was obliged to lecture to midwives in Hindi, to deal with Bengalis, and to study Urdu. It was compulsory for every officer of the Women's Medical Service to pass in Urdu before confirmation of service. I managed this with credit in two and a half months and then began to study Bengali, in order to understand the patients and help them to understand me. (cited in Hellstedt 1978, 39)

She moved on to work in Surat and later in Visakhapatnam. She kept learning the required languages of the areas in order to serve patients better as well as to train midwives and nurses who worked at the local hospitals and clinics. For a few years she also worked at the Lady Willingdon Medical School in Madras, and then returned to Visakhapatnam in 1922 when she was hired to help the hospital there overcome financial difficulties. She had good organizational and administrative skills and was well qualified to assume in 1940 the position of principal of the Lady Hardinge Medical College in New Delhi. She held this position for three years and later became chief of the Women's Medical Service for India. She remained in this post until 1947 and then became the superintendent of Vellore Medical College as it entered a transitional phase of coeducation.

She remained active in the administration of hospitals after she retired from Vellore in 1950. She also served for a time as professor at the Andrha Medical College in Visakhapatnam and worked to better the facilities.

References: Hellstedt, Leone McGregor, *Women Physicians of the World: Autobiographies of Medical Pioneers,* Washington, DC: Hemisphere (1978); Lazarus, Hilda, "Message from India," *Journal of the American Medical Women's Association* 3, no. 6 (June 1948): 250; Lovejoy, Esther Pohl, *Women Doctors of the World,* New York: Macmillan (1957); Ogilvie, Marilyn, and Joy Harvey, eds., *The Biographical Dictionary of Women in Science: Pioneering Lives from Ancient Times to the Mid-20th Century,* New York: Routledge (2000).

L'Esperance, Elise Depew Strang
1878–1959

Elise L'Esperance opened the first clinic in the United States for cancer detection.

Born in Yorktown, New York, in 1878, she was the third daughter of Albert Strang and Kate Depew. Her father wanted a physician in the family and, not having a son to follow in his footsteps, encouraged his third daughter to pursue medical studies.

Elise attended school in Albany, New York, at St. Agnes Episcopal School before attending the Women's Medical College of the New York Infirmary for Women and Children. She graduated in 1900 with her medical degree and married David A. L'Esperance.

L'Esperance served as a pediatrician in both New York and Detroit but decided more clinical research was needed on many of the child illnesses she saw and treated. She left private practice after several years to join the Tuberculosis Research Commission in New York.

Her interest in pathology developed when she later worked with James Ewing at Cornell University Medical School. She studied tumors and cancerous cells and realized cancer could be detected in its early stages. In 1917, she moved on to the New York Infirmary for Women and Children. She worked there for over thirty years while also working as an instructor at various hospitals and as an assistant professor at Cornell.

When her mother died in 1930, she opened the Kate Depew Strang Tumor Clinic with the help of her sister, May Strang, at the New York Infirmary. The clinic focused on cancer detection in women and children as opposed to treatment of the illness. L'Esperance felt strongly that malignant cancers could many times be prevented if physicians knew what to look for. Her clinic later expanded to include male patients and became so successful that she opened another one in 1940.

She became an expert on cervical cancer, and research at her clinic led to the Pap smear for detecting cervical cancer and the proctoscope for detecting colon and rectal cancer. She encouraged women physicians to stay in the field and was a leader in educating women about their health, the importance of routine examinations, and cancer prevention. She passed away in Pelham Manor, New York, on January 21, 1959.

References: Perry, Marilyn Elizabeth, "L'Esperance, Elise Strang," *American National Biography,* vol. 13, New York: Oxford University Press (1999); Shearer, Benjamin F. and Barbara S. Shearer, *Notable Women in the Life Sciences,* Westport, CT: Greenwood Press (1996).

Levi-Montalcini, Rita
1909–

Rita Levi-Montalcini was the 1986 Nobel Prize recipient, along with Stanley Cohen, for discovering the nerve growth factor (NGF), which is vital for the growth and stimulation of nerve cells.

Born in Turin, Italy, on April 22, 1909, to Adele Levi and Adamo Levi, an electrical engineer, Rita, who had a twin sister and two other siblings, decided early on that she wanted to study medicine. She was disappointed in her early education because it lacked what she would need in the way of science studies.

She took it upon herself to study under tutors in Greek, Latin, and math for several months before she took her medical school entrance exams. She passed and, along with a cousin, attended the University of Turin, receiving her M.D. in 1936. She stayed and worked as an assistant to Giuseppe Levi, at the time a well-known professor of histology.

Levi "inspired Rita's expert skill in the study of tissue structure. Under his direction at the Institute of Anatomy, she mastered a new technique that involved staining chick neurons with chrome silver to highlight the nerve cells in infinitesimal detail" (Van der Does and Simon 1999, 142). She continued studying chick embryos and their nervous systems by dissecting them and examining motor neurons.

Neither Levi nor Levi-Montalcini could hold an official position at the university because the Fascist regime in Italy was quite strong at the time and they were Jews. Her family went south when the Nazis invaded.

As the war closed in on her family, they had to flee again, this time going to Florence with false identification.

Once the war was over, Levi-Montalcini vowed to work with the survivors as a doctor. She worked with the Allied health service, persevering during a typhoid epidemic. "The risk of contagion, to which I was at every moment exposed, diminished my never entirely alleviated sense of guilt for not having taken a more active part in the partisan resistance" (Levi-Montalcini 1988, 108).

While treating a young girl, Levi-Montalcini became attached to her and her parents. The girl's death caused Levi-Montalcini to doubt her competence as a physician: "My sense of impotence in this case contributed

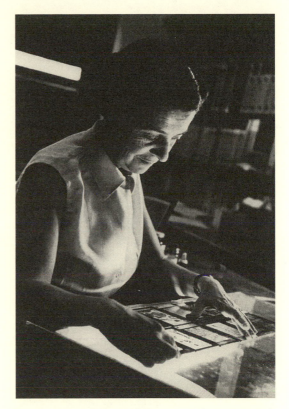

Rita Levi-Montalcini (Herb Weitman/U.S. National Library of Medicine)

to the decision I later took not to practice the profession. I lacked, in fact, the detachment that allows a doctor to face the suffering of a patient without creating an emotional involvement damaging to both parties" (Levi-Montalcini 1988, 108). She later devoted her energies to research on the nervous system.

She went to the United States in 1947 to work with Viktor Hamburger at Washington University in St. Louis. She served as an associate professor in zoology and in 1958 as a professor of neurobiology. It was during this time that she worked on identifying the nerve growth factor (NGF). She and Hamburger published some papers together, but she wasn't able to isolate and identify NGF until Stanley Cohen came to St. Louis and worked with her. Together they would discover NGF.

They began by studying mouse tumors and later snake venom. Both produced many nerve fibers. It wasn't until Cohen deduced that the saliva gland produced nerve growth factor that they were able to purify it. Levi-Montalcini continued to work on NGF after Cohen left Washington University in 1959. She felt strongly that the scientific community did not realize the importance of the discovery.

She left in 1961 to return to Rome and established the Laboratory of Cellular Biology. She continued her work there, and as time passed, her discovery attracted more attention. By the mid-1980s, many neurobiologists were aware of the importance of growth factors. It became clear "that the nerve growth factor keeps cells from dying in their early embryonic stages. Without nerve growth factors, half of some kinds of cells would die; with NGF, they survive. NGF affects particular kinds of cells, whether they are in the central nervous, the peripheral nervous system, or the brain. It also appears to link the immune and the nervous systems of the body" (McGrayne 1998, 220).

In 1986, she and Cohen received the Nobel Prize in physiology or medicine for their discovery. Some scientists were surprised that Viktor Hamburger was excluded. Levi-Montalcini's defense of the Nobel committee's decision to give the award to her and Cohen strained her relationship with Hamburger, who received the national Medal of Science in 1989.

She had served in Rome as the director of the Institute of Cell Biology from 1969 to 1979. After winning the Nobel Prize, she became a national celebrity and continued to work as much as she could on NGF, later taking an interest in degenerative diseases. She served as president of the Italian Multiple Sclerosis Association for many years.

References: Levi-Montalcini, Rita, *In Praise of Imperfections: My Life and Work,* New York: Basic Books (1988); McGrayne, Sharon Bertsch, *Nobel Prize Women in Science: Their Lives, Struggles, and Momentous Discoveries,* Secaucus, NJ: Carol (1998); Shearer, Benjamin F., and Barbara S. Shearer, *Notable Women in the Life Sciences: A Biographical Dictionary,* Westport, CT: Greenwood Press (1996); Van der Does, Louise Q., and Rita J.

Simon, *Renaissance Women in Science,* Lanham, MD: University Press of America (1999).

Longshore, Hannah Myers
1819–1901

Hannah Longshore was the first female faculty member in a medical college of the United States and the first to practice in Philadelphia. Longshore was an early pioneer in women's medical education in the United States.

She was born on May 30, 1819, in Sandy Spring, Maryland, to Samuel Myers and Paulina Oden Myers. She married Thomas E. Longshore in 1841 and had two children. Her brother-in-law, Joseph Longshore, tutored Hannah privately to prepare her for entrance to the Female Medical College of Pennsylvania (renamed the Women's Medical College of Pennsylvania in 1867). Joseph Longshore was a physician and, with some other male doctors, had played a vital role in the establishment of the college. Hannah graduated in 1851 and became a demonstrator of anatomy there, the first woman in the United States to hold a faculty position in a medical school.

Hannah also taught for a year at the New England Female Medical College in Boston. After Joseph Longshore was ostracized by the faculty at the Female Medical College of Pennsylvania for wanting to teach water cures and other eclectic therapies, he founded the Pennsylvania Medical University. Hannah taught anatomy there from 1853 to 1857.

Her private practice thrived to the point that she eventually gave up teaching and lecturing to spend all her time with the 300 families under her care. She died on October 18, 1901, in Philadelphia, Pennsylvania.

See also: Medical College of Pennsylvania
References: Kaufman, M., "Longshore, Hannah E. Myers," *Dictionary of American Medical Biography,* Westport, CT: Greenwood Press (1984); Ogilvie, Marilyn, and Joy Harvey, eds., *The Biographical Dictionary*

of Women in Science: Pioneering Lives from Ancient Times to the Mid-20th Century, New York: Routledge (2000).

Lopez, Rita Lobato Velho
1866–19?

Rita Lopez was the first woman doctor who graduated from a medical school in Brazil. She received her degree in 1887 from the University of Bahia.

References: Lovejoy, Esther Pohl, *Women Doctors of the World*, New York: Macmillan (1957).

Lovejoy, Esther Clayson Pohl
1870–1967

Esther Lovejoy was the first woman to head a city health department. She raised the issue of public health in the schools and established school health inspections, became a leader of women in medicine by establishing the Medical Women's International Association, and was instrumental in documenting numerous medical women's events and accomplishments.

She was born November 16, 1870, in Seabeck, Washington. Her parents, Edward and Annie Quinton Clayson, moved around to make a living. Esther first lived in a logging camp where her father worked, then in a hotel her parents managed, and later on a farm. Her early education was in Seabeck; later she had a professor as a tutor. She worked to earn money for medical school.

She attended the University of Oregon Medical School and became the second woman graduate in 1894. She married Emil Pohl, a surgeon, later that year, and did postgraduate work at the West Side Post Graduate School in Chicago, where she studied obstetrics and gynecology. In 1898, they went to Alaska, where her brothers lived, to set up practice, and they were instrumental in setting up Union Hospital.

Her brother Fred Clayson mysteriously disappeared while she lived there, and two men he had been traveling with were found murdered. Some of the local people suspected her brother of murdering them for a dog sledge. Speculation mounted, and a few months after the snow had melted, her brother's body was also found—shot like the others. The mystery was partly solved, but Esther could no longer bear to stay in Alaska. She moved and set up a private practice in Portland, Oregon, and commuted to Skagway in order to visit her husband.

When their son was born in 1901, Emil moved to Portland as well and set up a practice. Lovejoy became involved with the Portland Board of Health in 1905, becoming the first woman to head such a department in 1907. She witnessed numerous child illnesses due to unhealthy school conditions and contaminated milk. Frederick, her only child, died in 1908 from what she believed to be the result of contaminated milk. She fought and won the battle for advanced sanitation standards, and a milk ordinance was eventually passed. Her husband died three years after she lost her son. In 1913, she married George Lovejoy; they divorced in 1920.

Much of her later career focused on organizational activities in order to promote women as able physicians and to provide channels for women to lend aid to those in need. This work led to the establishment of the American Women's Hospital Service (AWH) in 1917, which she helped direct. With her organizational skills, fundraising ability, and tireless effort, the AWH was able to work in numerous countries in cooperation with the Red Cross. She also helped found the Medical Women's International Association to help women physicians and also soldiers and victims of war, famine, and epidemics around the world. She wrote a great deal about women in the medical field and their contributions.

Lovejoy died in New York on August 17, 1967.

References: Bass, Elizabeth, "Esther Pohl Lovejoy, MD," *Journal of the American Medical Women's Association* 6, no. 9 (September 1951): 354–355; Burt, Olive Woolley, *Physician to the World: Esther Pohl Lovejoy*, New York: J. Messner (1973); Dodds, G. B., "Lovejoy, Esther Pohl," *Dictionary of Ameri-*

can *Medical Biography,* Westport, CT: Greenwood Press (1984); Lovejoy, Esther Pohl, *Women Doctors of the World,* New York: Macmillan (1957); Perry, Marilyn Elizabeth, "Lovejoy, Esther Pohl," *American National Biography,* vol. 14, New York: Oxford University Press (1999).

Luisi, Paulina
1875–1950

Paulina Luisi was the first female physician of Uruguay. She devoted most of her life to ridding Uruguay of the slave trade in women and children.

Born in 1875, Luisi graduated from the University of Uruguay Medical School in 1908 and became both a teacher and a surgeon. Early on she became involved in the fight against the trade in women and children. She represented her country at the League of Nations, wrote on the importance of hygiene, and was active in the women's rights movement in her country. She died in Montevideo in 1950.

References: "Outstanding Uruguayan Women," http://www.correo.com.uy/filatelia/frames/MujeresDestacadas_ingles.htm; Sapriza, Graciela, "Clivajes de la Memoria: Para una Biografía de Paulina Luisi," in *Uruguayos Notables,* Montevideo: Fundación BankBoston (1999).

Lyon, Mary Frances
1925–

Mary Lyon is a geneticist who proposed the well-known Lyon hypothesis, which states that females have two X chromosomes, one inactivated early in an embryo's life. This hypothesis has led to a better understanding of sex-linked diseases and opened the door to research on numerous genetic issues and hereditary traits.

She was born in Norwich, England, on May 15, 1925, to Louise Frances Kirby Lyon

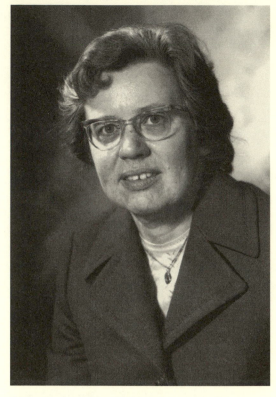

Mary Frances Lyon (Godfrey Argent Studio)

and Clifford James Lyon. She grew up in various locations in England and graduated from Cambridge with a degree in zoology in 1946.

Lyon was fascinated by the emerging field of embryology, an interest that led to her work in genetics. She studied under R. A. Fisher and Conrad H. Waddington in England, receiving both her M.A. and her Ph.D. in 1950. Upon completion of her Ph.D., Waddington offered her a position at the Medical Research Council in the United Kingdom, where she has carried out most of her work and where she formed her Lyon hypothesis.

References: Grinstein, Louise S., Carol A. Biermann, and Rose K. Rose, eds., *Women in the Biological Sciences: A Biobibliographic Sourcebook,* Westport, CT: Greenwood Press (1997); Parry, Melanie, *Chambers Biographical Dictionary,* Edinburgh: Chambers (1997).

M

Mabie, Catharine Louise Roe
1872–1963

Catharine Mabie was an early medical missionary to the Congo. She battled tuberculosis, infections, sleeping sickness, and superstition to become a trusted physician among various tribes.

Born in Rock Island, Illinois, she was determined early on to become a missionary. She frequented Methodist revivals and was baptized in a Baptist church. When she was only ten she ventured out to neighborhoods in Chicago in an effort to reach troubled youth with religion.

She received her medical training and degree at Rush Medical College, where, she felt, most of her professors were not biased about women in class.

> Saturday mornings from 8 to 1:30 all classes were in surgical clinic. At the opening session several men who could not take it were carried out but never one of the girls. We girls were a very small minority and not welcomed by the men students. For the most part our professors were neutral. Our anatomy professor, however, definitely did not like having us in his class and dissecting room. He made a point of trying to make us jittery, asking us to demonstrate difficult complex combinations of muscular action and reaction. One by one he called us into his office for oral examinations. One of mine on the twelve pairs of cranial nerves lasted well over an hour. Luck-

ily I had concentrated on them, both in dissecting them and in Gray's *Anatomy*, so I got off with a good grade. (Mabie 1952, 21)

Upon her graduation, the Woman's Baptist Foreign Missionary Society (WBFMS) appointed her to serve in the Democratic Republic of the Congo (formerly known as the Belgian Congo and later as Zaire) in 1898. She did much of her work at the Banza Manteke Hospital. Mabie was deeply involved in trying to change local attitudes toward illness and healing:

> The Congo knows very little about anatomy, and has no sane notions whatever concerning physiology, hygiene, pathology, or therapeutics. With his animistic notions he attributes all his physical and mental ailments to spirit interference through an intermediary or to direct interposition. In dreams his own spirit wanders apart from the body, and if too rudely awakened may fail to return. To dream of the dead gives rise to great anxiety, and much importance is attached to interpretation of dreams. Whenever serious illness occurs, the person bewitching the patient is sought, and before the white man interfered trial of witches was frequent and usually fatal. Delirium is greatly feared; another spirit than the sufferers is in possession and speaking strange things. Epileptic seizures, insanity, and all mental aberrations are diagnosed as due to direct spirit possession. Witch-

doctors and fetishes were their chief reliance in sickness. (Mabie 1917, 23)

Mabie died in 1963.

References: Anderson, Gerald H., *Biographical Dictionary of Christian Missions*, New York: Macmillan Reference USA (1998); Franklin, James Henry, *Ministers of Mercy*, New York: Missionary Education Movement of the United States and Canada (1919); Hume, Edward Hicks, *Doctors Courageous*, New York: Harper (1950); Mabie, Catharine Louise Roe, *Congo Cameos*, Philadelphia: Judson Press (1952); Mabie, Catharine L., *Our Work on the Congo: A Book for Mission Study Classes and for General Information*, Philadelphia: American Baptist Publication Society (1917), as reproduced in the *History of Women Collection*, no. 7541.1, New Haven, CT: Research Publications (1976).

Macklin, Madge Thurlow
1893–1962

Madge Macklin was a leading genetics researcher of the early twentieth century. She advocated tirelessly for the inclusion of a curriculum that included medical genetics at all medical schools. She also wrote vociferously on eugenics and the repercussions of a decline in the offspring of the intellectually fit. She was a controversial spokesperson for sterilization of the mentally ill.

Born in Philadelphia, Pennsylvania, on February 6, 1893, to Margaret De Grofft and William Harrison Thurlow, she attended Goucher College in Baltimore and received an A.B. degree in 1914. She was briefly an outspoken suffragist before going to Johns Hopkins Medical School and receiving her medical degree in 1919. While in medical school she met Charles Macklin, a Canadian anatomist. They married in 1918.

Both Macklin and her husband went to the University of Western Ontario in London, Canada, in 1921 when Charles was offered a position as head of the Department of History and Embryology. Madge worked for low pay teaching both histology and em-

bryology. Her early publications, some with her husband, concerned anatomy, but by 1926 she had become very interested in medical genetics. She studied heredity in relation to mental retardation and to cancer and other diseases.

She utilized data from a Canadian mental hospital to validate her belief in eugenics and the consequences of persons with mental illness procreating. She wrote several papers on the topic and later became the director of the Eugenics Society of Canada. At the same time, she began advocating medical genetics as a valid part of the curriculum in all medical schools.

Her views were not well received by some, particularly late in the 1930s and the 1940s, as the public became aware of Hitler's attempts to exterminate the mentally ill and create an elite race. Because of her views, she lost her position at the University of Western Ontario in 1945.

In 1946 she obtained a position as a cancer researcher at Ohio State University, the first medical school to have a medical genetics course. Her research there focused on heredity and breast cancer. Her husband remained at the University of Western Ontario, and she commuted back and forth for many years. They had three daughters.

Macklin died in Toronto on March 14, 1962.

References: Rechnitzer, Peter A., "Macklin, Madge Thurlow," *American National Biography*, vol. 14, New York: Oxford University Press (1999); Shearer, Benjamin S., and Barbara S. Shearer, *Notable Women in the Life Sciences*, Westport, CT: Greenwood Press (1996).

Macnamara, Dame Annie Jean
1899–1968

Jean Macnamara was an Australian scientist who did research on polio, helping to discover that there was more than one strain of the polio virus. In an unrelated interest, she was also instrumental in lobbying for use of the controversial virus myxomatosis to control Australia's rabbit population.

Born in Beechworth, Victoria, on April 1, 1899, she gained a medical education from Melbourne University, graduating in 1922 and becoming one of the first female residents at Melbourne Hospital. Several Melbourne hospitals had for years refused to take on women, blaming their lack of toilets; Melbourne Hospital installed toilets.

Jean encountered many polio victims and worked to alleviate the crippling effects of infantile paralysis with traditional methods that sometimes were at odds with the experimental treatments of Elizabeth Kenny. In the poliomyelitis epidemic of 1925 she introduced a serum with limited success. She then traveled to the United States and Canada to do further research. Back in Australia she worked with Sir Macfarlane Burnet, and together they discovered there was more than one strain of the polio virus. This discovery would eventually help in the development of the Salk vaccine. She also is responsible for introducing the first artificial respirator in Australia.

She married Ivan Connor, a dermatologist, in 1934, and they had two daughters, Joan and Merran. She traveled throughout Europe, the United States, Australia, New Zealand, and Canada to speak about myxomatosis to control rabbits and also about polio treatments. She passed away on October 13, 1968.

See also: Kenny, Elizabeth

References: Crystal, David, *The Cambridge Biographical Encyclopedia,* Cambridge: Cambridge University Press (1998); Muir, Hazel, *Larousse Dictionary of Scientists,* Edinburgh: Larousse (1994); Sherratt, Tim, "No Standing Back: Dame Jean Macnamara," *Australasian Science* 13, no. 4 (Summer 1993): 64; Zwar, Desmond, *The Dame: The Life and Times of Dame Jean Macnamara, Medical Pioneer,* South Melbourne: Macmillan (1984).

Mahoney, Mary Eliza
1845–1926

Mary Mahoney was the first black professional nurse in the United States. She was a leader in nursing and was instrumental in organizing black nurses and pursuing equal opportunities for black women interested in nursing as a profession. She was central to the success of the National Association of Colored Graduate Nurses (NACGN).

Born in Dorchester, Massachusetts, on May 7, 1845, she was the daughter of Charles Mahoney and Mary Jane Stewart Mahoney. She had one brother, Frank, and two sisters, Ellen and Louise. Louise died at an early age.

For a time she attended the Phillips Street School in Boston. She worked for several families as a private nurse before she entered the School of Nursing at the New England Hospital for Women and Children. She did well and received her diploma on August 1, 1879. Linda Richards had received her diploma in 1873, becoming the first professional nurse in the United States.

Like most black nurses of her era, Mahoney entered private-duty nursing because most hospitals would not hire black nurses. She realized early on that black nurses must organize in order to have a voice in nursing affairs. She was able to become a member of the Nurses Associated Alumnae (later the American Nurses Association); however, she realized many other blacks could not become members because a requirement for joining that organization was membership in their state nursing associations, which were often closed to blacks.

She was a gifted speaker, welcoming all to the first convention of the NACGN in 1908, and a good organizer. She remained active in the NACGN all her life. In 1911 she became the supervisor at the Howard Orphan Asylum for Black Children, located on Long Island in Kings Park. She worked until 1922, when she retired.

Mahoney never married. She died of progressive breast cancer on January 4, 1926. She was buried at Woodlawn Cemetery in Everett, Massachusetts. Her grave was uncovered and restored during a ceremony on August 15, 1973, and a monument was placed at the gravesite. She was inducted into the Nursing Hall of Fame in 1976, and an award is still given in her name to honor nurses who have made significant contributions to the field.

See also: Richards, Linda

References: Davis, Althea T., *Early Black American Leaders in Nursing: Architects for Integration and Equality*, Boston: Jones and Bartlett (1999); Hine, Darlene Clark, *Black Women in America: An Historical Encyclopedia*, Brooklyn, NY: Carlson (1993); Miller, Helen S., *Mary Eliza Mahoney, 1845–1926: America's First Black Professional Nurse*, Atlanta: Wright (1986).

Malahlele, Mary Susan

Mary Malahlele of the Bapedi Nation was the first female native South African physician. She received her degree at the University of the Witwatersrand in 1947 with an interest in African children's diseases and worked for McCord Hospital in Durban.

References: Hume, Edward Hicks, *Doctors Courageous*, New York: Harper (1950); Lovejoy, Esther Pohl, *Women Doctors of the World*, New York: Macmillan (1957).

Mandl, Ines
1917–

Ines Mandl was an early biochemist. Her understanding of chemistry and its application to biomedical problems helped advance knowledge in the areas of enzymes and pulmonary emphysema.

Born on April 19, 1917, in Vienna, Austria, she was the daughter of Ernst Mandl and Ida Bassan Hochmuth. She attended both state-supported schools and a private school and then, as was customary, married.

In 1938 she and her family moved to England because the National Socialists were on the rise in Austria. When World War II broke out, they moved to Ireland. Ines went to the National University of Ireland in Cork and graduated with a degree in chemistry, specializing in biochemistry. She then followed her parents to the United States and later met a fellow Jew, Carl Neuberg, who was doing research in the new field of biochemistry. She joined him at New York University doing research and, with his encouragement, enrolled at the Polytechnic Institute of Brooklyn. There, she earned a master's in science and in 1949 became the first woman to earn a doctorate at that institution.

She published with Neuberg on research with fructose and sugar derivatives and continued to stay in touch with him after she went to work at Columbia University. She joined Delafield Hospital as director of the obstetrics and gynecology labs and began focusing on human tissue and the enzymes involved in its breakdown, as well as the enzymes that are present in tumors found in the reproductive system.

She later studied the effects of tobacco on the lungs and found that smoke damaged elastin and thus led to the deterioration of lung tissue. She was known worldwide as a pioneer in applying chemistry to many biomedical problems. She received the Garvan Medal in 1982.

References: Shearer, Benjamin F., and Barbara S. Shearer, *Notable Women in the Physical Sciences*, Westport, CT: Greenwood Press (1997).

Manley, Audrey Forbes
1934–

A physician and college president, Audrey Manley has been a leading black medical administrator. She served as the acting surgeon general in 1995.

Born on March 25, 1934, in Jackson, Mississippi, she obtained her bachelor's degree from Spelman College in Atlanta in 1955 and continued on toward her medical degree at Meharry Medical College. She completed her residency at Cook County Children's Hospital in Chicago. She became the first African American woman to become chief resident of that hospital.

Manley also sought neonatology training at the University of Illinois Abraham Lincoln School of Medicine. She also earned a degree in public health from Johns Hopkins University. She has been a professor at several medical schools, but her chief contributions have been in the field of public health.

She rose to become the deputy assistant secretary for health within the U.S. Department of Health and Human Services.

Manley has encouraged women and minorities to go into education and careers in the sciences. She is currently the president of Spelman College.

References: Manley, Albert E., *A Legacy Continues: The Manley Years at Spelman College, 1953–1976*, Lanham, MD: University Press of America (1995); "Manley, Audrey Forbes," *Who's Who of American Women*, 22d ed., New Providence, NJ: Marquis Who's Who (2000).

McClintock, Barbara
1902–1992

Barbara McClintock received the 1983 Nobel Prize in physiology or medicine for discovering that genes could move from one place to another on plants, thus changing future generations. Although researchers had long believed the "jumping genes" theory, there was no hard evidence of the phenomenon until McClintock proved it to be true.

Born in Hartford, Connecticut, on June 16, 1902, McClintock was the third of three daughters of Sara Handy and Dr. Thomas Henry McClintock. She always had a distant relationship with her mother, who had wanted a boy when Barbara was born and, with the son born after Barbara, had four small children to raise. When Barbara was young, her mother sent her to spend a lot of time with an aunt and uncle in rural Massachusetts, where she enjoyed collecting insects and studying them, fixing machinery, and going about with her uncle, who sold fish. Her father raised his daughters no differently than he did his son. Both parents supported Barbara's activities even when they differed from the norm. She was an independent child who spent a lot of time outdoors and alone.

Barbara did well in school and loved science and math at Erasmus Hall High School in Brooklyn, New York. When she was ready for college, she told her mother she wanted to go to Cornell. Her father was away in the Army Medical Corps, and her mother refused. When her father returned, he allowed her to enroll in Cornell's College of Agriculture. She graduated in 1923 after having already done graduate work and stayed on at Cornell to earn an M.S. in 1925 and a Ph.D. in 1927. She majored in cytology and minored in genetics and zoology.

Barbara's mother was worried she would never marry and become a professor instead. McClintock felt marriage would be a mistake because she was such a dominant person, and she never wed.

McClintock worked long hours while at Cornell and later at the University of Missouri. Before she obtained her Ph.D., she "developed a method of studying individual chromosomes of Indian corn (maize) under a microscope. This discovery allowed concurrent study of the chromosomes and the physical traits of maize" (Shampo and Kyle 1995, 448). McClintock published on the genetics of corn in the late 1920s and early 1930s.

While at the University of Missouri she discovered that after X rays break chromosomes, the chromosomes repair themselves, sometimes fusing together in rings. This discovery came well before the study of DNA in the 1950s, at which time some scientists were observing the damage-and-repair process and others still believed that chromosomes were stable. McClintock received a Guggenheim Fellowship and used it to visit Germany in 1933. She was so distressed to find the scientific community in disarray as a result of Hitler's ridding the universities of the Jews that she immediately returned to Cornell. With the depression on, she was able to secure two years at Cornell only with the help of the Rockefeller Foundation.

Unable to obtain a full-time faculty position at Cornell because of her gender, she took a faculty position, her first, at the University of Missouri in 1936. She was unconventional (she did not wear dresses, did not work well in organized settings, and did not like to teach as well as she liked doing research), and did not last long there. In 1942, she obtained a position with the Carnegie Foundation working at Cold Spring Harbor, an environment that suited her temperament and her work ethic. She stayed there over forty years.

It was at Cold Spring Harbor that she made the discovery of "jumping genes," or transposable elements. She announced her finding in 1951 and later published her research, but the scientific community was skeptical and she got little notice. She continued working on other projects, and in 1983, she won the Nobel Prize for her work thirty years prior.

Part of the reason for the delayed recognition was that the Nobel Prize was not given for botany research until it was clear the work had significance for human well-being. "The discovery of transposable genetic systems and genetic regulation anticipated the findings of bacterial geneticists by 15 years and explained how the resistance to antibiotic drugs can be passed from one type of bacteria to another through 'jumping genes'" (Shampo and Kyle 1995, 148).

Her "ideas, like her discoveries, truly span the century of genetics. Some were timely and quickly recognized. Others were well ahead of their time, but eventually caught on. Some still pull us into the future" (Fedoroff 1992, 3). Barbara McClintock died on September 2, 1992.

References: Comfort, Nathaniel C., *The Tangled Field: Barbara McClintock's Search for the Patterns of Genetic Control*, Cambridge, MA: Harvard University Press (2001); Fedoroff, Nina, and David Botstein, eds., *The Dynamic Genome: Barbara McClintock's Ideas in the Century of Genetics*, Cold Spring Harbor, NY: Cold Spring Harbor Laboratory Press (1992); Keller, Evelyn Fox, *A Feeling for the Organism: The Life and Work of Barbara McClintock*, San Francisco: W. H. Freeman (1983); McGrayne, Sharon Bertsch, *Nobel Prize Women in Science*, Secaucus, NJ: Carol (1998); Shampo, Marc A., and Robert A. Kyle, "Barbara McClintock—Nobel Laureate Geneticist," *Mayo Clinic Proceedings* 70, no. 5 (1995): 448; Van der Does, Louise Q., and Rita J. Simon, *Renaissance Women in Science*, Lanham, MD: University Press of America (1999).

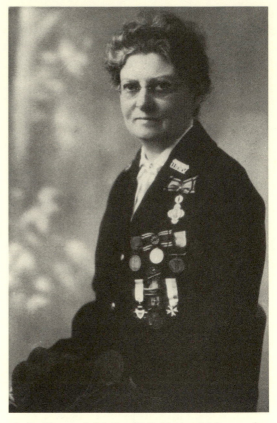

Anita Newcomb McGee (U.S. National Library of Medicine)

McGee, Anita Newcomb
1864–1940

Anita McGee was the founder of the U.S. Army Nurse Corps. She heightened public awareness of the importance of an organized nursing unit for the military.

Born in Washington, D.C., on November 4, 1864, McGee was the daughter of Caroline Hassler and Simon Newcomb. Her father served as an astronomer at the Naval Observatory. She received her early education, along with two sisters, at private schools and with tutors. She spent some time in Europe with her mother and studied various subjects, including languages and art. She took some classes at the University of Geneva and also Cambridge University.

She did a great deal of research on her forebears and became one of the early members of the Daughters of the American Revolution (DAR). She also wrote articles for an encyclopedia, was active in politics, and had an interest in science. In 1888 she married William John McGee; they had three children. She decided to attend medical school the year after her marriage and enrolled at Columbian College (now called George Washington University).

During her last year, the college decided to refuse admittance to future female applicants. She fought this decision but to no avail; women were not admitted after she graduated. She went on to intern at the Washington, D.C., Women's Clinic and later opened a private practice. Following the death of her son in 1895, she joined the staff of the Women's Dispensary.

War with Spain seemed inevitable in 1898, and McGee used her influence to persuade the army to allow the DAR to assist in placing trained nurses in the military and setting criteria for nurses' qualifications. However, her work with organizing nurses put her in a negative light with the Red Cross, which felt slighted when it was not selected to be in charge of military nurses.

McGee was instrumental following the war in drafting legislation to form the Nurse Corps as a part of the Army Medical Corps. She was determined to see nurses as part of both the Army Medical Corps and the reserves. "In addition to this permanent force, definite provision should be made for war reserves. The Army and National Guard will supply corps men for the arduous field service, but they cannot maintain a large enough corps to fill the needs of war emergency, with its large Army and large percentage of sick, and neither can they turn recruits into competent nurses in a few weeks" (McGee 1977, 6).

She was active in the Russo-Japanese War, training nurses and inspecting hospitals overseas. She believed that nurses deserved a higher professional status and that the military deserved nurses as well qualified as those who served civilians.

Her husband died in 1912, and she spent time with her children and lecturing on various health topics. She died on October 5, 1940, and was buried with honors at Arlington National Cemetery.

References: McGee, Anita Newcomb, *The Nurse Corps of the Army,* Carlisle, PA: Association of Military Surgeons (1902), reprinted in *History of Women Collection,* no. 10001, New Haven, CT: Research Publications (1977); Reeves, Connie L., "McGee, Anita Newcomb," *American National Biography,* vol. 15, New York: Oxford University Press (1999).

McKinnon, Emily H. S.
1873–1968

Emily McKinnon was the first female to become a physician in New Zealand. She graduated from the University of Otago in 1896. More information on her life is at the Alexander Turnbull Library in Wellington.

References: Lovejoy, Esther Pohl, *Women Doctors of the World,* New York: Macmillan (1957).

Medical Act of 1858

The British Parliament passed the Medical Act of 1858 to restrict the medical profession to those who were perceived to be qualified. The law excluded women from British medical schools. The act was overturned by the Russell Gurney Enabling Act of 1876, which gave women the same rights as men to enter medical schools and earn their M.D. degrees.

See also: Jex-Blake, Sophia Louisa; Russell Gurney Enabling Act of 1876
References: Waddington, Ivan, *The Medical Profession in the Industrial Revolution,* Dublin: Gill and Macmillan (1984).

Medical College of Pennsylvania
1850–

The Medical College of Pennsylvania was originally founded by Quakers in Philadelphia in 1850 as the Female Medical College of Pennsylvania. In 1867, it became known as the Women's Medical College of Pennsyl-

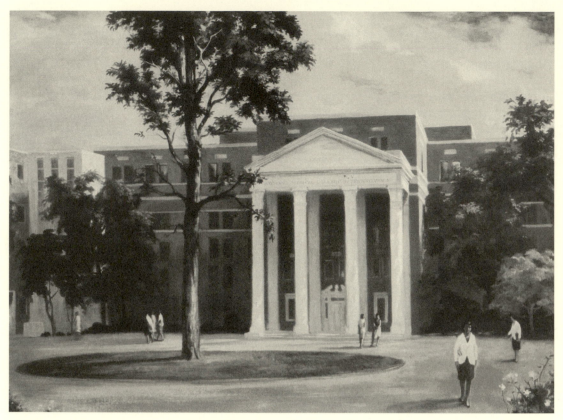

Medical College of Pennsylvania (Lucius Crowell/U.S. National Library of Medicine)

vania. In 1969, it became coeducational. During the 1920s and 1930s it was the only medical college for women that survived. Struggling financially at times, it stayed a course that would ensure a permanent place in Philadelphia history and in the history of women in medicine around the world.

References: Peitzman, Steven J., *A New and Untried Course: Women's Medical College and Medical College of Pennsylvania, 1850–1998*, New Brunswick, NJ: Rutgers University Press (2000).

Medical Women's International Association (MWIA)
1919–

The Medical Women's International Association, created by members of the American Medical Women's Association and their foreign guests in October 1919, was the first organization to unify women physicians worldwide. The Medical Women's Federation of Great Britain was the only other large association in existence at the time; it was organized in 1917.

The association grew out of a recognized need for international cooperation on health care and medical education for women. Women health care workers had been overwhelmed during World War I by the conditions in some countries, especially regarding the health of women and children and general nutrition. The war opened the world's eyes to the needs of the underdeveloped countries.

Today the MWIA has over 20,000 members in seventy countries. The majority of members are from affiliated national associations; a small number of members are individual women who come from countries that do not have a national association.

They continue to strive for equal opportunities in medical education for women, to disseminate information on various health issues, and to attempt to overcome gender discrimination in the medical field.

The MWIA has maintained an affiliation with the World Health Organization (WHO) since 1954 and has recently collaborated with WHO on women's health, AIDS, and immunization. It has also worked with UNESCO and other national and international agencies in providing information on various health care issues. MWIA's home office is in Dortmund, Germany.

References: Lovejoy, Esther Pohl, *Women Physicians and Surgeons: National and International Organizations,* Livingston, NY: Livingston Press (1939), http://www.who.int/ina-ngo/ngo/ngo143.htm.

Mendenhall, Dorothy Reed
1874–1964

Dorothy Mendenhall was a physician who helped discover the cells important for the diagnosis of Hodgkin's disease. Both she, an American, and Carl Sternberg, from Austria, gave the most thorough descriptions of the cells (Sternberg in 1898 and Mendenhall in 1902), now called Reed-Sternberg cells.

Mendenhall was born on September 22, 1874, in Columbus, Ohio. Her parents were William Pratt Reed and Grace Kimball. The family had a certain amount of financial security even though her father, a shoe manufacturer, passed away when she was a child. She was able to obtain a good education at home.

She went to Smith College in Northampton, Massachusetts, in 1891. She became interested in biology and discovered that a medical career was possible through Johns Hopkins. She obtained her degree from Smith and then went to the Massachusetts Institute of Technology to better her understanding of chemistry. She also began a correspondence with Dr. William Welch of Johns Hopkins and later enrolled. One of her classmates was Florence Sabin. "The study of medicine itself and its many nu-

ances satisfied her need to be challenged mentally that went all the way back to the days when she had been tutored by Anna Gunning. It incorporated her love of biology that she had discovered at Smith and allowed her to escape from the social pressures placed on her while she was at home" (Halamay 2000, 54).

Her mother had not managed the finances of the family well enough to support her well in college, and she became more interested in a career. After her sojourn at Johns Hopkins, where she discovered the Reed-Sternberg cells, she worked for four years at Babies Hospital in New York under Dr. Emmett Holt.

She married Charles Elwood Mendenhall in 1906, and they had four children. The first died in childbirth, and this tragedy affected Mendenhall for the rest of her life. She blamed the death on poor obstetrical care and afterward worked on exploring the problems of infant mortality and the importance of nutrition. She became an active public health physician, working for the U.S. Department of Agriculture, the Children's Bureau, and the Wisconsin State Board of Health.

Mendenhall was a rarity in her time. For the most part, a woman either had a career or had a husband and children. "Dorothy Reed Mendenhall represented a third type that is not present in the usual depiction of early twentieth century women. She was a professional woman who married and had children, *and* who managed to pursue a career after her marriage. A study of her life allows us to see that some women did exist during the late nineteenth and early twentieth centuries who, even in the face of vehement opposition, used innovation and ingenuity to carve out new lives and, in so doing, found fulfillment" (Halamay 2000, 137).

Mendenhall published several reports about children's health and childbirth issues and remained active until her retirement. She died in Chester, Connecticut, on July 31, 1964.

References: Halamay, Kate Elizabeth, "'I Like Everything about Medicine, Except . . .': Dorothy Reed Mendenhall and the

Issues Confronting Women Physicians in the Early Twentieth Century," Ph.D. dissertation, Smith College (2000); Mauch, Peter M., et al., *Hodgkin's Disease*, Philadelphia: Lippincott, Williams, and Wilkins (1999); Morantz-Sanchez, Regina, "Mendenhall, Dorothy Reed," *American National Biography*, vol. 15, New York: Oxford University Press (1999).

Mendoza-Gauzon, Marie Paz
18?–19?

Marie Mendoza-Gauzon was the first female physician of the Philippines. She graduated from the College of Medicine at the University of the Philippines in 1912 and married Dr. P. Gauzon, who was head of Philippine General Hospital's Department of Surgery. She served as a professor of pathology at the university.

References: Lovejoy, Esther Pohl, *Women Doctors of the World*, New York: Macmillan (1957).

Mergler, Marie Josepha
1851–1901

Marie Mergler was an early gynecological surgeon who became dean of the Women's Medical College of Chicago in 1899. Her example and teaching influenced a number of women pursuing medical careers in the late nineteenth century. She was well-known and respected among the male physicians of her day. She was born in Mainstockheim, Bavaria. Her family moved to Illinois when she was a child. Her mother was Henrietta von Ritterhausen and her father, a physician, was Francis R. Mergler.

She gained an education from her father during her childhood and eventually helped him in his medical work. She trained for a teaching career, however, because of the numerous obstacles facing women who wanted a medical career. She taught high school for a time before deciding to enter the Women's Medical College of Chicago in 1877. She graduated with honors and was allowed to

compete with men for a position at the Cook County Insane Asylum. She did well, but the hospital board prevented her from taking the position. She then chose to do postgraduate work in Zurich, Switzerland.

She later became an assistant in Chicago to William H. Byford, a gynecologist. The following year she gained a position at the Women's Medical College and gradually rose to become its dean. She also worked at Cook County Hospital, the Women's Hospital of Chicago, Wesley Hospital, and the Chicago Hospital for Women and Children. Mergler died in Los Angeles, California, on May 17, 1901.

References: Fine, Eva, "Mergler, Marie Josepha," *American National Biography*, vol. 15, New York: Oxford University Press (1999); Southgate, M. Therese, "Women in Medicine II," in John Walton, Paul B. Beeson, and Ronald Bodley Scott, eds., *The Oxford Companion to Medicine*, Oxford: Oxford University Press (1986).

Miller, Jean Baker
1927–

A pioneering psychiatrist, Jean Miller broke new ground in understanding women and their psychological needs with the publication in 1976 of *Toward a New Psychology of Women*. She continues her work today at the Jean Baker Miller Institute at Wellesley College in Wellesley, Massachusetts.

She was born in New York City on September 29, 1927. She graduated from Sarah Lawrence College in Bronxville, New York, in 1948 with a B.A. and then went to Columbia University, where she obtained her M.D. in 1952. She was an intern and later a resident at Montefiore Hospital and then studied and was a resident in psychiatry at Bellevue Medical Center. Miller expressed some of the feelings that prompted her to write her first book:

Well, for years I was practicing psychotherapy, and also teaching psychiatry, and it seemed to me that something was fundamentally wrong with the formulations about women, which were based upon traditional psychoanalytic theories. I thought that they were wrong, but I didn't have a framework for an alternate way of thinking. Also, in addition to thinking that these formulations were wrong, I always felt that the women whom I was seeing in my practice had a lot of strengths. These capabilities, such as making relationships and knowing how to do that, or helping the whole family survive and flourish a little, were extraordinarily valuable. However, in our culture, the women themselves could never really perceive them as being strengths, and so these strengths did not help them anywhere near as much as they should. (Welch 1995, 336–337)

Toward a New Psychology of Women reexamined women's roles as workers, mothers, and wives, as well as women's strengths. She says that these strengths derive in part from women's subservient roles throughout history and that they can be used toward becoming proactive participants rather than passive victims. Her book "has had a profound impact on the development of psychological theory and practice concerning gender roles. The book has helped to deconstruct and reconstruct the questions and methods of psychological research and has played a major role in the development of new psychology, not only of women but of human behavior generally" (Antler 1988, 63).

Miller has been a professor or lecturer at many institutions with long stays at the Upstate Medical Center at the State University of New York, Albert Einstein College of Medicine, Harvard Medical School, Wellesley College, and Boston University School of Medicine. Miller currently is the director of the Jean Baker Miller Training Institute in Wellesley, Massachusetts, and clinical professor of psychiatry at Boston University School of Medicine. She is married and has two children. She has continued her writing and has emphasized that "studying women's lives offers us a crucial key to thinking about societal transformation—and that this transformation is essential" (Miller and Stiver 1997, 62).

References: Antler, Joyce, "Book Review: *Toward a New Psychology of Women*," *Social Policy* 18, no. 3 (Winter 1988): 63–64; Bowman, John S., *The Cambridge Dictionary of American Biography*, Cambridge, MA: Cambridge University Press (1995); Kester-Shelton, Pamela, ed., *Feminist Writers*, Detroit: St. James Press (1996); Miller, Jean Baker, *Toward a New Psychology of Women*, Boston: Beacon Press (1976); Miller, Jean Baker, and Irene Pierce Stiver, *The Healing Connection: How Women Form Relationships in Therapy and in Life*, Boston: Beacon Press (1997); Welch, Amy S., "Learning from Women," *Women and Therapy* 17, nos. 3–4 (1995): 335–346.

Minoka-Hill, Lillie Rosa
1876–1952

Lillie Minoka-Hill was the second Native American woman to become a physician. She served the Oneida community in Wisconsin for many years.

She was born August 30, 1876, on the St. Regis Reservation in New York. Her mother was a Mohawk and her father was Joshua Allen, a physician. She received an education at Grahame Institute in Philadelphia before attending the Women's Medical College of Pennsylvania, obtaining her medical degree in 1899. She interned at the Women's Hospital in Philadelphia and then had a private practice.

She married Charles Abram Hill in 1905 and had six children. They moved to Oneida, Wisconsin, where Minoka-Hill maintained an informal practice for many decades. After the death of her husband in 1916, she had to work harder as a physician, attending to friends, relatives, and neighbors and taking whatever they could afford to pay. In 1934 she took the state medical exam and passed it, allowing her to receive government reimbursement for some of her desperately needed services.

Minoka-Hill had a great deal of respect for traditional Indian medicinal cures but also used Western medications and health care practices to further the welfare of the people she served. She passed away on March 18, 1952, in Fond du Lac, Wisconsin.

References: Apple, R. D., "Minoka-Hill, Lillie Rosa," *Dictionary of American Medical Biography,* Westport, CT: Greenwood Press (1984); Perry, Marilyn Elizabeth, "Minoka-Hill, Lillie Rosa," *American National Biography*, vol. 15, New York: Oxford University Press (1999); Thomas, David Hurst, Betty Ballantine, and Ian Ballantine, *The Native Americans: An Illustrated History*, Atlanta: Turner (1993).

Mission Work

Church missions provided women in the medical field with another professional opportunity. As the twentieth century approached, there were still few professions open to women. Nursing and teaching were the most common, with physician work a possibility for a small number of women who had the tenacity to gain admission to a medical school and the endurance to graduate and become licensed. The women's movement fueled the fight late in the nineteenth century, and the various religions proved a good ally because they were beginning to see the need for female medical missionaries about the same time. Thus there was finally another route for women to take if they had a medical degree but could not find employment. This opportunity also convinced some schools that educating women in the medical field had real merit.

Church leaders had early on perceived the need to spread Christianity to foreign lands. By the 1800s, the push was coming from Europe and the United States. In the 1880s the American Medical Missionary Society (AMMS) published a pamphlet, *A Great Field for Women*, in which the society urged women to become medical missionaries. Realizing that some cultures forbade women to seek out male physicians for advice, they turned to women for help. "These millions of women cannot be reached by male missionaries. The doors are shut and locked against such. Nor can Christian women, ordinarily, gain entrance to them. But the female Medical Missionary is able to do it, for her professional acquisition is a key. She can unlock the doors and secure for herself a welcome" (AMMS 1977).

Mission work had gone on for centuries in large part due to the Catholic Church. At the close of the eighteenth century, however, Catholic missions were somewhat at a standstill for various reasons. In the sixteenth through the eighteenth centuries, there was some movement on the part of Protestants as well. "Zealous Protestant missionaries, fueled by the Pietist movement of continental Europe and the evangelical awakenings in England and North America, had established pockets of believers in the coastlands of Asia, India, Africa, and the Middle East. These areas already were occupied by significant communities of Roman and Orthodox Catholics" (Terry, Smith, and Anderson 1998, 199).

In Canton, China, Protestant medical missionary work was well under way before 1850. The Canton Hospital, which opened in 1835, was China's first Western medical establishment. By 1879 local Cantonese women were taking classes at the nearby Canton Medical Missionary Hospital. The goals of the missions were varied, but in Canton the church was open to educating the local females in medical care as well as having able female physicians treat native females.

When a rift between two of the head physicians split loyalties there in 1899, the women were left out. This prompted Mary Fulton to work to establish an educational setting for the local women. In 1902 it took the name Hackett Medical College due to a donation from Mr. E.A.K. Hackett of Indiana.

In Persia the Church Missionary Society of the Church of England realized early on that offering medical treatment was the best means of establishing a relationship with Iranian women. "During the period between 1891 and 1934 many women worked as missionary nurses and doctors in Iran" (Ward and Stanley 2000, 97). The fact that Iranian women could not consult males for medical treatment gave early impetus to promoting medical education for women. "Female workers were necessary in order to gain easier access to Iranian women who lived largely in seclusion. As the number of women missionaries began to increase, the tasks they carried out were divided into three distinct categories: education, medicine, and evangelism" (Ward and Stanley 2000, 96). Physician Emmeline Stuart arrived in 1897 and very effectively oversaw the female medical staff in Persia, where the society opened hospitals and set some standards for the future.

Ida Scudder made enormous headway in India when she opened a school for nursing in 1909 in Vellore in southern India; the Vellore Medical College followed in 1918. Both were extremely successful at training Indian women to become nurses and physicians. Missionaries like Scudder who found themselves in rural areas and had to work with local governments to get things done had to be accomplished in diplomacy as well as health care. In 1950 the Vellore Medical College began accepting male students and became affiliated with Madras University.

In Egypt, Mary Louisa Whately established a medical mission after establishing two schools for Muslim children. In Africa, David Livingstone's explorations of the continent and medical missionary work greatly aided all missionaries. The large growth in African missions was due in large part to the desire of African Americans recently freed during the American Civil War to reach out to their ancestors in Africa. Another factor that helped within the mission community as a whole was the formation of several women's missionary groups. Before they became active, most church donations for evangelical work in foreign fields were designated for preaching. Pastors' wives worked in health care, but few single women had substantial support. "Before the formation of these women's organizations, mission funds had been collected by ministers and other church leaders, most of whom emphasized parish work or home missions to the Indians or freedmen. What money was spent on foreign missions was under the control of exclusively male foreign mission boards that were uniformly uneasy about the radical new idea of sending independent, unmarried women out into the mission field" (Tucker 1990, 363).

Hospitals grew in number in India, China, Africa, Japan, and the Middle East as the nineteenth century unfolded. At the beginning of the twentieth century, the missionary movement was well aware of the growing need for women with physician credentials. Many women left their own countries to serve as medical missionaries; others stayed home to serve the underserved populations in the countries where they lived.

See also: Fulton, Mary Hannah; Guangzhou, China; Scudder, Ida Sophia; Whately, Mary Louisa

References: American Medical Missionary Society (AMMS), *A Great Field for Women*, Chicago: American Medical Missionary Society (1880?), reprinted in *History of Women*, reel 939, no. 8277, Woodbridge, CT: Research Publications (1977); Drake, Fred W., *Ruth V. Hemenway, MD: A Memoir of Revolutionary China, 1924–1941*, Amherst: University of Massachusetts Press (1977); Fleming, Leslie A., *Women's Work for Women: Missionaries and Social Change in Asia*, Boulder, CO: Westview Press (1989); Jeffrey, Mary Pauline, *Dr. Ida: India; The Life Story of Ida S. Scudder*, New York: Fleming H. Revell (1938); Jordan, Louis Garnett, *Up the Ladder in Foreign Missions*, Nashville, TN: National Baptist Publishing Board (1903); Laurie, Rev. Thomas, *Women and the Gospel in Persia*, New York: Fleming H. Revell (1887); Rubinstein, Murray A., *The Origins of the Anglo-American Missionary Enterprise in China, 1807–1840*, Lanham, MD: Scarecrow Press (1996); Terry, John Mark, Ebbie Smith, and Justice Anderson, *Missiology: An Introduction to the Foundations, History, and Strategies of World Missions*, Nashville, TN: Broadman and Holman (1998); Tucker, Sara W., "Opportunities for Women: The Development of Professional Women's Medicine at Canton, China, 1879–1901," *Women's Studies International Forum* 13, no. 4 (1990): 357–368; Ward, Kevin, and Brian Stanley, *The Church Mission Society and World Christianity, 1799–1999*, Grand Rapids, MI: William B. Eerdmans (2000); Whately, Elizabeth Jane, *The Life and Work of Mary Louisa Whately*, London: Religious Tract Society (1890).

Montoya, Matilde

Matilde Montoya was the first female physician of Mexico. She graduated from the University of Mexico in 1887.

References: Lovejoy, Esther Pohl, *Women Doctors of the World*, New York: Macmillan (1957).

Morani, Alma Dea
1907–2001

Alma Morani was the first female plastic surgeon in the United States. She had to fight to go to medical school and to be able to practice surgery. She began early in her career to speak up for women in medicine.

Born in New York City, she attended New York University and later the Women's Medical College of Pennsylvania, earning her M.D. in 1931. She interned in Newark, New Jersey, at St. James Hospital, followed by a residency in surgery at Women's Medical Hospital in Philadelphia. She served at Roxborough Memorial Hospital in Philadelphia for over forty years and was a professor at the Medical College of Pennsylvania for fifty years.

Morani had a desire early on "to take up

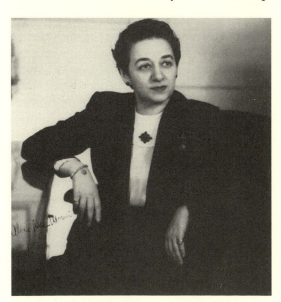

Alma Dea Morani (U.S. National Library of Medicine)

plastic surgery—against tremendous odds. 'What I wanted to be doing was the surgery of repair, not the surgery of despair'" ("Profile" 1983, 137). Morani died on January 27, 2001.

References: Morani, A. D., "Reflections," *Clinics in Plastic Surgery* 10, no. 4 (October 1983): 669–670; "Profile: Alma Dea Morani, MD," *Journal of the American Medical Women's Association* 38, no. 5 (September–October 1983): 137; *Who's Who in America, 1990–1991*, 46th ed., Wilmette, IL: Marquis Who's Who (1990).

Murray, Flora

Flora Murray was a British physician and surgeon charged with the first British military unit of medical women during World War I. She established, with the help of Dr. Louisa Garrett Anderson, daughter of Dr. Elizabeth Garrett Anderson, the Women's Hospital Corps in Paris to prepare for the wounded of World War I.

Born in England, she worked at the hospital on Endell Street in Paris, where she and the other women physicians carried a heavy workload: "The surgeons spent all their mornings in the wards, and most of their afternoons in the operating theatre, where it was not unusual to have a list of twenty or thirty cases on each operating day" (Murray 1920, 162).

She and the other women treated soldiers from many countries. "Racial characteristics were very evident. The English were slow and phlegmatic, satisfied with theaters, billiards and the football news. The Scots were friends with the librarian and always pushing to get well enough to see London. The Irish brought grace and charm into the ward" (Murray 1920, 149).

See also: Anderson, Elizabeth Garrett
References: Murray, Flora, *Women as Army Surgeons: Being the History of the Women's Hospital Corps in Paris, Wimereux and Endell Street, September 1914–October 1919*, London: Hodder and Stoughton (1920).

N

Neufeld, Elizabeth Fondal
1928–

An authority on genetic diseases, Elizabeth Neufeld became the first female to head a department at UCLA's School of Medicine. Her major contributions have been in research on inherited disorders such as Hurler and Sanfilippo syndromes.

She was born in Paris, France, on September 27, 1928, to Jacques and Elvira Fondal, Russian refugees. The family moved to New York while she was still a child, and she attended a New York high school before going on to Queens College and obtaining a B.S. degree in 1948. She later worked in Bar Harbor, Maine, at the Jackson Memorial Laboratory and decided on graduate study at the University of Rochester.

She later moved to Baltimore and briefly worked at the McCollum-Pratt Institute of Johns Hopkins University before entering the University of California, Berkeley, to study for her Ph.D. in 1952. She received her doctorate in comparative biochemistry in 1956.

She worked as a biochemist for the National Institute of Arthritis and Metabolic Diseases in Bethesda, Maryland, from 1963 to 1973. It is associated with the National Institutes of Health (NIH). She worked in various other positions at NIH, focusing on research in genetic diseases. Her work involved the study of arthritis, metabolism, diabetes, and kidney diseases as well as rare disorders such as Hurler syndrome, Sanfilippo syndrome, and other mucopolysaccharide (MPS) disorders.

In 1994 Neufeld received the National Medal of Science. Currently she is chair of the Biological Chemistry Department at UCLA's School of Medicine. She married in 1951 and has two children. Her research on rare diseases has prompted others in the medical community to find cures for MPS disorders. She continues to teach and do research.

References: *American Men and Women of Science,* 20th ed., vol. 5, New York: Bowker (1998); Grinstein, Louise S., Carol A. Biermann, and Rose K. Rose, *Women in the Biological Sciences: A Biobibliographic Sourcebook,* Westport, CT: Greenwood Press (1997); Shearer, Benjamin F., and Barbara S. Shearer, *Notable Women in the Life Sciences,* Westport, CT: Greenwood Press (1996).

New England Female Medical College
1848–1874

The New England Female Medical College was founded in Boston in 1848 by Samuel Gregory, who initiated the effort to provide this educational institute for women because he believed that male midwives and physicians were offensive to women in labor.

Because Gregory had limited funds, he began by organizing a class with two male physicians teaching twelve women. Most of these women were preparing to become midwives. Because of initial difficulties regarding the new institution's charter, for a time the college collaborated with faculty from the Female Medical College of Pennsylvania.

By 1852 the college offered women a full course of studies and a medical degree and was officially recognized as the New England Female Medical College. The first female professor was Hannah Longshore. In 1859, Marie Zakrzewska came from New York to plan and run a hospital and serve as professor of obstetrics and diseases of women and children.

The first hospital operated only a few years. On July 1, 1862, with a permanent location found for the hospital, Zakrzewska became the attending physician at the New England Hospital for Women and Children.

The hospital was an extremely beneficial adjunct to the college because it provided the students with clinical training. Nurses also trained there.

Numerous financial woes, administrative struggles between the board and faculty, a troubling relationship between Zakrzewska and Gregory, and arguments over some of the educational requirements were all typical of nineteenth-century medical education. The college continued despite lean years during and immediately following the Civil War but merged officially with Boston University in 1874. Today it is Dimock Community Health Center, one of Beth Israel Deaconess Medical Center's community health centers.

See also: Longshore, Hannah Myers; Zakrzewska, Marie Elizabeth
References: Waite, Frederick Clayton, *History of the New England Female Medical College*, Boston: Boston University School of Medicine (1950).

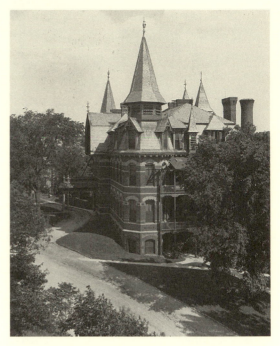

New England Hospital (Library of Congress)

New England Hospital
1862–1969

Founded initially as the New England Hospital for Women and Children in Boston in 1862, the New England Hospital, which changed its name in 1949, was one of the first hospitals for women and children staffed by female physicians. Few of the women's medical colleges at the time had clinical training facilities, and Marie Zakrzewska, the hospital's founder, gave women physicians the opportunity to gain clinical experience. She also wanted to provide women and children with a place to be treated by women physicians.

As more men's medical colleges began to open their doors to women, some questioned the need for the hospital's continued existence. Elizabeth Blackwell, whom Zakrzewska had trained with at the New York Infirmary for Women and Children, had seen no further need for her medical school once Cornell opened its doors in 1899. She closed the Women's Medical College of the New York Infirmary and saw this step as a positive one. Many women agreed. The traditional schools were bigger and had better facilities. Women who had fought for integration saw victory at hand.

Some held to the idea of a women's hospital for women. Zakrzewska was a proponent until her death in 1902, and her hospital continued to appeal to women through the trying years following the Flexner Report, which caused many of the all-female medical colleges to close because of a lack of credentials.

Though more and more women questioned the need for separatism, and many would have preferred the hospital to hire men as well as women, the hospital remained as its founder had intended for over 100 years. It will always be remembered by those interested in the history of women in medicine. "Indeed, the general shift from sexual separatism to integration, the emergence of a modern medical profession, and the erosion of Victorian moralism by the rise of a science of society in America were enacted in the lives of the women doctors at the New England Hospital. These important social changes constantly presented the women doctors with new problems and challenged them to find novel solutions. As the story of the women doctors at the New England Hospital so vividly shows, a woman's struggle to become a doctor was but the first step in her more enduring struggle to be a doctor" (Drachman 1984, 15). The hospital closed in 1969.

See also: Blackwell, Elizabeth; Flexner Report; Zakrzewska, Marie Elizabeth
References: Drachman, Virginia G., *Hospital with a Heart: Women Doctors and the Paradox of Separatism at the New England Hospital, 1862–1969*, Ithaca, NY: Cornell University Press (1984).

New Hospital for Women and Children
1872–

Founded by Elizabeth Garrett Anderson, this hospital grew out of a dispensary she started in 1866 in London. The hospital continued to grow over the years, serving as a place where women physicians could gain experience. It is still in existence today, known as the Elizabeth Garrett Anderson Hospital.

See also: Anderson, Elizabeth Garrett
References: Manton, Jo, *Elizabeth Garrett Anderson*, New York: Dutton (1965).

Nielsen, Nielsine Mathilde
1850–1916

The first woman physician in Denmark, Nielsine Nielsen read about women practicing medicine in the United States and applied to the University of Copenhagen, graduating in 1885. She continued her medical education in London, Bern, and Paris. She returned to Denmark and developed a large gynecology practice.

References: Lovejoy, Esther Pohl, *Women Doctors of the World*, New York: Macmillan (1957).

Nightingale, Florence
1820–1910

Undoubtedly the most famous nurse in world history, Florence Nightingale set a precedent of nursing excellence, efficiency, duty, honor, and love of humanity. She wrote extensively, founded hospitals worldwide, inspired millions of young women, and cared for thousands of people around the world who were victims of pestilence, war, malnutrition, and abuse. The field of military nursing was officially born after her undaunted performance during the Crimean War.

She was born in Florence, Italy, on May 12, 1820. Her parents, William Edward Nightingale and Frances Smith Nightingale, were wealthy landowners. As a child, Florence was frequently ill. She grew up in the family homes in Derbyshire, Hampshire, and London. She had one sister, Frances Parthenope, who was a year older than Florence.

Nightingale's father was a well-educated man who felt women's minds could hold an education as well as a man's. He tutored Florence at home in many subjects including science, mathematics, history, and philosophy. He and her mother had also encouraged Florence's love of animals, and she had a gift for nursing them when they were injured.

When she was a young woman, in 1837, she received what she felt was a call from

God to serve humanity and the working classes. Initially her parents were not supportive of her turning her attention away from the more traditional aspirations of finding a suitable husband and raising a family. They also were concerned about the dangers to her health of working among the sick.

She enrolled in the Deaconess Institution at Kaiserswerth on the Rhine in Germany in 1851. This Protestant institution reflected all her beliefs. She had already learned much by visiting the sick near her family's homes and hospitals in other countries. She worked among the poor with Pastor Fliedner, often accompanying him on his rounds.

In the few years following her Kaiserswerth days, Nightingale worked in France and England, first traveling to Paris and working with the Sisters of St. Vincent de Paul. She also observed surgeries in the hospitals. Back in England she became the superintendent at the Establishment for Gentlewomen during Illness, reorganizing the home to provide better care. "The Home had been languishing through mismanagement and lack of funds, and its new superintendent set to work with characteristic method. She got donations from her friends, inspired old subscribers with a new confidence, and managed to get the institution on its feet again, but not without a serious strain of overwork" (Tooley 1914, 85).

When the Crimean War broke out in 1854, William Howard Russell, who wrote for the London *Times*, called for more nurses to tend to British soldiers. French women were already in the field helping French soldiers, but the British had no organization and no trained staff. Nightingale offered her services to the British secretary of war, Sydney Herbert, who at the same time was writing a letter to her seeking her services. She accepted a position as the superintendent of nurses and had a group ready by the end of the week.

Nightingale's thirty-eight nurses were from both Catholic and Protestant backgrounds; their home churches were in agreement that all would have to obey Nightingale as their superior in the field. "The Roman Catholic bishop at once agreed

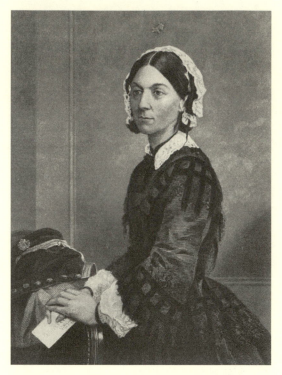

Florence Nightingale (U.S. National Library of Medicine)

to the regulations laid down, and signed a paper agreeing that the sisters of mercy joining the expedition should give entire obedience to Miss Nightingale, and that they should not enter into religious discussion except with the soldiers of their own faith. Mutual arrangement was made that the Roman Catholic sisters should attend on the soldiers of their own faith, and the Protestant sisters on those of their faith" (Tooley 1914, 118).

The expedition set out for Turkey on October 21, 1854, from London en route to Scutari. Upon arrival at the hospital, Nightingale

made her first round of the wards at Scutari. The beds were reeking with infection and the 'sheets,' she relates, 'were of canvas, and so coarse that the wounded men begged to be left in their blankets. It was indeed impossible to put men in such a state of emaciation into those sheets. There was no bedroom furniture of any kind, and only empty beer or wine bottles for candlesticks.' In addition to the miseries entailed by overcrowding, the men lying on the floors of the corridors were tormented by vermin and their limbs attacked by rats as they lay helpless in their pain. (Tooley 1914, 126–127)

The medical men already there felt the women would be more of a hindrance than a help. Less than a day later the wounded soldiers from the Battle of Inkerman began arriving, overwhelming a staff that had not had the time to clean and organize. In the crowded conditions, the wounded were placed in the mud outside the hospital.

Nightingale set about tending the wounded and assigning tasks to everyone who could help, including untrained, wounded soldiers. Some got drunk on the brandy that was for the patients. Many of the men were dragged to the "dead house" while they were still alive.

Nightingale saw, however, that it was not so much the incompetence of those tending the sick that led to the state of general despair but the lack of organization. She began organizing the staff, securing medical supplies, and instituting a regimen to ensure sanitary conditions. Later in her famous *Notes on Nursing*, she would again stress organization and cleanliness. If a nurse "allow[s] her sick to remain unwashed, or their clothing to remain on them after being saturated with perspiration or other excretion, she is interfering injuriously with the natural processes of health just as effectually as if she were to give the patient a dose of slow poison by the mouth" (Nightingale 1975, 93).

The doctors chose their surgical patients based on their chances of survival, separating those patients they felt would die. Many of the latter survived under Nightingale's care. She made her rounds at night carrying a little lamp, and many later referred to her as the Lady with the Lamp.

By 1855, the hospital at Scutari was functioning well. Nightingale's parents had given some financial help, Nightingale had used her own monies, and the British government was forthcoming with supplies once she had explained the hospital's needs.

She had set up a kitchen and laundry and sanitation guidelines. She would later teach that organization and management have a huge role in nursing care: "All the results of good nursing, as detailed in these notes, may be spoiled or utterly negatived by one defect, viz.: in petty management, or in other words, by not knowing how to manage that what you do when you are there, shall be done when you are not there" (Nightingale 1975, 35).

On May 2, 1855, Nightingale left Scutari, Turkey, and set sail for the Crimea and Balaclava. It was her duty as superintendent to inspect all hospitals, and she was anxious to see how the wounded in other hospitals were faring. She was by now a household word in England, and in the Crimea, soldiers had heard about her work at Scutari.

She inspected some hospitals but then suddenly became ill. Word spread quickly that she was dying; even the press in England reported this. However, she recovered enough to decide to stay on in her war duties.

On September 9, 1855, Sebastopol fell, and the Russians retreated. With the end of the war, Nightingale remained with the remaining wounded who needed treatment.

Nightingale's detailed notes and letters on conditions in the field led to many reforms as time went on and benefited many future soldiers in Britain and around the world.

Florence Nightingale knew how to get results. Against the backdrop of the Victorian era, when most women of high birth were relegated to the drawing room, she changed the face of health care forever. She championed sanitary practices, such as hand washing and improving sanitation in health care institutions. She launched social and health care reforms in England and abroad. She performed statistically based research and used innovative pie chart diagrams to illustrate her data. ("Tracing Nightingale's Steps" 2001, 44)

Upon returning to England, Nightingale was "haunted by the memories of the thousands of soldiers who had died because of the glaring deficiencies and unpreparedness of the army's Medical Department. Of the 97,800 soldiers who had fought in the Crimean War, 4,500 had died of battle-related causes, but nearly four times as many—17,600—had died of disease and exposure" (Dossey 2000, 186).

Following the Crimea, she turned her attention to India. After the Sepoy Rebellion, there were many reports of unsanitary conditions in India, and British soldiers were again subject to poor medical care in the field. From her home, Nightingale gathered statistics for reports to the government. In a short time, her reports led to a reduction in the mortality rate of the wounded. Eventually her efforts aided in the establishment of a sanitary department with great authority in India.

In 1860 the Nightingale Home and Training School opened as part of St. Thomas's Hospital. It had been one of Nightingale's goals from the beginning to provide better training for nurses that included setting fractures, preparing medications, and basic chemistry as well as instilling a professionalism that had been lacking in the field of nursing. Her training facility did not grow quickly, but her methods rapidly caught on in Australia, Canada, and the United States, and over the years nursing schools were built around her teachings.

Often ill, some believe from a fever she had contracted in the Crimea, Nightingale continued to plan and write from her home. She proposed many changes that eventually became a reality, for example separate facilities for the insane, children, and those with infectious diseases. Many of her initiatives are now protocols in hospitals, nursing schools, and nursing homes. She continued her advocacy for better health care for all and a sound education for nurses. In 1907 she received the Order of Merit from King Edward VII; she was the first female so honored. She also received the Norwegian Red Cross, the Cross of Merit from Germany, and the gold medal of Secours aux Glessés from France, among other honors. She passed away on August 13, 1910.

References: Andrews, Mary Raymond Shipman, *A Lost Commander: Florence Nightingale,* Garden City, NY: Doubleday, Doran (1929); Baly, Monica E., *Florence Nightingale and the Nursing Legacy,* London: Croom Helm (1986); Cook, Sir Edward, *The Life of Florence Nightingale,* London: Macmillan (1925); Dossey, Barbara Montgomery, *Florence Nightingale: Mystic, Visionary, Healer,* Springhouse, PA: Springhouse (2000); Nightingale, Florence, *Notes on Nursing: What It Is, and What It Is Not,* New York: D. Appleton (1860), reprinted in *History of Women,* reel 343, no. 2366, New Haven, CT: Research Publications (1975); Snodgrass, Ellen, *Historical Dictionary of Nursing,* Santa Barbara, CA: ABC-CLIO (1999); Tooley, Sarah A., *The Life of Florence Nightingale,* London: Cassell (1914); "Tracing Nightingale's Steps," *Nursing* 31, no. 1 (January 2001): 44; Woodham-Smith, Cecil, *Florence Nightingale, 1820–1910,* London: Constable (1950).

Novello, Antonia Coello
1944–

Antonia Novello was the first woman to become the surgeon general of the United States. She was also the first Hispanic to serve in that capacity. Her focus on AIDS awareness, injury prevention in children, and health care for minorities contributed to public awareness of the challenges to come.

Born in Fajardo, Puerto Rico, on August 23, 1944, she was the eldest of the three children of Antonio Coello and Ana Delia Coello. She was born with an abnormally large colon that malfunctioned until she was eighteen and had surgery to correct it. Before and after the operation, her ailment led to numerous hospital stays.

Novello's mother and her aunt, who was a nurse, encouraged her in her ambition to become a pediatrician, a goal she had formed in part to keep other children from suffering so long with a similar ailment. Her pediatrician and her gastroenterologist, who, she felt, were good examples of caring physicians, also influenced her.

Novello attended the University of Puerto Rico in Rio Piedras and graduated in

1965 with a B.S. She earned her medical degree in 1970 from the University of Puerto Rico's Medical School in San Juan. She married a navy flight surgeon, Joseph Novello, and they both went to the University of Michigan in Ann Arbor to continue their medical studies. She concentrated on pediatrics and nephrology.

Novello also earned a master's degree in public health from Johns Hopkins University in 1982. In 1976 she had opened a private practice in Springfield, Virginia, but she empathized with her patients and their parents to the degree that she felt she had to move on and closed the practice after two years. In 1978 she joined the National Institutes of Health and quickly rose in the ranks to become the deputy director of the National Institute of Child Health and Human Development.

During the 1980s she was very active in tackling some issues of major concern to minorities, children, and women. She fought for better warning labels on tobacco products, better education on AIDS prevention, and health care for the Hispanic community. She also played a major role in the realization of the National Organ Transplant Act of 1984, which would lead to better organization and a network for acquiring organs needed for transplantation.

She became the fourteenth surgeon general of the United States and thus the "doctor for all Americans" on March 9, 1990, after being nominated by President George Bush in 1989. She broadened her focus to many other public health concerns, including domestic abuse and underage drinking. She brought a clever, intelligent, well-informed persona to the mission of the surgeon general.

Novello served until Joycelyn Elders was appointed in 1993 after being nominated by President Bill Clinton. She is currently the New York state health commissioner and has recently been involved with state efforts to keep the West Nile virus under control.

References: Associated Press, "NY Battle Plan: Less Spraying; Plan's Emphasis on Prevention," *Newsday* (New York) (25 April 2001): A17; "Novello, Antonia," *Current Biography* 53, no. 5 (May 1992): 45–49.

Nusslein-Volhard, Christiane
1942–

Christiane Nusslein-Volhard received the Nobel Prize in physiology or medicine in 1995 along with Edward B. Lewis and Eric F. Wieschaus for discovering how genes control early embryo development.

Born October 20, 1942, during World War II, she is the daughter of an architect, Rolf Volhard, and Brigitte Haas Volhard of Frankfurt, Germany. She is the second of five children.

She loved nature and knew she wanted to be a biologist by the time she was twelve. She didn't do well in some subjects in school but excelled at science while attending Frankfurt's Schiller School. She had an interest in evolution and genetics. School in post–World War II Germany involved discussion of Hitler, anti-Semitism, and guilt. Many children like Nusslein-Volhard were shocked and horrified by what had taken place.

Her father died just before she entered the Johann-Wolfgang-Goethe-University in Frankfurt. She stayed there two years before moving to the University of Tübingen, which had just started a biochemistry program. She received her diploma in 1968 in biochemistry and continued her studies there in order to earn a Ph.D. in biology with a concentration in genetics in 1973.

While studying for her Ph.D., she worked as a research associate at the Max Planck Institute, where she wanted to study cells and the role genetics plays in embryo development. She spent hours in the lab studying the mutation of fruit flies, their eggs, and other characteristics, believing these studies would be key to dealing with more difficult questions.

In 1978 she moved to Heidelberg to head the European Molecular Biology Laboratory (EMBL). She and Eric Wieschaus studied random gene mutations in the drosophila, or fruit fly, and were able to identify fifteen genes that control early embryo development. "The genes identified by Nusslein-Volhard and Wieschaus also influence formation of the body axis and specialization of individual segments of the development of the human embryo. About 40 percent of idiopathic congenital malformations may be due to mutations in genes discovered by Nusslein-Volhard and Wieschaus" (Raju 2000, 81).

Nusslein-Volhard moved on to zebra fish, thinking they might be able to solve more of the puzzle of cell development.

When Leonard Zon, associate professor of pediatrics at Children's Hospital in Boston studied dozens of Nusslein-Volhard's mutants that failed to form red blood cells in the usual fashion, he found that some of the mutants had the fish equivalent of various human blood disorders, including thalassemia and a type of congenital anemia. "We owe Janni a tremendous debt," Zon says; "Her zebra fish mutants have provided not only a fantastic system for studying the whole process of blood formation, they're also providing critical insights into human disease. We could never have gotten to this level without her." (Ackerman 1997, 42)

Nusslein-Volhard is divorced and has no children. She is currently the director of the Max Planck Institute for Developmental Biology's Genetics Division in Tübingen.

References: Ackerman, Jennifer, "Journey to the Center of the Egg," *New York Times*, sec. 6 (12 October 1997): 42; McGrayne, Sharon Bertsch, *Nobel Prize Women in Science*, Secaucus, NJ: Carol (1998); Nusslein-Volhard, Christiane, and Jorn Kratzschmar, eds., *Of Fish, Fly, Worm, and Man: Lessons from Developmental Biology for Human Gene Function and Disease*, Berlin: Springer (2000); Raju, T. N., "The Nobel Chronicles," *Lancet* 356, no. 9223 (1 July 2000): 81.

Nutting, Mary Adelaide
1858–1948

Mary Nutting contributed to a higher standard of nursing practice in the United States. She was the first nurse to become a university professor.

Mary was born in Frost Village, Quebec, on November 1, 1858. The family soon moved to Waterloo, where she grew up. She was the daughter of a seamstress, Harriet Sophia Peasley Nutting, and a county clerk, Vespasian Nutting. She had three older brothers, Charles, Arthur, and Jim, and one younger sister, Harriette Armine.

They were poor but received an education at the local schools. The oldest, Charles, eventually graduated from law school at McGill University. The girls attended the Shefford Academy. Mary Adelaide also attended Bute House, a private school in Montreal, and developed some proficiency in music. Later the girls' mother moved with them to Ottawa, where her son Jim was already settled and working and she felt they would have more opportunities. Vespasian chose to stay behind.

They enjoyed Ottawa, but their financial situation was still grim. Mary Adelaide taught music and did seamstress work as she could find it. She nursed her mother during a brief illness that took her life in 1884. Increasingly lonely and in search of a job, Mary Adelaide remembered reading about Florence Nightingale and discovered there was a training school for nurses at Johns Hopkins. She applied and was accepted in 1889. She excelled in nursing and graduated in 1891 at the top of her class. Once the medical school opened in 1893, there was a great need for expanded hospital activity, and upon Isabel Hampton's resignation, Nutting became the assistant superintendent of nurses.

In 1894 she became full superintendent and worked to change students' nursing responsibilities. As in many schools and as had been the case in Nutting's student days, student nurses were many times overworked as nurses in associated hospitals instead of being given the needed time for study.

In a speech in 1896 to the American Society of Superintendents of Training Schools for Nurses, she stressed that it was time for

"people [to realize] that training schools were educational institutions." She pointed out the dangers of reducing students to servitude. Fearlessly she asserted that in many instances it was not for the purpose of giving more and better training that they were kept on duty so long, but rather that the amount of service to the hospital might be increased and the working force of the institutions be kept at a minimum. As a rule the number of student nurses was less than proportionate to the number of patients. Such attempts at economy were detrimental to student nurses and patients alike. (Marshall 1972, 73)

She advocated eight to nine work hours per day as a maximum. She used statistical data from national surveys to show that many student nurses were working fifteen and seventeen hours in some cases and then were expected to study and go to class. As she became more efficient in administrative and organizational matters, she worked to obtain an endowment for the training school, thus separating its budget from the hospital's. She also enlarged the curriculum to three years instead of two because nurses needed to be familiar with an ever-increasing number of medical specialties.

Nutting was instrumental in changing the public's and the physician's view of nursing. She provided leadership in establishing it as a profession with many requirements, thus giving more weight to a nursing degree. She realized that practical experience was requisite but not without the fundamentals of instruction.

She served on many committees and boards concerned with nursing education and helped draft the first nursing-practice law in Maryland in 1904. She became a professor of nursing in 1907 at Teachers College in New York, which needed an authority to teach courses to graduate nurses. She remained at Teachers College until her retirement.

One of her greatest and timeliest achievements was completing and publishing the *Standard Curriculum for Schools of Nursing* in 1917 for the National League of Nursing Education (NLNE) just as the United States was getting involved in World War I. It helped nursing to move forward in obtaining professional status. Nursing schools in many parts of the United States scrutinized and implemented her methods. Nutting passed away on October 3, 1948, in White Plains, New York.

See also: Robb, Isabel Hampton
References: Drachman, V., "Nutting, M[ary] Adelaide," in Martin Kaufman, Stuart Galishoff, and Todd L. Savitt, eds., *Dictionary of American Medical Biography*, Westport, CT: Greenwood Press (1984); Marshall, Helen E., *Mary Adelaide Nutting: Pioneer of Modern Nursing*, Baltimore, MD: Johns Hopkins University Press (1972); Snodgrass, Mary Ellen, *Historical Encyclopedia of Nursing*, Santa Barbara, CA: ABC-CLIO (1999).

Ockett, Molly
1750?–1816

An early Abenaki healer in Maine, Molly Ockett was the only medical help available for most people. She used herbs and encouraged mineral waters for ailing whites and Indians alike.

Not much is known about her life, but numerous stories abound about her, many fictitious. A noted criminal of the day, Henry Tufts, included her good deeds in his autobiography, which historians believe to be an accurate description of life in the region and of the people, both whites and Indians. Ockett treated Tufts for a knife wound around 1772, for which he was forever grateful. She died in 1816 and is buried in Andover, Maine.

References: Lecompte, Nancy, "The Last of the Androscoggins: Molly Ockett, Abenaki Healing Woman" (August 1997), http://www.avcnet.org/ne-do-ba/bio_moly.html; Tufts, Henry, *The Autobiography of a Criminal*, New York: Duffield (1930).

Ogino, Ginko
1851–1913

Ginko Ogino was the first woman licensed to practice Western medicine in Japan. She persevered against continual rejections of her efforts to gain a medical education.

Born in Saitama Prefecture, she graduated from the Women's Normal School, now known as Ochanomizu Women's University, and also from a private medical school, Kojuin. The latter was an all-male school, and she had difficulty gaining entrance. After she graduated, the government resisted allowing her to take the examinations that were a prerequisite to legally practicing medicine. After three years, in 1885, she was allowed to take the examinations and passed. She worked at the Meiji Girls' School and later went to Hokkaido to practice.

She contracted a venereal disease from her first husband that left her unable to bear children. She divorced him on these grounds and later married Shikata Shizen. She returned to Tokyo after his death and died in 1913.

References: Ogilvie, Marilyn, and Joy Harvey, eds., *The Biographical Dictionary of Women in Science: Pioneering Lives from Ancient Times to the Mid-20th Century*, New York: Routledge (2000); "Ogino Ginko," *Kodansha Encyclopedia of Japan*, vol. 6, Tokyo: Kodansha (1983).

Osborn, June Elaine
1937–

June Osborn is an epidemiologist, pediatrician, and professor. She has continued to lead and advise in the AIDS awareness and prevention movement and assists in public policy development regarding AIDS treatment both nationally and internationally.

Born on May 28, 1937, in Endicott, New York, she attended Oberlin College in Ohio, receiving a B.A. in 1957. She continued on to medical school at Case Western Reserve University and earned her medical degree in 1961. She has worked in several capacities at various medical schools and hospitals around the United States, concentrating in pediatrics and epidemiology as well as being deeply involved in all issues surrounding HIV and AIDS.

She has published numerous scientific and public policy papers. Her early work focuses on many research areas, particularly those concerned with vaccines and immunology. In the past couple of decades she has concentrated more on AIDS as a social as well as a medical problem.

Osborn has urged education about HIV. "We've seen a shocking disinclination to become involved at all in the care of people with HIV. 'Risk' is cited as an excuse, but the risk is far lower from HIV than from many other hazards in the health care workplace. Ignorance is offered as another excuse—but the proper response to ignorance on the part of a professional is to learn, not to walk away" (Osborn 1992, 64). Osborn is currently president of the Josiah Macy, Jr. Foundation in New York.

References: *American Men and Women of Science,* 20th ed., New York: Bowker (1998); Osborn, June Elaine, "AIDS and the Politics of Compassion," *Hospitals* 66, no. 18 (20 September 1992): 64; Osborn, June Elaine, "Infections," *Journal of Urban Health* 75, no. 2 (June 1998): 251–257.

P

Paget, Mary Rosalind
1855–1948

Mary Rosalind Paget was an English nurse and midwife who in 1881 founded the Midwives Institute, later known as the Royal College of Midwives. The health of England lay in increasing the birth rate, and midwives did not have proper training. The Royal College of Midwives continues to operate. Paget was born on January 4, 1855, in Greenbank, Liverpool, to Elizabeth Rathbone Paget and John Paget, a police magistrate. Early on she seemed to be pulled toward public service, and she went to Westminster Hospital to train as a nurse. In 1882 she went to the London Hospital and later to the British Lying-In Hospital. It was during this initial training that she became very concerned with infants and the inadequate training opportunities for those practicing as midwives.

She and a small group of women founded the Midwives Institute in 1881, and she worked hard to get the House of Commons to pass a bill requiring the registration and certification of midwives. This effort met with resistance for several years from those who believed the legislation would prevent birthing mothers from getting help from neighbors. The bill finally passed as the Midwives Act of 1902. The Central Midwives Board was established, which Paget served on for years. She was also the first queen's nurse, appointed by Queen Victoria in 1891.

Many in the decades before World War I concerned themselves with the moral character of unwed mothers and mothers of low socioeconomic status. Paget fought hard to ensure equal care for women and children regardless of the mother's socioeconomic, professional, or marital status. "When several Queen's nurses expressed confusion about whether or not they should attend only respectable married women, Rosalind Paget was clear that the health and safety of the mother and child were paramount and that the mother's marital status was irrelevant" (Hannam 1997, 91).

She founded and was the editor of *Nursing Notes* (later *Midwives' Chronicles*) for many years. She played a large part in advancing women's midwifery skills, fighting for better pay, and ensuring better prenatal care. Paget never married. She passed away on August 19, 1948, in Bolney, Sussex.

References: Hannam, June, "Rosalind Paget: The Midwife, the Women's Movement and Reform before 1914," in Hilary Marland and Anne Marie Rafferty, eds., *Midwives, Society, and Childbirth: Debates and Controversies in the Modern Period*, London: Routledge (1997); Pye, E. M., "Paget, Dame (Mary) Rosalind," *Dictionary of National Biography, 1941–1950*, London: Oxford University Press (1959); Snodgrass, Mary Jane, *Historical Encyclopedia of Nursing*, Santa Barbara, CA: ABC-CLIO (1999).

Pak, Esther Kim
1877–1910

Esther Pak was the first woman physician to practice Western medicine in Korea. She graduated from the Women's Medical College of Baltimore in 1900, afterward returning to Korea to work with women and children. She has served as an inspiration for other young women who wanted to become physicians.

References: "Doctor Esther Kim Pak," http://www.chass.utoronto.ca/~youngran/WomenScientists/esther.htm; Lovejoy, Esther Pohl, *Women Doctors of the World,* New York: Macmillan (1957); Pak, Rhoda Kim, "Medical Women in Korea," *Journal of the American Medical Women's Association* 5, no. 3 (March 1950): 116–117.

Parrish, Rebecca
1869–1952

Rebecca Parish was the first female physician to practice in the Philippines. After receiving a medical education at the Medical College of Indiana, she traveled to the Philippines in order to work as a Methodist medical missionary. She served there from 1905 to 1933. In 1906, she established a dispensary in Manila, where leprosy was prevalent because of the tropical climate. "Health is always a problem in the tropics; water is not safe, unless artesian wells are drilled. In the old days, with decaying fruits and vegetables, insects, especially mosquitoes, insufficient fresh milk for the babies, and the prevalence of cholera, smallpox, malaria, leprosy, dysentery, and tropical ulcers and eruptions, there was a serious health question" (Parrish 1936, 26). After a time she received money from an American philanthropist and established the Mary Johnston Hospital for women and children. It became an important medical facility over the next several decades and was restored after damage restricted its operation during World War II. Parrish died in Indianapolis, Indiana, on August 22, 1952.

References: "Dr. Rebecca Parrish: Medical Missionary," *New York Times* (24 August 1952): 89; Lovejoy, Esther Pohl, *Women Doctors of the World,* New York: Macmillan (1957); Ogilvie, Marilyn, and Joy Harvey, eds., *The Biographical Dictionary of Women in Science,* New York: Routledge (2000); Parrish, Rebecca, *Orient Seas and Lands Afar,* New York: Fleming H. Revell (1936).

Pearce, Louise
1885–1959

Louise Pearce was a physician and pathologist who helped develop the drug tryparsamide in order to treat trypanosomiasis (sleeping sickness). She tested it on humans in the Belgian Congo in 1920 and 1921 and obtained great success that was recognized with the Order of the Crown of Belgium award.

She was born in Winchester, Massachusetts, on March 5, 1885, to Charles Ellis Pearce and Susan Elizabeth Hoyt Pearce. She received her education at the Girls' Collegiate School in Los Angeles and then went to Stanford University and earned a bachelor's in physiology and histology in 1907. She went to Boston University's School of Medicine and taught before she was admitted to the Johns Hopkins University School of Medicine in 1909. She received her medical degree in 1912 and proceeded to the Rockefeller Institute, where she remained most of her career.

She and two other researchers, Walter A. Jacobs and Wade Hampton Brown, worked together to find a treatment for sleeping sickness. They found that tryparsamide was effective in treating rabbits with the disease. She then traveled to the Belgian Congo and treated humans with tryparsamide, and it was effective in overcoming the *Trypanosoma* parasite in the bloodstream. She treated patients with mild to severe cases in a clinic in Leopoldville and was given access to a government laboratory. Pearce's treatment was an important milestone in battling the illness, which is carried by the tsetse fly and is still an enormous problem today. It can be deadly if untreated. The Rockefeller Institute eventually patented the tryparsamide compound and worked on improving it.

Pearce also studied syphilis, cancer, and hereditary diseases while at the Rockefeller Institute and later as she continued her research while serving as the president of the Women's Medical College of Pennsylvania from 1946 to 1951. She lived with the novelist Ida White in Skillman, New Jersey, when she retired. She died in New York City in 1959.

References: Bailey, Martha J., *American Women in Science: A Biographical Dictionary*, Santa Barbara, CA: ABC-CLIO (1994); Lovejoy, Esther Pohl, *Women Doctors of the World*, New York: Macmillan (1957); Ogilvie, Marilyn, and Joy Harvey, eds., *The Biographical Dictionary of Women in Science*, New York: Routledge (2000); Rose, Kenneth W., *A Survey of Source at the Rockefeller Archive Center for the Study of Twentieth Century Africa*, North Tarrytown, NY: Rockefeller Archive Center (1996).

Perez, Ernestina

Along with Eloiza Diaz, Ernestina Perez attended the University of Chile. She was among the first women to obtain medical degrees in Latin America. Perez graduated in 1887 and practiced in Chile working very hard during the cholera epidemic following graduation. She continued her interest in the advances of medicine by traveling abroad in order to keep up with current medical practices.

See also: Diaz Inzunza, Eloiza
References: De Vargas, Tegualda Ponce, "Women Doctors of Chile," *Journal of the American Medical Women's Association* 7, no. 10 (October 1952): 389; Lovejoy, Esther Pohl, *Women Doctors of the World*, New York: Macmillan (1957).

Perozo, Evangelina Rodriguez
1898?–19?

Evangelina Perozo was the first woman to graduate from the oldest university in North America, the University of Santo Domingo. She graduated in 1919 and became the first woman physician of the Dominican Republic.

References: Heureaux, Mercedes A., "Oldest University in America," *Journal of the American Medical Woman's Association* 10, no. 7 (July 1955): 249; Lovejoy, Esther Pohl, *Women Doctors of the World*, New York: Macmillan (1957).

Petermann, Mary Locke
1908–1975

Mary Petermann was instrumental in isolating ribosomes. Her work helped researchers to better understand protein synthesis and RNA. Born in Laurium, Michigan, on February 26, 1908, Petermann attended Smith College and majored in chemistry, then pursued graduate study at the University of Wisconsin. She obtained her Ph.D. in 1939 in physiological chemistry. She was an early pioneer in the study of the relationship of chemistry and physiology in animals and humans.

Most of her career was spent in New York City at the Sloan-Kettering Institute for Cancer Research. She also served as a professor at nearby Cornell University's Medical College for many years. Her research focused on ribosomes, which "catalyze protein synthesis in all of the organisms in our biosphere; indeed, they are at one and the same time universal, essential, and complicated. The ribosomal proteins and the ribosomal nucleic acids provide the specific binding sites (for messenger RNA, transfer RNA, and initiation and elongation factors) and the catalytic activities required for the synthesis of a protein" (Wool 1997, 623).

Petermann was able to isolate animal ribosomes and better characterize them. She also studied the physical and chemical properties of proteins. In 1963 she received the Sloan Award in cancer research, and three years later the American Chemical Society honored her with the Garvan Medal. She died December 13, 1975.

References: *American Men and Women of Science*, 12th ed., New York: Bowker (1972); Bailey, Martha J., American *Women in Science: A Biographical Dictionary*, Santa Barbara, CA: ABC-CLIO (1994); "Petermann,

Mary PhD." [obit], *New York Times* (16 December 1975): 42, col. 3; Wool, Ira G., "Ribosomes," *Encyclopedia of Human Biology*, 2d ed., vol. 7, San Diego: Academic Press (1997).

Pickett, Lucy Weston
1904–1997

Lucy Pickett was an award-winning chemist. She did research on X-ray crystallography and studied organic molecules using spectroscopy.

Born on January 19, 1904, in Beverly, Massachusetts, she was the daughter of Lucy Weston and George Ernst Pickett. She attended school in Beverly and went on to Mount Holyoke College in South Hadley, Massachusetts, graduating in 1925 with honors and a degree in both math and chemistry. She continued her chemistry studies and in 1927 obtained a master's from Mount Holyoke.

Pickett taught for a year at Goucher College in Maryland before entering the Ph.D. program at the University of Illinois, which she completed in 1930. Her early work included the effects of X rays on chemical reactions and the use of X rays in determining molecular structure. She was invited to become a member of the faculty at Mount Holyoke upon completion of her doctorate and remained there her entire career.

She went to Europe briefly and studied X-ray crystallography with Sir William Bragg. When she returned to Mount Holyoke, she joined an active research team that included Mary Sherrill and Emma Perry Carr and began exploring molecular structures using spectroscopy. She was able to work with some very gifted scientists during her day, including Robert S. Mulliken and Linus Pauling.

For recognition for her work in spectroscopy she received the Garvan Medal from the American Chemical Society in 1957. She also established a fund upon her retirement to bring noted speakers to campus. She passed away on November 23, 1997, in Bradenton, Florida.

References: "Expert on Cell Surfaces to Deliver Lucy W. Pickett Lecture November 20," *College Street Journal* (Mount Holyoke College) (17 November 2000), http://138.110.28.9/offices/comm/csj/111700/pickett.shtml; Shearer, Benjamin F., and Barbara S. Shearer, *Notable Women in the Physical Sciences*, Westport, CT: Greenwood Press (1997).

Pittman, Margaret
1901–1995

Margaret Pittman helped standardize vaccines for typhoid, cholera, and whooping cough. She contributed as well to the understanding of the bacteria that cause meningitis.

Pittman was born in Prairie Grove, Arkansas, in 1901. She attended Hendrix College in Conway, Arkansas, and received an A.B. degree in 1923. She did graduate work at the University of Chicago and received her master's in 1926, followed by a Ph.D. in 1929. Her primary interest was bacteriology.

She worked for the Public Health Service and the National Institutes of Health, studying influenza types and helping to develop vaccines. "In her work with *Haemophilus influenzae* type b, Dr. Pittman was the first to identify capsular type b as one of the six types of *H. influenzae* responsible for most childhood meningitis. As a result of Dr. Pittman's work in *H. aegyptius*, with NIAID director Dorland Davis, the cause of epidemic conjunctivitis was identified. Working with Salmonella typhi, she made key observations that led to the development of a Vi-based vaccine. Dr. Pittman is believed to have been the first woman laboratory chief at the NIH" ("NIH Lectures" 2002).

Pittman was recognized internationally as an expert in bacteriology. She was a frequent consultant for government agencies and international organizations. She died in 1995.

References: Bailey, Martha J., *American Women in Science: A Biographical Dictionary*, Santa Barbara, CA: ABC-CLIO (1994); Kroll,

J. Simon, and Robert Booy, "*Haemophilus influenzae*: Capsule Vaccine and Capsulation Genetics," *Molecular Medicine Today* 2, no. 4 (April 1996): 160–165; "NIH Lectures," http://www1.od.nih.gov/oir/sourcebook/ir-communictns/lecture-info. htm#Pitt(2002); Proffitt, Pamela, *Notable Women Scientists*, Detroit: Gale Group (1999).

Pool, Judith Graham
1919–1975

Judith Pool was a major figure in the treatment of hemophilia and in establishing a standard procedure for isolating the antihemophilic factor in blood. Her method for blood transfusions greatly advanced therapy for hemophiliacs and was adopted widely as a standard around the world.

Born in 1919 in New York City, she obtained her Ph.D. in physiology at the University of Chicago. Her early studies focused on muscle physiology. In later decades she studied blood coagulation and looked for better ways to transfuse blood for those suffering with hemophilia.

She worked on many scientific committees and was

> a member of several working groups dealing with the translation of research findings to practical application, including preparation of factor VIII concentrates, assay procedures and standards for factor VIII, and analysis of inhibitors. Her analytical mind combined with good judgment made her a valued member of all groups with whom she worked. Her ability to sort out complex findings and to come out with clear statements with questions for future investigation was an attribute much admired. (Brinkhous 1976, 269)

Pool died on July 13, 1975.

References: Bailey, Martha J., *American Women in Science*, Santa Barbara: ABC-CLIO (1994); Brinkhous, K. M., "Judith Graham Pool, Ph.D. (1919–1975): An Appreciation," *Thrombosis and Haemostasis* 35, no. 2 (30 April 1976): 269–271.

Possanner-Ehrenthal, Garbrielle

Garbrielle Possanner-Ehrenthal was the first woman physician in Austria. She graduated from the University of Zurich in 1893 and was an assistant to Professor Friedrich Schauta, who held graduate clinics in obstetrics and gynecology in Vienna that were attended by medical students the world over. Much of her work was with poor women and children.

References: Lovejoy, Esther Pohl, *Women Doctors of the World*, New York: Macmillan (1957).

Preston, Ann
1813–1872

Ann Preston became the first female to hold the position of dean of a medical school. She graduated from the Female Medical College of Pennsylvania in 1851 and successfully lobbied for equal medical education for women, particularly clinical experience, which was being denied to so many. She helped establish a hospital connected to the college in 1861.

Born on December 1, 1813, in West Grove, Pennsylvania, she was the daughter of Amos and Margaret Smith Preston. She helped her mother, who was in poor health, raise the seven siblings that had survived infancy: Joseph, Simpson, Smith, Levi, Charles, Rebecca, and Howard. Joseph was the oldest and Ann was only two years younger, so many of the early chores fell to her. Her father had a large agriculture and dairy trade that kept the family busy.

Strong Quakers, the family was well respected in the area. Her father was influential in the community and concerned about the social issues of the day. The family was active in the abolition and temperance movements of the day, and their home was many times used to hide runaway slaves.

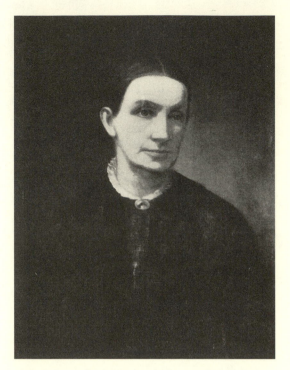

Ann Preston (U.S. National Library of Medicine)

When it was time for her to consider her education, Preston became interested in health and hygiene for young ladies and gave lectures in her community. With some encouragement, she decided to apply for medical school. No one would accept her until she applied at the new Female Medical College of Pennsylvania in Philadelphia, which Quakers had founded. She graduated and became a professor there.

Preston realized early on that her education was not adequate. The lack of a training hospital in which to observe and practice was a hindrance to many women physicians. She "had long recognized that clinical observations and instruction were necessary adjuncts to didactic lectures and theoretical treatises" (Foster 1984, 316). This is why she so diligently worked for a women's hospital when it was apparent most hospitals in the United States were not going to allow women to work as physicians. She accomplished her task, and the Women's Hospital of Philadelphia opened on December 16, 1861, with Emeline Cleveland as the resident physician.

The Female Medical College had temporarily closed due to financial woes created by the Civil War outbreak. About the same time, Preston suffered greatly from a bout of rheumatic fever and exhaustion, ailments that would plague her all her life. She was confined for three months at the insane asylum of Pennsylvania Hospital in order to rest and recuperate. She recovered fully and returned to work.

Shortly thereafter, there was a rift in the college over Edwin Fussell's refusal to award a student, Mary Putnam Jacobi, a medical degree. Preston disagreed with his decision, as did most of the faculty, since Jacobi had the necessary qualifications. Following this incident, Fussell resigned, and in 1865 Preston was named dean of the college.

She continued to speak out for equal education for women and also encouraged women of all races to work at receiving an education. Without her support, Rebecca Cole, the first black woman to graduate from the college, may never have become a physician.

In 1867 the Pennsylvania legislature was asked to change the name "Female" to "Women's." The latter seemed more acceptable at the time, and Preston supported the change. She continued to speak out for women despite opposition from males such as those belonging to the Medical Society of Philadelphia. In a letter published in the *Medical and Surgical Reporter* in 1867 she defused all their previous arguments, which were typical of the period, and asserted that women would insist on their entry into the medical field "in the sacred name of our common humanity, against the injustice which places difficulties in our way, not because we are ignorant, or pretentious, or incompetent, or unmindful of the code of medical or Christian ethics, but because we are women" (Preston 1867, 394).

Preston died on April 18, 1872, after having one of the strongest and most positive influences on nineteenth-century women physicians and medical education. "A woman of patience and determination, Ann Preston repeatedly withstood the hostilities vented upon her gender by the medical establishment and worked tirelessly to provide better opportunities and better training for the women who would follow her into the medical field" (Ford 1995, 1487).

See also: Cleveland, Emeline Horton; Cole, Rebecca; Jacobi, Mary Putnam; Medical College of Pennsylvania

References: Ford, Bonnie L., "Ann Preston," in Frank N. Magill, ed., *Great Lives from History: American Women Series,* vol. 4, Pasadena, CA: Salem Press (1995); Foster, Pauline Poole, *Ann Preston, M.D. (1813–1872): A Biography; The Struggle to Obtain Training and Acceptance for Women Physicians in Mid-Nineteenth Century America,* Pittsburgh: University of Pennsylvania Press (1984); Ohles, Frederik, Shirley M. Ohles, and John G. Ramsay, *Biographical Dictionary of Modern American Educators,* Westport, CT: Greenwood Press (1997); Preston, Ann, "The Status of Women-Physicians," *Medical and Surgical Reporter* 16, no. 18 (4 May 1867): 391–394, reprinted in *American Periodical Series II 1800–1850,* new series, reel 1200; Wells, Susan, *Out of the Dead House: Nineteenth-Century Women Physicians and the Writing of Medicine,* Madison: University of Wisconsin Press (2000).

Public Health and Women

What is a health which merely makes people ripe to be damaged, abused, and shot at again?

—Ernst Bloch

Early in the twentieth century, few women with a medical education had the option of working in private practice or in hospitals or clinics. The emerging field of public health offered opportunities for many.

Pasteur's late-nineteenth-century discoveries on contagious diseases and their causes were the beginning of serious public health initiatives. In 1946 the World Health Organization was established in Geneva, Switzerland, and the Communicable Disease Center (now known as the Centers for Disease Control and Prevention) was born in the United States. The Pan American Health Organization evolved through various names from 1902 on. They all emerged from the growing knowledge that disease had wiped out entire populations in the past and that the new medicines would not be effective unless they were distributed equitably and efficiently.

During the Civil War, women volunteered to help with the wounded. Once home, many put their energies into their local communities. "Institutions for the deaf, blind, insane, and orphaned had been built or expanded during the 1850s, giving women many opportunities to become involved in social welfare efforts and networks of voluntary associations" (Sivulka 1999, 2). Their gender still restricted them, however, to unpaid volunteer work.

In 1850, Lemuel Shattuck laid out some public health concerns in his *Report of the Sanitary Commission of Massachusetts,* more commonly known as the Shattuck Report. He made many recommendations concerning the containment of diseases, accurate records on causes of death, physicians who were better trained in sanitation and hygiene, and societal organization. Yet "there was very little effective public health work going on in America in 1879" (Smillie 1955, 443). "The whole trend of the century was to limit the teaching of medical students to the intensely practical fields, of diagnosis and treatment" (Smillie 1955, 444). Because women physicians were finding little public acceptance, they turned to the emerging field of public health, just as they had turned in the past to nursing as a way to enter the medical profession. Male physicians of the time took little interest in the field, preferring the more lucrative private practice, and thus women were welcome.

Following World War I, many women found that their competence in times of crisis was not rewarded with compensated employment. The frustration of women who worked during the war with the Scottish Women's Hospitals, now disbanded, reflected the feelings of many: "For many of the women there was no option but to return to the constrained middle-class existence they had known before the war. Rose West, who fearlessly drove over Macedonian mountain tracks as head of Motor Transport for the America unit, was not allowed to have her own car when she got home" (Leneman 1994, 213). Thus women again turned their attention to social issues and their energies to charitable work.

Sara Josephine Baker, a physician who tried private practice but could not make a living at it, contributed much as a public health administrator to the welfare of the poor in early-twentieth-century New York City. Baker realized that legislation recognizing the right of every individual to health care was as important as the need for physicians.

Even after legislation was passed, however, numerous problems with organization remained. Dr. Leslie Haden-Guest, a British physician and social reformer, wrote in 1912 that there were no "standards of cleanliness and decency with regard to premises and methods of serving the meals. I have myself seen school dinner centres in London, at which the food was served out of a bucket, and hundreds of plates and bowls 'washed up' between batches of children in one small tub of filthy water!" (Haden-Guest, 1912, 3–4). Many public health educators agree that five women were giants in the field in the twentieth century: Alice Hamilton, Sara Josephine Baker, Lillian Wald, Clara Barton, and Dorothea Dix. Ellen Swallow Richards had done much work in the late nineteenth century on sanitary issues and food safety as well (Smillie 1955, 479).

Another huge issue of the early twentieth century was the modern birth control movement, initiated by Margaret Sanger. Prior to her efforts, it was against the law for physicians and others to provide information on contraception. A public health nurse, Sanger was aware of the detrimental effects of frequent childbirth on both children and mothers.

These women were all pioneers in the field when public health education was not taken very seriously in medical schools. Charles-Edward Amory Winslow, the father of the public health movement in the early twentieth-century United States, wrote,

> Public Health is not a concrete intellectual discipline, but a field of social activity. It includes applications of chemistry and bacteriology, of engineering and statistics, of physiology and pathology and epidemiology, and in some measure of sociology, and it builds upon these basic sciences a comprehensive program of community service. . . . Preventive medicine must come, as a reality and not a pious phase, through a fundamental change in the attitude of the physician and through a fundamental change in the attitude of the medical school where he is trained. (Winslow 1923, 1, 64)

Eventually there were graduate degrees offered in public health. In 1917, Baker became the first female to hold such a doctorate degree.

In spite of increasing evidence, much of it gathered firsthand by Florence Nightingale, that sanitation and hygiene played a crucial role in health and growing recognition of the importance of the public health field, private practice or surgery continued to command greater respect. Public health was a "marginal" area of medicine (Glaser 1987, 98).

Although physicians today are increasingly aware of phrases such as "population-based health care," which refers to better cost management in order to adequately serve their communities, they need to be better informed in prevention and public health issues.

> Unfortunately, the medical and public health communities have worked separately from each other since the turn of the century. Medicine has taken a biomedical or bioengineering approach to medical care, stressing the achievement of health through disease reduction. The public health profession strongly draws from a social model of health care that emphasizes health promotion and disease prevention and understands health determinates as economic and cultural, as well as molecular and biochemical. Many clinicians have little understanding of basic public health tools, and many public health practitioners have little experience in making their knowledge relevant to the clinical domain. (Ambrose 1997, 1722)

As the AIDS epidemic continues to overwhelm some countries and as bioterrorism continues to be a serious threat to populations, those persons who go into the field will feel a higher obligation than ever, and the women who broke new ground with discoveries, data gathering, and administrative skills will possibly be more appreciated.

See also: Baker, Sara Josephine; Barton, Clara; Dix, Dorothea Lynde; Hamilton, Alice; Nightingale, Florence; Richards, Ellen Henrietta Swallow; Sanger, Margaret; Wald, Lillian D.

References: Ambrose, Paul, "Uniting Public Health and Medicine," *JAMA* 278, no. 21 (3 December 1997): 1722; Bloch, Ernst, *The Principle of Hope*, vol. 2, Cambridge, MA: MIT Press (1986); Delmege, James Anthony, *Towards National Health; or, Health and Hygiene in England from Roman to Victorian Times*, New York: Macmillan (1932); "From the Centers for Disease Control and Prevention. Achievements in Public Health, 1900–1999: Family Planning," *JAMA* 283, no. 3 (19 January 2000): 326–327, 331; Glazer, Penina Migdal, and Miriam Slater, *Unequal Colleagues: The Entrance of Women into the Professions, 1890–1940*, New Brunswick, NJ: Rutgers University Press (1987); Haden-Guest, Leslie, *Votes for Women and the Public Health*, London: Women's Freedom League (1912); Leneman, Leah, *In the Service of Life: The Story of Elsie Inglis and the Scottish Women's Hospitals*, Edinburgh: Mercat Press (1994); Sivulka, Juliann, "From Domestic to Municipal Housekeeper: The Influence of the Sanitary Reform Movement on Changing Women's Roles in America, 1860–1920," *Journal of American Culture* 22, no. 4 (Winter 1999): 1–7; Smillie, Wilson George, *Public Health: Its Promise for the Future; A Chronicle of the Development of Public Health in the United States, 1607–1914*, New York: Macmillan (1955); Tobey, James Alner, *Riders of the Plagues: The Story of the Conquest of Disease*, New York: C. Scribner's Sons (1930); Williams, Ralph Chester, *The United States Public Health Service 1798–1950*, Washington, DC: Commissioned Officers Association, U.S. Public Health Service (1951); Winslow, Charles-Edward Amory, *The Evolution and Significance of the Modern Public Health Campaign*, New Haven, CT: Yale University Press (1923).

Q

Quimby, Edith Hinkley
1891–1982

Edith Quimby was a radiation physicist who was a pioneer in the use of radioisotopes for medical purposes as well as for addressing safety issues in the handling of radioactive materials. She helped bring about the age of radiotherapy and nuclear medicine and enabled later generations to better utilize these methods in cancer treatments and disease diagnosis.

Born on July 10, 1891, in Rockford, Illinois, she was the daughter of Harriet Hinkley and Arthur S. Hinkley. As a child she lived in Illinois, Alabama, and Idaho. She studied mathematics and physics at Whitman College in Walla Walla, Washington.

Quimby taught for a couple of years before pursuing graduate studies in physics at the University of California at Berkeley. She graduated in 1916 and continued to teach. She met and married her husband in 1915, and they both moved to New York City when he accepted a position at Columbia. She became a researcher at the New York City Memorial Hospital for Cancer and Allied Diseases and started studying X rays, correct dosages for the treatment of tumors, and radium, about which not much was known. From 1920 to 1940 she studied radiation and its effects on humans and published her findings. She measured the amount of radiation to which people were being exposed during medical treatment, and the best dosages for treating illness while preventing unnecessary harm to the patient.

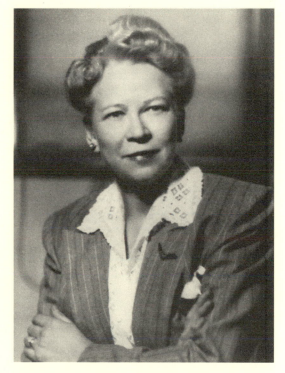

Edith Hinkley Quimby (U.S. National Library of Medicine)

In 1941, Quimby began teaching radiology at Cornell University Medical College, and by 1943 she had moved to Columbia University and was looking into using radium as a tool to conduct research on the circulatory system, thyroid problems, and cancer. She used her knowledge in the development of the atomic bomb during World War II when she worked on the Manhattan Project.

Following the war she became more involved in the safety issues surrounding the handling of radioactive materials. Even after she retired, she continued to be a consultant and to write. She died in New York City on October 11, 1982.

References: Bailey, Martha J., *American Women in Science: A Biographical Dictionary*, Santa Barbara, CA: ABC-CLIO (1994); Carey, Charles W., Jr., "Quimby, Edith Hinkley," *American National Biography*, vol. 18, New York: Oxford University Press (1999).

R

Ramsey, Mimi
1953–

Mimi Ramsey is a nurse and an activist. She was instrumental in influencing the U.S. government to recognize the practice of female genital mutilation (FGM) as child abuse and outlaw its use.

Ramsey was born in Ethiopia. Like many other young girls in the region, she suffered from the emotional trauma and physical pain of FGM. After coming to the United States and after a time of dealing with her personal distress over the experience, she became a vocal advocate of outlawing the practice, which was ongoing in the United States among African immigrants.

Many of the immigrant mothers who are making these decisions about their daughters know little or nothing about their own anatomy. They are told that if the clitoris is left alone, it will grow and drag on the ground; that if their daughters are left uncircumcised, they will be wild, and will crave men; that no man from their home country will marry them uncircumcised (although many African men say that they prefer uncircumcised women for sex and marriage); that circumcision aids in menstruation and childbirth (although the opposite is true in both cases); and that it is a religious—usually Islamic—requirement (although none of the major Islamic texts calls directly for FGM). And so these women and their husbands come to the United States

filled with misinformation, and remain blindly dedicated to continuing this torturous tradition. (Burstyn 1995, 30)

Ramsey has been of great help in counseling many who have been through the experience. The U.S. government banned the practice in 1998. It is also banned in many other countries but is still practiced widely around the world.

See also: Female Genital Mutilation
References: Burstyn, Linda, "Female Circumcision Comes to America," *Atlantic Monthly* 276, no. 4 (October 1995): 28–35; Jensen, Rita Henley, "Mimi Ramsey," *Ms.* 6, no. 4 (January 1996): 50–52.

Remond, Sarah Parker
1826–1894

An active abolitionist in the nineteenth century, Sarah Remond became a physician late in life. She went to Europe, where there was more acceptance of professional black women, to pursue her studies. By leaving the United States, she likely accomplished more as a physician and for women's and blacks' rights than if she had stayed in her home country.

She was born in Salem, Massachusetts, on June 6, 1826. Both her parents, John Remond and Nancy Lenox, were activists in the movement to abolish slavery and influenced her early on to become involved as well. She attended local schools until blacks were forced out in 1835. Her family moved to Newport, Rhode Island, for a time after that, returning to Salem in 1841.

In the 1840s and 1850s, she lectured in the United States and Europe on women's rights and antislavery. Because of her American background, audiences composed of both men and women were allowed to attend her lectures in England. She had great popularity with both the social elite and the working class.

Her brother Charles, a well-known abolitionist, was a proponent of women's rights and encouraged her to participate actively in the cause. "Sarah's decision to join her brother was a courageous one given the prevailing gender expectations held by many black men involved in abolitionism" (Brownlee 1997, 109).

She went to France and settled in Florence, Italy, in 1866. She attended the Santa Maria Nuova Hospital from 1866 to 1868 and became a professional medical practitioner. She was well respected as a black physician. She died on December 13, 1894, and is buried at the Protestant cemetery in Rome.

References: Brownlee, Sibyl Ventress, "Out of the Abundance of the Heart: Sarah Ann Parker Remond's Quest for Freedom," Ph.D. dissertation, Amherst (1997); Hunt, Karen Jean, "Remond, Sarah Parker," *American National Biography*, vol. 18, New York: Oxford University Press (1999); Porter, Dorothy, B., "Remond, Sarah Parker," in Rayford W. Logan and Michael R. Winston, eds., *Dictionary of American Negro Biography*, New York: Norton (1982).

Richards, Ellen Henrietta Swallow
1842–1911

Ellen Richards was a chemist who led the effort for better sanitation in homes and is commonly known as the mother of home economics for the twentieth century. Her work in educating institutions on sanitation, the proper handling of foods, and the importance of water quality fueled the emergence of ecology and home economics as serious disciplines.

Born on December 3, 1842, in Dunstable, Massachusetts, she was the daughter of Peter Swallow and Fanny Gould Taylor Swallow. She went to school at Westford Academy and entered Vassar College, which had been founded in 1861 for women. She graduated in 1870 and decided to go to the Massachusetts Institute of Technology for further studies in chemistry. She was the first woman admitted to MIT, but her tuition was waived because the university did not want a woman on its roster. Richards attended as an "experimental" case. She graduated in 1873 with a B.S. in chemistry and became the first woman to graduate from MIT. She became a laboratory assistant at MIT after the school discouraged her pursuit of a Ph.D.; officials did not want the first Ph.D. in chemistry to go to a woman.

She married Robert Hallowell Richards and continued her career at MIT, teaching sanitation chemistry. She conducted a huge survey of drinking water in Massachusetts in order to check for pollution. While teaching, she also was very active in advocating equal educational rights for women, particularly in the sciences. By the 1890s she was developing the field of home economics.

She was a very practical woman. When friends considered a location for a home or summer cottage, "Mrs. Richards's contribution, or shall we say her part of the housewarming, would almost invariably be a thorough investigation of the water supply. When we consider how many people fall victims to typhoid fever during their summer outings, we realize how valuable this contribution was" (Hunt 1912, 106). Richards continued her work until her death on March 30, 1911.

References: Hunt, Caroline Louisa, *The Life of Ellen H. Richards*, Boston: Whitcomb & Barrows (1912); Stage, Sarah, "Richards, Ellen Henrietta Swallow," *American National Biography*, vol. 21, New York: Oxford University Press (1999).

Richards, Linda
(Melinda Ann Judson)
1841–1930

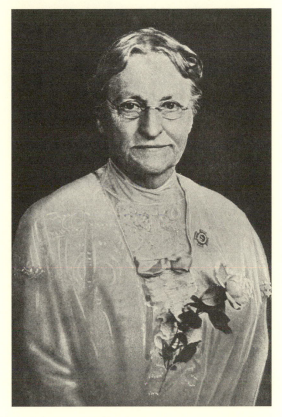

Linda Richards (U.S. National Library of Medicine)

Linda Richards was the first trained nurse in the United States. She was a pioneer in nursing-education reforms and differed significantly from other reformers of her day. From her early experience, she felt nurses needed to be self-sacrificing as well as competent. Unlike many of her colleagues, who felt physicians were hostile to the nursing profession, she was content with the current subjugation of nursing to the authority of hospitals and physicians, whom she trusted. She developed schools with an emphasis on nurses in this subservient role.

Born on July 27, 1841, near Potsdam, New York, she was the daughter of Betsy Sinclair and Sanford Richards. Her family and she were deeply religious, and she began by helping the sick and poor in the community. Before long she was asked to help out in hospitals and was astonished to find such low standards in the nursing field. She found many nurses to be insensitive to patients as well as poorly educated. She was determined to change this state of affairs and embarked on a nursing career.

She graduated in 1873 from a nurses' training course at the New England Hospital for Women and Children, thus becoming the first trained nurse in the United States. The next year she was superintendent of nurses at a Boston training school that later became the Massachusetts General Hospital Training School of Nursing. A few years later she founded the Boston City Hospital Training School for Nurses and disturbed some of her contemporaries by not giving authority for the school to a board of women, which had become the norm. Instead she gave the hospital authority.

She went abroad in order to see the hospitals of Europe. In 1877 she met with Florence Nightingale. "Miss Nightingale showed the truest interest in our American training schools, and it was a marvel to me how she went to the very bottom of everything concerning their needs and the relative value of American methods in compar-

ison with those used in the English and Scotch hospitals. How kindly were all her criticisms, and how carefully did she question me concerning all I had seen while in England and Scotland! Her advice to me concerning the future was absolutely invaluable" (Richards 1915, 52–53).

From 1885 to 1890 she was very involved in the mission field and founded a Japanese nurses' training school in Kyoto. In her many years of service to the nursing profession, Richards oversaw four major hospitals and many small hospitals and mental hospitals and was part of the Visiting Nurses' Service. Other nursing educators who were beginning to form training schools also consulted her on a regular basis. Richards died on April 16, 1930, at the New England Hospital for Women and Children in Boston.

References: Baer, Ellen D., "Richards, Linda," *American National Biography*, vol. 18, New York: Oxford University Press (1999);

Richards, Linda, *Reminiscences of Linda Richards, America's First Trained Nurse*, Boston: Whitcomb & Barrows (1915).

Robb, Isabel Hampton
1860–1910

Isabel Robb was a nursing leader and educator who advocated an undergraduate nursing curriculum in universities as the best way to train nurses. She believed nurses should have an academic education rather than learning in hospital wards alone.

Born on August 26, 1860, in Welland, Ontario, she was the daughter of Samuel Hampton and Sarah Mary Lay. She did very well in school and taught upon completion. She was gifted early on at getting others to work together. She sought tutoring and was very ambitious to do something besides teach. In 1881 she went to New York City to train as a nurse. She graduated from Bellevue Hospital Training School for Nurses in 1883.

Her early experience was quite varied. She first worked at New York's Women's Hospital, then traveled to Rome to work at a small hospital that provided care for travelers. She also worked for various wealthy patients, traveling with them if needed. After returning to the United States, she took a position as superintendent of nurses at the Illinois Training School for Nurses at Cook County Hospital, Chicago.

In 1889 she moved to the newly opened Johns Hopkins Training School for Nurses. She and her assistant, Lavinia Lloyd Dock, began to work toward raising the status of the nursing profession by instituting higher standards and more stringent requirements. She and Dock helped with the organization of the American Society of Superintendents of Training Schools for Nurses of the United States and Canada.

She married Hunter Robb in 1894 and left Johns Hopkins and worked at various nursing occupations in Cleveland, Ohio, where she had three children, one who died in infancy. Five years later she was organizing a

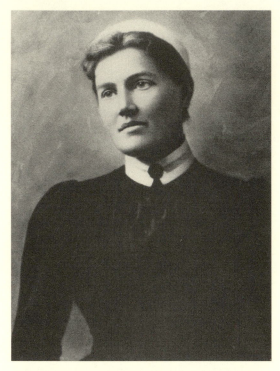

Isabel Hampton Robb (U.S. National Library of Medicine)

graduate training program for nurses at Columbia University in New York. She published books and lectured extensively. She was an able administrator, organizer, and writer.

Robb felt nurses needed to possess personal domestic skill.

> Every woman before entering upon hospital work should be a thoroughly trained housekeeper. Practical household economy should be a part of her home education, for in hospital wards the nurses are the stewards, the caretakers of the hospital property, and upon their thrift and careful ordering must depend the economical outlay of the hospital funds. I cannot dwell upon this practical household economy with too great emphasis, for experience has shown me to a painful extent how this branch of woman's work is neglected or superficially understood by so many women in all ranks of life. A total lack of or appreci-

ation for the principles that govern such work will inevitably be followed by a deficiency in thoroughness and system. (Robb 1985, 28)

Robb's devoted work for the nursing profession was prematurely cut short when she died in a streetcar accident in Cleveland on April 15, 1910.

See also: Dock, Lavinia Lloyd
References: Noel, Nancy L., "Robb, Isabel Hampton," *American National Biography,* vol. 18, New York: Oxford University Press (1999); Robb, Isabel Hampton, *Educational Standards for Nurses,* New York: Garland ([1907] 1985).

Rodriguez-Dulanto, Laura Esther
18?–19?

Laura Rodriguez-Dulanto was the first female physician in Peru. She graduated from the University of San Marcos at Lima in 1900.

References: Lovejoy, Esther Pohl, *Women Doctors of the World,* New York: Macmillan (1957).

Russell Gurney Enabling Act of 1876

The Russell Gurney Enabling Act of 1876, passed by the British Parliament, overturned the Medical Act of 1858, which excluded women from medical schools. The Russell Gurney Act gave women the same rights as men to enter medical schools and receive a medical education. The bill was proposed by Russell Gurney, a member of Parliament in London who supported equal education for both sexes, and Sophia Jex-Blake. Those who wanted women excluded from medical schools and the practice of medicine opposed the act. With its passage, Jex-Blake was able to finally obtain her license to practice medicine from the Irish College of Physicians.

See also: Jex-Blake, Sophia Louisa; Medical Act of 1858
References: Roberts, Shirley, *Sophia Jex-Blake: A Woman Pioneer in Nineteenth Century Medical Reform,* London: Routledge (1993).

Ruys, A. Charlotte
1898–1980?

Charlotte Ruys was a professor of microbiology. She served as dean of the medical faculty at the University of Amsterdam.

Born December 21, 1898, in Dedemsvaart, the Netherlands, she was one of eight children. She was interested in medicine at an early age and went to Utrecht University. During her final years there women were experiencing sexual harassment, so she chose to transfer to the University of Groningen, where she graduated in 1924.

She worked for the Public Health Service as a physician beginning in 1928. "It was wonderful to be able to combine practice and research," she said of the experience.

My first real success was when I was able to demonstrate that microscopic examination of specimens from children with vulvovaginitis often led to a false diagnosis of gonorrhea. In studying typhoid fever, we found that contaminated water was frequently the source of infection. The new methods of typing bacteria made possible a more thorough study of the epidemiology of many infectious diseases. In the 1930s I gave courses of lectures on food hygiene to girls studying at a school of social science. (Hellstedt 1978, 165)

Ruys saw both world wars. During World War II, medical supplies and even food were hard to come by. She tended both Germans and Allied soldiers but was an active member of the resistance movement.

"In February of 1945 I was arrested because I was in contact with a radio transmitter of the Allies. A colleague bacteriologist and three others who were also arrested were shot a few days later. As I was a woman, I had to be shot in Germany. I was in prison with two other women condemned on the same charge. We were not moved, as transport to Germany was impossible; the Allies had blocked all the roads. The day after the German surrender, we were set free" (Hellstedt 1978, 166).

She married Guus Defresne in 1945 and they were together until his death in 1961. Ruys served as dean of the medical faculty at the University of Amsterdam from 1949 to 1953 and later worked with the Government Advisory Commission for Health until 1966. She resigned from the university in 1969 when she was seventy years old.

References: Hellstedt, Leone McGregor, *Women Physicians of the World: Autobiographies of Medical Pioneers*, Washington, DC: Hemisphere (1978); Lovejoy, Esther Pohl, *Women Doctors of the World*, New York: Macmillan (1957).

S

el Saadawi, Nawal
1931–

Nawal el Saadawi is known for her writings, which reveal the hardships many young girls and women endure in some Arab cultures. A physician and psychiatrist, Saadawi has been persecuted many times for her advocacy of women's sexual rights, and she has worked to educate others on the harmful medical and emotional consequences of female circumcision.

She was born on October 27, 1931, in Kafr Tahla, Egypt, to el Sayed and Zeinab. She attended Cairo University and earned a medical degree in 1955 and a master's in public health (M.P.H.) from Columbia University in 1966. She used her education to gain employment as the director of health education with the Egyptian government's Ministry of Health. In 1971 she was dismissed from her job due to her outspoken views on women's rights.

In *The Hidden Face of Eve: Women in the Arab World*, Saadawi gives a graphic description of her and her sister being circumcised when she was six years old. That experience, as well as seeing innumerable little girls in her clinic who were suffering from the physical and psychological effects of circumcision—effects that sometimes included death—changed her focus. She lost interest in a medical career and became more involved in speaking out against the continuing tragedy.

"As a rural doctor I lived close to village people, shared their experiences, learnt about their lives, witnessed what the triple scourge of poverty, ignorance and sickness did to them. Women bore a double burden since they also suffered from the oppression exercised on them by fathers and husbands, brothers and uncles and other men. I saw young girls burn themselves alive, or throw themselves into the waters of the Nile and drown, in order to escape a father's or a husband's tyranny" (Saadawi 1999, 290–291).

Saadawi found that one physician could not fix the bigger problem and turned to writing in order to better help those who suffered.

"I was not attracted to the medical profession. It seemed unable to do much in face of the sufferings imposed on people. I realized how sickness and poverty are linked to politics, to money and power, that medical practice was removed from our everyday life. Writing became a weapon with which to fight the system, which draws its authority from the autocratic power exercised by the ruler of the state, and that of the father or the husband in the family. The written word for me became an act of rebellion against injustice exercised in the name of religion, or morals, or love" (Saadawi 1999, 291–292).

Saadawi has most recently been a visiting professor at Duke University. She has two children.

References: Hiro, Dilip, *Dictionary of the Middle East*, New York: St. Martin's Press (1996); "Nawal El Saadawi," *Contemporary Authors Online*, Gale Group (2001); Saadawi, Nawal, *A Daughter of Isis: The Autobiography of Nawal El Saadawi*, London: Zed Books

(1999); Saadawi, Nawal, *The Hidden Face of Eve: Women in the Arab World*, Boston, MA: Beacon Press (1982).

Sabin, Florence Rena
1871–1953

Florence Sabin was the first woman elected to the National Academy of Sciences. Her extensive research in embryology and histology led to the discovery that blood cells and the lymphatic system develop in the veins and not in the tissue of the embryo. She was also the first woman faculty member of Johns Hopkins University School of Medicine.

Born in Central City, Colorado, November 9, 1871, she was the daughter of George K. Sabin and Serena Miner Sabin. Her father was a mining engineer, and she had one older sister. Her mother died when she was very young, and she was raised in part by an uncle in Chicago, then moved to Vermont to attend the Vermont Academy in Saxton's River.

She originally wanted to become a musician but later decided to take college preparatory courses. Her sister, Mary, went to Smith College in 1887, and Florence joined her in 1889. She excelled at science and determined to be a doctor even though her father and sister were not supportive. She was encouraged by news that Johns Hopkins was going to allow women to enter its new medical school and tutored to earn the tuition. She graduated from Smith College in 1893, and then taught for three years, entering medical school in 1897.

Women students had become the norm by the time Sabin entered Johns Hopkins, and scholastic requirements were high. She did very well and was influenced and encouraged by Franklin Mall, a well-known anatomist at Johns Hopkins University. She gained an internship upon completing her studies and later became the first full-time woman professor at Johns Hopkins. She did much research in embryology and histology and was one of the earliest researchers to use supravital staining as a technique for studying blood cells. She wrote extensively in the medical literature. One of her works,

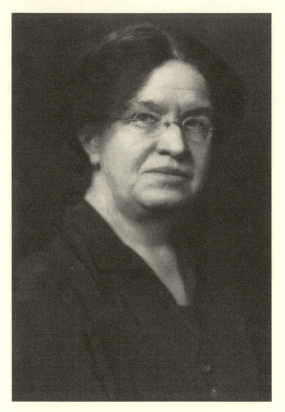

Florence Rena Sabin (U.S. National Library of Medicine)

the *Atlas of the Medulla and Midbrain*, published in 1901, served for many years as a standard medical textbook.

Her major contribution to medicine was discovering that "the lymphatics arise from veins by sprouts of endothelium, and next that these sprouts or buds connect with each other as they grow outwards from the veins toward the periphery, so that the entire system is derived from already existing vessels. Further, she showed that the peripheral ends of the lymphatics are closed and that they neither open into the tissue spaces nor are derived from them" (McMaster and Heidelberger 1960, 279). She left Johns Hopkins in 1925 to join Simon Flexner at the Rockefeller Institute. She was the first woman to head the American Association of Anatomists and in 1925 was elected to the National Academy of Sciences, the first female to be so honored.

Sabin joined her sister in Colorado in 1938 and eventually became immersed in public health issues. She became very well-known in Colorado during her day as a public health proponent and did much to encourage better funding, conditions, and legislation. She died in Denver, Colorado, on October 3, 1953. Her statue is in the U.S. Capitol.

See also: Johns Hopkins University
References: Bluemel, Elinor, *Florence Sabin: Colorado Woman of the Century*, Boulder, CO: University of Colorado Press (1959); Delaney, James J., Jr., "Roy Cleere and Florence Sabin," *Colorado Medicine* 80, no. 2 (February 1983): 46–47; Harvey, Abner McGehee, "A New School of Anatomy: The Story of Franklin P. Mall, Florence R. Sabin and John B. MacCallum," *Johns Hopkins Medical Journal* 136, no. 2 (February 1975): 83–94; McMaster, Philip D., and Michael Heidelberger, "Florence Rena Sabin," *Biographical Memoirs* 34, New York: National Academy of Sciences (1960); Morantz-Sanchez, Regina, "Sabin, Florence Rena," *American National Biography*, vol. 19, New York: Oxford University Press (1999).

Salber, Eva Juliet
1916–1990

Eva Salber was a South African physician who worked with her husband in public and community health care in South Africa, the United Kingdom, and the United States. She advocated ceaselessly for equal health care for minorities, those in rural communities, and the elderly.

Born in Cape Town, South Africa, on January 5, 1916, Salber was the daughter of Moses Salber and Fanny Srolowitz Salber. She married Harry Tarley Phillips in 1939, and they had four children. She received her education at the University of Cape Town, earning a medical degree in 1955. She worked in South Africa at the Sir Henry Elliott Hospital in Umtata, the Cape Town Free Dispensary, and the Institute of Family and Community Health in Durban. In London she worked at the Queen Elizabeth Hospital for Children.

In 1956 she went to the United States and became naturalized in 1961. She worked in Boston at the Children's Hospital Medical Center and the Martha Eliot Health Center for several years before moving to the Duke University School of Medicine. Her interests lay in rural health care and equal care for the poor in both urban and rural settings. She taught her students with enthusiasm and tried to give them a sense of what poor people had to go through to obtain proper care.

The discrimination Salber faced as a woman and a Jew did not deter her from success as both a physician and a mother. In her autobiography she says, "I believe that being a mother made me a gentler, more sympathetic doctor and that being a doctor made me a more loving and understanding mother. It isn't easy for women to combine motherhood and work outside the home, and we often feel guilty, but reviewing my life enabled me to acknowledge that my well-being depended not only on the love of my family but also on the satisfaction I got in being useful to some of society's disregarded people" (Salber 1989, 273). Salber passed away on November 18, 1990.

References: Salber, Eva Juliet, *The Mind Is Not the Heart: Recollections of a Woman Physician*, Durham, NC: Duke University Press (1989); Salber, Eva Juliet, "Payment for Health Care in the United States: A Personal Statement," *Journal of Public Health Policy* 4, no. 2 (June 1983): 202–206; *Who's Who of American Women*, 17th ed., Chicago: Marquis Who's Who (1991).

Salpêtrière Asylum
1656–1970

Louis XIV established the Salpêtrière Asylum in order to house poor men and women in Paris. It is best known for the work of Phillippe Pinel in establishing more humane methods for dealing with and treating the mentally ill who were placed there in the late nineteenth century. It had significance for many women desiring medical training because the Salpêtrière Asylum allowed them to work there when traditional hospitals turned them away. It became a traditional hospital in 1970—Hospital de la Pitié Salpêtrière (where Princess Diana died in 1997).

References: Guillain, Georges, and Pierre Mathieu, *La Salpêtrière*, Paris, France: Masson (1925).

Sanger, Margaret
1879–1966

Margaret Sanger was a nurse who crusaded early in the twentieth century for women's rights to birth-control information. She fought state and federal laws prohibiting contraceptive information and forced the issue into the public. Her work as a visiting nurse to New York City's poor gave her insight into the toll frequent childbirth had on families.

She was born on September 14, 1879, in Corning, New York, to Michael Hennessey Higgins and Anne Purcell Higgins. She had ten siblings and felt that her mother's death at a young age was due to her having and caring for so many children. Margaret decided early on that she wanted an education and attended Claverack College, Hudson River Institute, and White Plains Hospital. She worked toward her registered-nurse degree but quit when she married. She and her husband, William Sanger, moved to Westchester, New York, and had three children.

They returned to New York in 1911, and Sanger became involved in the radical activism of New York that preceded World War I. She began writing on topics such as venereal disease, sex education, and contraception and had several run-ins with the postal authorities, who considered her information obscene. Such information was, in fact, obscene according to the laws of the time.

Sanger later wrote,

The following spring found me still seeking and more determined than ever to find out something about contraception and its mysteries. Why was it so difficult to obtain information on

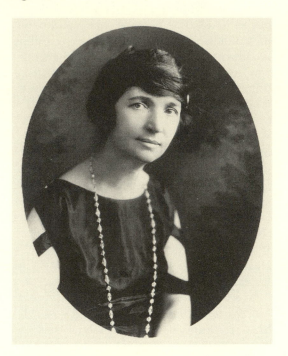

Margaret Sanger (Underwood and Underwood/ Library of Congress)

this subject? Where was it hidden? Why would no one discuss it? It was like the missing link in the evolution of medical science. It was like the lost trail in the journey toward freedom. Seek it I would. If it was in existence it should be found. I would never give up until I had obtained it nor stop until the working women of my generation in the country of my birth were acquainted with its substance. (Sanger 1932, 58)

Sanger was indicted in 1914 for violation of the obscenity laws. She did not feel she could have a just trial, so she jumped bail and went to England. Her marriage to Sanger ended the same year. In England, she prepared her defense and was influenced by Havelock Ellis, who was challenging the views on sexuality long held by traditional Victorian society.

She returned to face the charges against her in 1915. "I was not afraid of the penitentiary. I was not afraid of anything except being misunderstood. That I dreaded. I did not want to go to jail for 'obscenity,' but I had no hesitation to go for a principle or as a challenge to the obscenity laws, providing my case could be properly heard" (Sanger 1932, 90).

Her daughter Peggy died that same year, and because she had the sympathy of much of the public, the government decided not to prosecute her. She then decided to travel and lecture. Eventually she turned her focus away from censorship issues and toward the availability of contraceptives for women. She felt they would liberate women physically, emotionally, and economically.

She opened the first birth-control clinic in the United States in October 1916. The authorities closed it several days later and arrested her. She continued to fight, and two years later physicians were able to prescribe birth control. She then aimed at ensuring women's rights to sexual information and birth control and at gaining government assistance for contraceptive services.

Over the next several decades Sanger organized, increased public awareness of the issues, and sought international assistance. The medical profession was mixed on the issue. She eventually sought better female contraceptives and helped raise the funds necessary for Gregory Pincus to develop the first birth-control pill.

She has been synonymous with the birth-control movement for decades, but she also was motivated from the beginning to give women the chance to live the healthy lives possible if they were aware of a means of limiting reproduction. Her efforts were geared toward lengthening lives, enabling women to have careers, helping children have better health, and affording men better socioeconomic situations by having fewer children to take care of. Sanger died on September 6, 1966.

References: Katz, Esther, "Sanger, Margaret," *American National Biography,* vol. 19, New York: Oxford University Press (1999); Sanger, Margaret, *My Fight for Birth Control,* London: Faber & Faber (1932).

Saunders, Cicely Mary Strode
1918–

Cicely Saunders is the English founder of the current-day hospice movement. The movement has revolutionized the way health care workers, counselors, families, and physicians look at death and dying, patients' rights, and the options of the terminally ill.

Born in the borough of Barnet, in Greater London, Saunders attended Roedean School and later St. Anne's College at the University of Oxford. She trained at the Nightingale School of Nursing as well as the St. Thomas Medical School. She was a medical student from 1951 to 1957. During this time, she witnessed the beneficial effects of many new drugs. She went on to St. Joseph's Hospice in London, where she worked until 1965. She saw firsthand the physical and emotional needs of terminal patients and their families and wrote and lectured a great deal.

In 1967 she founded St. Christopher's Hospice in Sydenham in an effort to help those with terminal illnesses die with dignity. She promoted sensitive nursing care for the dying, pain control, and the concept that death is a part of living rather than a medical failure. She continued educating others, particularly health practitioners, on the importance of palliative care.

Saunders feels it is very important to do research and have good physicians at St. Christopher's Hospice. She "has always been determined that St. Christopher's should be unrivalled medically; that in building a hospice as a protest against the shortcomings of modern high technology she would not lose the benefits that modern technology has to offer. To fulfill this aim she needed not only the best clinical physicians, she also needed a research team to establish and develop the scientific foundations on which their teaching is based" (Du Boulay 1984, 183). She became a DBE (Dame of the British Empire) in 1980 and received the Order of Merit in 1989. She lives in England.

References: Du Boulay, Shirley, *Cicely Saunders: Founder of the Modern Hospice Move-*

ment, New York: Amaryllis Press (1984); Parry, Melanie, ed., *Chambers Biographical Dictionary*, Edinburgh: Chambers (1997); Saunders, Cicely, "A Personal Therapeutic Journey," *British Medical Journal* 313, no. 7072 (21–28 December 1996): 1599–1601.

Scharlieb, Mary Ann Dacomb Bird
1845–1930

Mary Ann Dacomb Scharlieb was the first woman in England to be appointed to a medical position at a general hospital (Royal Free Hospital in London) and founded the Royal Victoria Hospital in India around 1884.

Born in London on June 18, 1845, she received her early education in Manchester. It wasn't until after her marriage in 1865 to William Scharlieb, and their move to India, that she became interested in medicine. Her husband was an attorney and while helping him with his practice, she found herself assisting the local women with childbirth after hearing about their reluctance to see male physicians if they had problems. She determined to study medicine and went to the Madras Medical College in India. Although she qualified for a medical license there, she returned to England to gain more medical education, receiving her M.D. from London University in 1888. She was the first woman to obtain a medical degree there, with the encouragement of Florence Nightingale and Elizabeth Garrett Anderson.

Eventually she began teaching at the Madras Medical College as well as continuing to build her own practice in India, becoming an able surgeon. Her husband died in 1891. Two of her three children became doctors. She died on November 21, 1930.

References: Cullis, W. C., "Scharlieb, Dame Mary Ann Dacomb," *Dictionary of National Biography, 1922–1930*, Oxford: Oxford University Press (1937); Haines, Catharine M. C., and Helen Stevens, *International Women in Science: A Biographical Dictionary to 1950*, Santa Barbara, CA: ABC-CLIO (2001);

Scharlieb, Mary Ann Dacomb Bird, *Reminiscences*, London: Williams and Norgate (1924), reproduced in the Gerritsen Collection of Women's History, no. 2518.2, Sanford, NC: Microfilming Corporation of America (1975–1977).

Scottish Women's Hospitals
1914–1919

Dr. Elsie Maud Inglis of Scotland founded the Scotland Women's Hospitals (SWH). They were established in order for women to serve as physicians and allied health practitioners in World War I.

During World War I, women who had training as physicians and nurses were barred from serving in regular medical units. Inglis raised the money and in late 1914 established the Scottish Women's Hospitals, made up of numerous units that served all over Europe until the close of World War I. The women of the Scottish Women's Hospitals not only served the war effort but proved that an all-woman medical unit could get the job done. Many lost their lives in service.

> This characteristic common to them all, of strength, reliability, and efficiency, has been impressed on each Unit largely by its chief medical officer. These last tragic years disclose in the ranks of the S.W.H., and many another organization, an unfailing supply of women with force of character, largeness of mind, and powers of leadership, combined with professional skill in various directions, who have devotedly given their services to humanity in noble and unselfish labour. This must be a source of profound joy to all who love their country. (McLaren 1919, 358)

The all-woman hospitals, using prisoners as orderlies, served Serb, Russian, French, Italian, German, British, Austrian, Turkish, Greek, Bulgarian, and Romanian soldiers and civilians. They traveled anywhere they were needed. They dealt with difficult terrain in all weather conditions and drove through explosions and gunfire to set up hospital units. They were a dependable, very competent, and courageous group of women who fought epidemics, typhus, tuberculosis, and dysentery and performed numerous surgical operations.

See also: Inglis, Elsie Maud
References: McLaren, Eva Shaw, *A History of the Scottish Women's Hospitals,* London: Hodder & Stoughton (1919).

Scudder, Ida Sophia
1870–1960

Ida Scudder was a pioneer medical missionary. She established a hospital and medical college in Vellore, India, and served for decades.

She was born in Ranipet, India, on December 9, 1870, to medical missionary John Scudder and Sophia Weld Scudder. She grew up in India and at times in the United States. In her early life she wanted to stay in the United States and not become a missionary like so many in her family before her, but she visited her parents in India in 1890 and had a life-changing experience.

One night when she and her father were in the mission, three men came to ask for help for their wives, who were in labor. John Scudder could not help because the Hindu religion forbade a man to see or examine a woman. Ida Scudder had no medical training and did not go. During the evening all three women died, and Ida Scudder determined that God wanted her to serve the women of India as a physician.

Scudder went to the Women's Medical College of Pennsylvania in 1895 and eventually decided to go to Cornell in New York when it opened to women. She obtained her medical degree in 1899 and went to India, deciding her father would be her best practical teacher.

Throughout her long and arduous training as a medical student, Ida did not swerve from her accepted purpose. India claimed a devotion that never wavered. To return to India, qualified by skill and science to be of service to her people, was the one absorbing ambition of this eager and impetuous, yet disciplined woman. The dream of one who had no sisters of her own was that the day would come when she might be a sister to others who, in seclusion, suffered pain that might be abated and died preventable deaths. Her busy brain seethed with great plans for the future. (Jeffery 1938, 57)

Before going to India, she raised money for a hospital in Vellore. She was on her own fairly soon after arriving, as her father died within the first year. She found herself in a very rural area, and many patients were hesitant to come to a woman doctor. Eventually they accepted her and sought out her help.

One of her endeavors was to help the rural population find transportation. She began a series of roadside clinics that became very popular. She was able to secure vehicles that typically

held ten people plus medicine boxes, powder bags, sterile dressings and instruments. There were ten stops on the Gudiyatham roadside and so great was the demand for medical attention that the car was often overcrowded. Waiting patients had to be taken to the hospital in Vellore for operations or better care and a chance visitor might find herself holding one or two passengers in her lap while the servant boy returned to Vellore, standing on the running board. Members of the staff in Vellore Medical College are now getting dusty on four roadsides every week. They scout, they preach, they prescribe, they operate on the roadsides, and they offer no apologies. (Jeffery 1938, 146)

Her biggest contribution was her dedication to rural health care and the implementation of the roadside clinics. Her faith and hard work inspired those who worked with her. The hospital in Vellore was built in a short time after she arrived and opened in 1902. As the workload increased she realized she would need to teach Indian women to care for the people. She opened a nursing school and eventually the Vellore Medical College.

Scudder stayed active in India most of her life, working, teaching, and caring for the people there. The friends and the patients she cared for were her family. She died on May 24, 1960, near her home in Kodaikanal.

References: Jeffery, Mary Pauline, *Dr. Ida: India—The Life Story of Ida S. Scudder,* New York: Fleming H. Revell (1938); Jumonville, Robert Stuart, "Scudder, Ida Sophia," *American National Biography,* vol. 20, New York: Oxford University Press (1999).

Seacole, Mary Jane Grant
1805–1881

Mary Jane Seacole was a Jamaican who served as a nurse with the British during the Crimean War. She received the Order of Merit posthumously in 1990.

Born in Kingston, Jamaica, to an African American woman and a Scottish soldier, Mary Jane became very successful running boardinghouses for soldiers, as her mother had done. While tending to the needs of her guests, she developed skills in treating wounds and tropical diseases and even performed minor surgeries.

She had married Edwin Horatio Seacole, but after his early death, she and a brother left Jamaica and went to New Granada (now known as Colombia, Ecuador, Panama, and Venezuela). She found herself treating people suffering from cholera. When cholera broke out in epidemic proportions in Jamaica in 1853, she returned and served people there in large part based on her experiences in New Granada.

She traveled to Haiti, Cuba, the Bahamas, and eventually to England, where she served in the Crimean War. She was a free black woman, unlike many of her contemporaries, and was able to make a significant contribution to the war effort.

Her autobiography was very successful in the years following the war. She wrote of the siege of Sebastopol: "A line of sentries forbade all strangers passing through without orders, even to Cathcart's Hill; but once more I found that my reputation served as a permit, and the officers relaxed the rule in my favour everywhere. So, early in the day, I was in my old spot, with my old appliances for the wounded and fatigued; little expecting, however, that this day would so closely resemble the day of the last attack in its disastrous results" (Seacole 1988, 170).

Some soldiers referred to her long after the war ended as the Crimean Heroine. She died on May 14, 1881, of a stroke.

References: Brice-Finch, Jacqueline, "Seacole, Mary," *Oxford Companion to African American Literature,* New York: Oxford University Press (1997); Seacole, Mary, *Wonderful Adventures of Mrs. Seacole in Many Lands,* New York: Oxford University Press ([1857] 1988); Snodgrass, Mary Ellen, *Historical Encyclopedia of Nursing,* Santa Barbara, CA: ABC-CLIO (1999).

Seibert, Florence Barbara
1897–1991

Florence Seibert was a scientist who helped develop the tuberculin test. She also contributed to implementing better safety standards for drug therapy.

Born on October 6, 1897, in Easton, Pennsylvania, Seibert survived polio at age three to graduate with high honors from high school. She attended Goucher College in Towson, Maryland, and majored in chemistry. After graduating in 1918 she worked during World War I at Hammersley Paper Mill as a chemist and then won a scholarship to Yale. She earned a doctorate in 1923 in biochemistry.

During her doctoral work she discovered that patients receiving drug therapy could develop fevers from contaminated distilled water. She developed a new method for distillation that killed all the bacteria. She continued her research at the University of Chicago and then taught and conducted re-

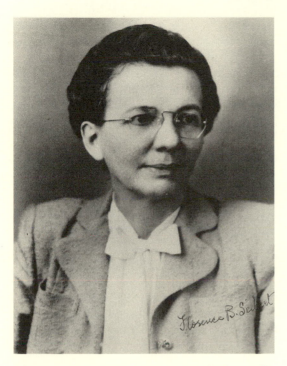

Florence Barbara Seibert (U.S. National Library of Medicine)

search at the Sprague Memorial Institute. It was there that she was involved in discovering "that the tuberculin protein, like other proteins, was an excellent antigen; that is, when, as a foreign substance it was injected into the body it stimulated the body to produce antibodies in the blood stream against it. Antibodies are known to be able to combine with the antigens that induced them and in this way frequently produce immunity and protect the body against any toxic action that the free antigens might have. Various aspects of these immunological reactions were studied" (Seibert 1968, 46). She later went with Dr. Esmond R. Long to the Henry Phipps Institute at the University of Pennsylvania.

She received a Guggenheim Fellowship and traveled to Sweden in 1937 to do research at Uppsala University. There she was able to isolate tuberculosis protein molecules and use the material to develop the skin test for infection. The tuberculin skin test is still used today. The United States adopted it as a standard in 1941 and the World Health Organization, in 1952.

Seibert taught at the University of Pennsylvania, becoming a full professor in 1955. She retired in 1958, at which time she became a consultant for the U.S. Public Health Service. She continued her research, focusing on cancer at the Cancer Research Laboratory in St. Petersburg, Florida. Seibert died on August 23, 1991, in St. Petersburg.

References: Lambert, Bruce, "Dr. Florence B. Seibert, Inventor of Standard TB Test, Dies at 93," *New York Times*, sec. 1 (31 August 1991): 12, col. 4; Seibert, Florence Barbara, *Pebbles on the Hill of a Scientist*, St. Petersburg, FL: St. Petersburg Printing (1968); Shearer, Benjamin F., and Barbara S. Shearer, *Notable Women in the Physical Sciences*, Westport, CT: Greenwood Press (1997).

Sewall, Lucy Ellen
1837–1890

Lucy Sewall was one of the few nineteenth-century female physicians who had a thriving practice as well as hospital responsibilities. She spent the majority of her professional career in Boston at the New England Hospital for Women and Children.

She was born in Boston, Massachusetts, on April 26, 1837, to Samuel E. Sewall and Louisa Maria Winslow. Her father was very supportive of women's rights, and she had a liberal education. In 1856 she met Marie Zakrzewska and became interested in medicine. She saw the need for female physicians, particularly their value for women and children's health.

She enrolled at the New England Female Medical College, and Zakrzewska also tutored her a great deal. She received her medical degree in 1862 and then traveled to Europe to gain valuable practical experience in clinics and hospitals. She returned to Boston in 1863 and became resident physician at the New England Hospital for Women and Children. She remained there the rest of her life and became very popular, many patients wanting to see only her. She also worked at building the hospital's training program for other women who needed clinical experience.

Sewall led the way for many other women to seek a medical education. She suffered from poor health off and on her entire life and died on February 13, 1890, in Boston from heart disease.

See also: New England Hospital; Zakrzewska, Marie Elizabeth

References: Kass, Amalie M., "Sewall, Lucy Ellen," *American National Biography*, vol. 19, New York: Oxford University Press (1999); Morantz-Sanchez, Regina Markell, *Sympathy and Science: Women Physicians in American Medicine*, New York: Oxford University Press (1985).

Shaibany, Homa
1913?–19?

Homa Shaibany was the first woman surgeon in Iran. She received a scholarship from the Persian government to attend London University in 1930. She was one of the fortunate few foreigners to gain admittance to one of the only two colleges that admitted women. She proved to have exceptional talent.

Shaibany was born in Tehran to the daughter of a Cambridge graduate and wanted to study medicine in order to help the women of her country. She was educated at a U.S. mission school before proceeding to London University. During "her pre-clinical years she proved so brilliant in human anatomy and morphology, embryology, and neurology, that her professors advised her to postpone clinical study and take a degree in these subjects" (Fahimi 1952, 272).

She subsequently stayed at London University and received her B.Sc. in anatomy and morphology. She obtained clinical experience in Dublin at the Rotunda Hospital and earned her licentiate from the Royal College of Physicians. Unfortunately she could not return to Iran when she received her M.B.B.S. in 1939, since World War II had started. She stayed in England, and since there was a need for physicians there, she worked in the Redlands Hospital for Women in Glasgow and then at the Nuneaton Emergency Hospital. After it was destroyed by bombing, she worked at numerous other British hospitals and operated during wartime conditions of bombings and heavy casualty loads.

After the armistice she remained in London at St. Leonard's Hospital until 1948, when she returned to Persia to finally serve her own country. She found much opposition from men and no possibility to teach or obtain a post at a university. However, she persevered because she knew Muslim women were forbidden to be seen by a male physician and thus needed her services.

She was eventually aided and encouraged by Princess Shamse, head of the Persian Red Cross. She established a hospital for the Red Cross and aided in its successful operation, always dealing with resentment from male physicians.

References: Fahimi, Miriam, "Homa Shaibany, M.B.B.S.: First Woman Surgeon of Iran," *Journal of the American Medical Women's Association* 7, no. 7 (July 1952): 272–273; Lovejoy, Esther Pohl, *Women Doctors of the World*, New York: Macmillan (1957).

Sheppard-Towner Act of 1921

The Sheppard-Towner Act of 1921 was passed by Congress under pressure from women physicians, particularly those of the U.S. Children's Bureau, to better educate women about prenatal care, regulate midwifery, and establish health centers. Many male physicians of the American Medical Association were convinced that the American Medical Women's Association had pressed for the act in order to show some political weight, as women had just obtained the right to vote. They felt that women were trying to control maternal health care and lobbied to overturn the act. The ensuing battle reflected both good intentions and political motivations, and Congress rescinded the act in 1929.

References: Barker, Kristin, "Women Physicians and the Gendered System of Professions: An Analysis of the Sheppard-Towner Act of 1921," *Work and Occupations* 25, no. 2 (May 1998): 229–255.

Sherrill, Mary Lura
1888–1968

Mary Sherrill worked on antimalarial drugs to replace quinine, which was impossible for countries in Southeast Asia to obtain during World War II. Some of the new drugs that came out of the research Sherrill headed are still used instead of quinine in many instances.

Born on July 14, 1888, in Salisbury, North Carolina, she was the daughter of Miles Sherrill and Sarah Bost Sherrill. The youngest of seven, she received her early education at the public schools before entering Randolph-Macon Women's College. She received her bachelor's degree in chemistry in 1909 and a master's in physics in 1911. She remained at Randolph-Macon for five years as a teacher.

In 1916 she went to the University of Chicago to work on her Ph.D. in chemistry. Before she obtained her degree she was asked to work with the Chemical Warfare Service during World War I. She eventually obtained her doctorate in 1923 while also working at Mt. Holyoke College in South Hadley, Massachusetts. She advanced to associate professor in 1924, full professor in 1931, and chair of the Department of Chemistry in 1946. Her research at Mt. Holyoke focused on antimalarials to replace quinine.

She also studied briefly with the physicist Johannes D. van der Waals in Amsterdam in order to learn more about synthesizing and purifying organic compounds. She received the Garvan Medal from the American Chemical Society in 1947. She retired in 1954 and after several years moved back to North Carolina. She died in High Point, North Carolina, on October 27, 1968.

References: Grinstein, Louise S., Carol Rose, K. Rose, and Miriam H. Rafailovich, *Women in Chemistry and Physics: A Biobibliographic Sourcebook*, Westport, CT: Greenwood Press (1993); Shearer, Benjamin F., and Barbara S. Shearer, *Notable Women in the*

Physical Sciences, Westport, CT: Greenwood Press (1997).

Siegemundin, Justine Dittrichin
1630–1705

Justine Siegemundin was a Silesian midwife. She wrote a text for midwives that was heavily utilized. She was self-taught and served the royal family of Prussia.

References: Ogilvie, Marilyn, and Joy Harvey, eds., *The Biographical Dictionary of Women in Science: Pioneering Lives from Ancient Times to the Mid-20th Century*, New York: Routledge (2000).

Solis, Manuela
18?–18?

Manuela Solis was the first female physician in Spain. She graduated from the University of Valencia. She did graduate study in Paris and returned to Valencia and enjoyed a successful practice. She later moved to Madrid and practiced obstetrics and gynecology.

References: Lovejoy, Esther Pohl, *Women Doctors of the World*, New York: Macmillan (1957).

Solis Quiroga, Margarita Delgado de
fl. 1926–1957

Margarita Solis Quiroga was an early Mexican physician. She also served as a physiology and biology professor at the University of Mexico.

References: Lovejoy, Esther Pohl, *Women Doctors of the World*, New York: Macmillan (1957); Ogilvie, Marilyn, and Joy Harvey, eds., *The Biographical Dictionary of Women in Science: Pioneering Lives from Ancient Times to the Mid-20th Century*, New York: Routledge (2000).

Spaangberg-Holth, Marie
1865–1942

Marie Spaangberg-Holth was the first female physician in Norway. She led the way for others shortly after the University of Norway opened its doors to women.

Born in 1865, Spaangberg-Holth received her medical degree from the University of Norway in 1893 and went to Germany to study obstetrics and gynecology. She began a private practice the following year in Oslo. The government then appointed her to work within the Department of Venereal Diseases, where she treated women primarily for syphilis.

She married ophthalmologist Soren Holth in 1897 and focused on diseases of the eye for the rest of her career. She raised three children. Spaangberg-Holth died in 1942.

References: Gundersen, Herdis, "Medical Women in Norway," *Journal of the American Medical Women's Association* 6, no. 7 (July 1951): 281; Lovejoy, Esther Pohl, *Women Doctors of the World*, New York: Macmillan (1957).

Spoerry, Anne
1918–1999?

Anne Spoerry was a female doctor in Kenya who became a regional legend. She piloted a small airplane, bringing medical services to a vast number of farmers in cooperation with the African Medical Research Foundation (AMREF).

Born in 1918 to a Swiss-Alsatian family, she wanted to study medicine from an early age and went to Paris. Her studies were disrupted by the Nazi occupation of Paris, and she and her brother François worked with the French Resistance and ran a safe house. The Gestapo arrested them in 1943 and sent them to Fresnes Prison and later on to Ravensbruck, a concentration camp where she tried to utilize the few medical skills she had to help the sick.

After liberation she had to recuperate before furthering her medical studies. She received a medical degree in tropical medicine after study in Paris and Switzerland. In Kenya, while helping farmers who needed a physician, the AMREF asked her to join and open flying clinics in northeastern Kenya. She made her rounds over a five-week period and became very familiar with spear and gunshot wounds, various diseases, and infection.

Spoerry sometimes had to take her patients by plane to a hospital. One patient was the only survivor of a family that had been murdered. Once in the plane,

> she began to yell at the top of her voice. She then undid her seat belt and tried to throw herself out of the door. I had to keep the plane steady with one hand, while, with the other, trying to keep her in her seat. I tried to reason with her but she did not speak Swahili. Finally I offered her something to eat. I think it was a biscuit and this seemed to pacify her. . . . Three months later I passed through Nakuru. At the hospital a woman called out to me. It was my patient, now fully recovered. She had acquired a little Swahili, sufficient for us to carry on a conversation. I said: "You are much better. Next month I shall be coming to take you home." She smiled, a very sweet smile. This time she had no qualms about flying. (Spoerry 1996, 137–138)

Spoerry strove to educate people on the importance of good hygiene and immunizations. Many in the area remember her as Mama Daktari, Swahili for Mother Doctor.

References: "Anne Spoerry Tribute," *AMREF Current News*, http://www.amref.org/ Spoerry.html; Spoerry, Anne, *They Call Me Mama Daktari*, Norval, ON: Moulin (1996).

Stern, Lina Solomonova
1878–1968

Lina Stern was a prolific writer on physiology and the first woman to be elected to the

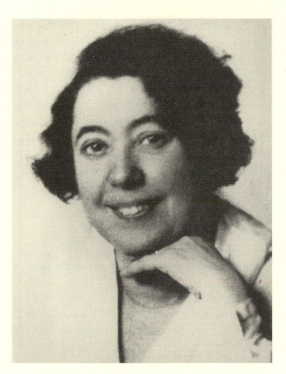

Lina Solomonova Stern (U.S. National Library of Medicine)

Academy of Sciences of the Soviet Union. She discovered the hematoencephalic barrier, which acts as a filtering membrane in order to protect spinal fluid and nerves from harmful substances.

Born in Latvia in 1878, Stern was taken to Switzerland at an early age. She graduated from the University of Geneva Medical Faculty in 1903 and eventually became a full professor of physiological chemistry there.

In 1925 she returned to the Soviet Union and Moscow to work at the Moscow Medical Institute and later became the director of the Moscow Institute of Physiology. Her studies involved the central nervous system and the effects of injecting medications into the nerve centers of the brain in order to bypass the hematoencephalic barrier. This treatment proved helpful for some illnesses and for shock victims during World War II. Stern died in 1968.

References: "Lina and the Brain," *Time* 49, no. 9 (3 March 1947): 45; "Prof. Lina Stern, Physiologist, 89," *New York Times* (9 March 1968): 29.

Steward, Susan Maria Smith McKinney
1847–1918

Susan Steward was the first African American physician in New York State. She was persistent in obtaining a medical degree and became the third black woman to become a physician in the United States.

Born in 1847 in Brooklyn, New York, she was the daughter of Ann Springstead Smith and Sylvanus Smith. She was of mixed black, Indian, and European descent. She had a prosperous family with nine siblings and enjoyed music, learning to play the organ at an early age.

In 1867, she entered the New York Medical College for Women, which was a homeopathic institution that welcomed women. Prior to her entering college, two of her brothers died during the Civil War, and a widespread cholera epidemic struck Brooklyn, resulting in numerous deaths. These events may have had an impact on her decision to become a physician.

She worked hard to get through medical school and clinical training at Bellevue Hospital and graduated at the top of her class in 1870. The private practice she opened after graduation grew very slowly at first, but eventually her reputation reached many in her community and she served both old and young as well as black and white.

Steward married William G. McKinney and had two children. He was a minister, and she was active as the organist while working to raise a family and practice as a physician. In 1892 her husband died.

In 1891, Steward cofounded the Brooklyn Women's Homeopathic Hospital and Dispensary, which served African Americans. She then received more medical education at the Long Island Medical College Hospital. From 1892 until 1896 she worked for the New York Medical College and Hospital for Women.

She married a U.S. army chaplain, Theophilus G. Steward, in 1896 and traveled with him to both Montana and Wyoming and practiced medicine in both states. She eventually joined the faculty at Wilberforce

University in Ohio, where she taught various health courses for over twenty years. She also was an excellent writer and orator who presented papers in the United States and overseas on various medical topics, especially the needs of black women for equal education and opportunity.

Steward was unusually successful relative to other black female physicians in the nineteenth century. Aspiring female physicians of the time greatly appreciated her intellectual gifts, musical talent, and oratory skills. She died on March 7, 1918.

References: Hayden, Robert C., "Steward, Susan Maria Smith McKinney," *American National Biography*, vol. 20, New York: Oxford University Press (1999); Hine, Darlene Clark, and Kathleen Thompson, *Facts on File Encyclopedia of Black Women in America*, vol. 11, New York: Facts on File (1997); Sammons, Vivian Ovelton, *Blacks in Science and Medicine*, New York: Hemisphere (1990).

Stewart, Alice
1906–

Alice Stewart is a British epidemiologist who uncovered the dangers of low-level radiation, particularly as it affected children with cancer. She has also fought for workers in high-risk occupations despite fierce opposition from the atomic energy industry.

Born in Sheffield, England, on October 4, 1906, she is the daughter of two physicians. Her father, Albert Ernest Naish, was an internist who taught at Sheffield University and her mother, Lucy Welburn Naish, was an anatomy teacher there. She had seven siblings and with her parents' support attended Cambridge University to become a physician. Three of her siblings also studied medicine.

She became a physician in 1931 and in 1941 took a position at Oxford University. During World War II she aided the British government in studying the harmful effects on workers of handling TNT during World War I. Following World War I, many munitions workers developed blood disorders, including liver disease, and the government wanted to study the safety of the munitions plants before they opened again for World War II. She concluded quickly that the handling of such substances as TNT would indeed impede a person's ability to form blood. The British government subsequently changed its manufacturing procedures.

Stewart became a very well-known epidemiologist and in 1956 turned her attention to low levels of radiation, finding that children who were exposed to more prenatal X rays died from cancer at twice the rate of those who received lower exposures. These findings were met with great opposition, but over the next two decades more studies verified that her findings were accurate. She testified in the late 1980s in U.S. congressional committees that the Department of Energy procedures for assessing radiation exposure and hazards were not adequate.

She also is a strong advocate of getting medical students more involved in the study of diseases.

> The medical profession is very gravely to blame for not putting more of its brain into epidemiology. I'm absolutely certain that the present system of teaching epidemiology just puts medical students off. They come to it too late. They should be introduced to the subject before they get gripped with the fascination of clinical medicine—which *should* grip them. I know the excitement someone has coming from clinical medicine. But if you get to students before they're seized with this passion and reach them with the excitement of looking at disease through the lens of the group, if you could attune them to think of the larger picture every time they looked at an individual disease, you could get them to see the fascination of epidemiology. (Greene 1999, 225)

Alice Stewart continues to speak to students and scientists about many public health issues and has been steadfast in her fight for better safety measures for workers in the nuclear energy industry.

References: Greene, Gayle, *The Woman Who Knew Too Much: Alice Stewart and the Secrets of Radiation*, Ann Arbor: University of Michigan Press (1999); Kay, Virginia, "Stewart, Alice," *Current Biography* 61 no. 7 (July 2000): 70–76; Schneider, Keith, "Scientist Who Managed to 'Shock the World' on Atomic Workers' Health," *New York Times*, sec. A (3 May 1990): 20, col. 1.

Stone, Emma Constance
1856–1902

Emma Stone was the first Australian female physician. She worked with poor women and children in Melbourne for many years and helped establish the Queen Victoria Hospital.

Stone was born on December 4, 1856. Her father was a London contractor who had settled in Tasmania. She received her education in the United States at the Women's Medical College of Pennsylvania in Philadelphia and in Canada at the University of Trinity College in Toronto. She received her M.D. in 1888 and obtained her licentiate from the Society of Apothecaries in 1889 in London, subsequently spending most of her life practicing medicine in Australia.

She worked with the poor most of her career and strove to raise the age for legal prostitution. She dedicated a large part of her life to establishing a hospital for poor women and children in Victoria. She maintained a private practice and worked at a free dispensary on a regular basis. Stone died on December 29, 1902, at the age of forty-six.

References: "Obituary," *British Medical Journal* 1, no. 2197 (7 February 1903): 343; Ogilvie, Marilyn, and Joy Harvey, eds., *The Biographical Dictionary of Women in Science*, New York: Routledge (2000).

Stowe, Emily
1831–1903

Emily Stowe was the first woman to practice medicine in Canada. She championed a woman's right to equal education in medicine, was an activist in the women's movement in Canada, and was antagonistic toward the male medical establishment of her day.

Born to Solomon and Hannah Jennings on May 1, 1831, Stowe was the eldest of six daughters. One brother died in infancy. The Jenningses were of Quaker background and felt that in many ways their daughters were equal to men. They lived in Norwich, Ontario, and educated their children at home, with Emily doing much of the teaching when she was in her teens. In 1846 she had a chance to fill in at the local school and taught many children of all ages.

After several years she desired more education herself. She was denied admission to Victoria College in Cobourg because she was female. She proceeded to the Provincial Normal School in Toronto in 1853 in order to complete a teacher-training course, which she did in 1854. She excelled at academics and became the first woman principal at an Ontario public school.

She married John Stowe in 1856 and had three children, Ann Augusta, John Howard, and Frank Jennings. By 1863 John Stowe was very ill with pulmonary tuberculosis and was separated from the family, probably in a sanatorium. During this time Emily decided to become a physician and support the family.

After being rejected by some Canadian schools, Stowe entered the New York Medical College and Hospital for Women, a homeopathic institution, and graduated in 1867. She set up a practice in Toronto without a license, feeling that she would have no chance at passing the examinations required because the examiners were not supportive of women. Also, like her great uncle Solomon, she felt it was all right to ignore the law if it wasn't fair, being confident that in time it would change. Her practice prospered.

John Stowe was well now and back with the family. Emily had met Jennie Trout, whom she had influenced to go into medicine, and they attended lectures at the Toronto School of Medicine. Trout decided to go to the Women's Medical College of Pennsylvania in 1872, and from that time forward there was friction between the Stowes and Trouts. This friction grew even more when Trout became licensed before Stowe, and they moved on in their careers and founded different medical schools for women.

Stowe was involved in a scandal in 1879 involving the death of Sarah Lovell, whom she had known and who had died from taking poison to abort her unborn child. Stowe denied giving Lovell any poison and was found innocent in two separate trials concerning the death. Soon thereafter, officials in the profession granted her a license to practice. Jennie Trout had gained her license in 1875; she was the only woman licensed to practice medicine in Canada until Stowe obtained her license in 1880.

Stowe helped found the Ontario Medical College for Women, which became the Women's College Hospital in Toronto.

She was a vocal and strong-willed proponent for women, especially those seeking medical education. Stowe passed away on April 30, 1903.

See also: Trout, Jennie Kidd
References: Duffin, Jacalyn, "The Death of Sarah Lovell and the Constrained Feminism of Emily Stowe," *Canadian Medical Association Journal* 146, no. 6 (15 March 1992): 881–888; Fryer, Mary Beacock, *Emily Stowe: Doctor and Suffragist*, Toronto: Hannah Institute; Dundurn Press (1990).

Sundquist, Alma
1880?–1940

Alma Sundquist was a Swedish physician active in the League of Nations. She specialized in the treatment of venereal diseases of women and children. Very active in establishing the medical women's organizations of her day, she served as president of the Medical Women's International Association in 1934.

Born in Sweden around 1880, Sundquist

attended the Karolinska Institute of Stockholm University and then organized and worked in free clinics in Stockholm. Her work brought the problems of venereal disease to the attention of the authorities, who needed to understand the importance of preventive methods and treatment. Sundquist became a well-respected physician in her lifetime. She died in January 1940.

References: *Journal of the American Medical Women's Association* 6, no. 1 (January 1951): 33–34; Lovejoy, Esther Pohl, *Women Doctors of the World*, New York: Macmillan (1957); Ogilvie, Marilyn, and Joy Harvey, eds., *The Biographical Dictionary of Women in Science*, New York: Routledge (2000).

Swain, Clara A.
1834–1910

Clara Swain was the first medical missionary to Asia in 1869. She worked diligently for the Methodists, who sent her from the United States to treat patients in India, teach medicine to women, and eventually open a large hospital to take care of the needs of the people of Bareilly.

Born on July 18, 1834, Swain was the daughter of John Swain and Clarissa Seavey. She was born in Elmira, New York, but her family moved to Castile when she was very young. She graduated from the Canandaigua Seminary and taught school for many years.

Many relatives encouraged her to become a nurse because she had a gift for caring for others who were ill. She decided to become a physician and worked at the Castile Sanitarium at the invitation of Dr. Cordelia Greene, who had founded the institution, until she earned her medical degree at the Women's Medical College of Pennsylvania in 1869.

During the 1860s many traditional churches were organizing to preach, teach, and lend medical aid in foreign countries. Swain's church had raised money to support a small mission in India, and Swain, who had just graduated and who was very religious, decided to serve.

In 1869, she left with another woman for India. She opened a small clinic and found herself very busy. The first year she made hundreds of visits to zenanas, the female part of Indian homes, and to other patients outside the clinic.

She began teaching classes in anatomy and diseases the next year, and later some of the women became licensed physicians. As more and more people came to the clinic, Swain realized they would need a hospital.

A donor gave her an estate with over forty acres to build a dispensary, and in 1874 the first women's hospital opened in India. "At first we find it a little difficult to persuade the women to let us examine them, even to get at their pulse or to see their tongue, but this reluctance soon wears off, and some of the women now in the hospital have lost a good deal of their shyness and meet us freely" (Swain 1977, 89).

The Indian men were also very grateful for a female physician. "Quite a number of native gentlemen have called to pay their respects, as they say. Some of them have told me that they appreciate my having left my native land and all my friends to come here to care for their women who can never see a physician of the other sex" (Swain 1977, 29).

As she was increasingly called on by the sick, she herself became ill and had to travel to the United States to recover. She continued to return to India and was asked to become the physician to the women of the palace for the rajah of Khetri. She remained in the palace for many years. Swain died on Christmas Day, 1910.

References: Beatty, William K., "Swain, Clara A.," *American National Biography*, vol. 21, New York: Oxford University Press (1999); Swain, Clara A., *A Glimpse of India: Being a Collection of Extracts from the Letters of Dr. Clara A. Swain, First Medical Missionary to India of the Woman's Foreign Missionary Society of the Methodist Episcopal Church in America*, New York: J. Pott (1909), reprinted in *History of Women Collection*, no. 6170, New Haven, CT: Research Publications (1977).

Sylvain, Yvonne
1907–1989

Yvonne Sylvain was the first female physician of Haiti. She is one of the most respected and admired Haitian women of all time. "She is an esthete and an aristocrat, a daughter of an elite, extraordinarily educated and accomplished family whose roots go back deep into Haiti's violent and stubbornly independent history. She is the best known woman in Haiti today" ("Doctor Number One" 1955, 93).

She received her medical degree in 1940 from the University of Haiti. She was the first woman accepted into the medical school, and following graduation she worked in clinics in Port-au-Prince, made house calls, educated people on hygiene and birth control, and worked on gaining proper therapies for cancer. She lived her life to serve others. She was active in the women's suffrage movement. Sylvain died in 1989.

References: "Doctor Number One," *Holiday* 17, no. 2 (February 1955): 92; Lovejoy, Esther Pohl, *Women Doctors of the World*, New York: Macmillan (1957).

T

Taussig, Helen Brooke
1898–1986

Helen Taussig was a pioneer in pediatric cardiology. Her work with Alfred Blalock led to the "blue-baby operation," which revolutionized cardiac surgery and gave hope to hundreds of parents who had children with cardiac problems. She also was instrumental in avoiding a national tragedy by helping to keep thalidomide off the market. This drug causes phocomelia, or shortened limbs.

One of four children, she was born May 24, 1898, in Cambridge, Maine. Her mother, Edith Guild, died when she was still a child. Her father, Frank W. Taussig, was a very well-known professor who helped establish the Harvard Graduate School of Business Administration and is regarded as one of the founding fathers of economics in the United States. She received an education at the Cambridge School for Girls and went on to Radcliffe in 1917. After two years she was ready to get out from under her father's shadow and transferred to the University of California at Berkeley.

Upon graduation in 1921 she told her father she wanted to become a doctor. He advised her to go into public health, but she wasn't interested. She chose to go to Johns Hopkins, which admitted women, to study cardiology. She obtained her M.D. degree in 1927 and stayed at Johns Hopkins Hospital to train in cardiology and pediatrics.

In 1930 she began her career as head of the Children's Heart Clinic at Johns Hopkins University and would remain there until her retirement in 1963. She determined early on that something could be done for children suffering from tetralogy of Fallot, which results in a lack of oxygen in the blood. She was one of the first doctors to really understand congenital heart malformations.

Because a person with one congenital anomaly not infrequently has others, some of Taussig's children with tetralogy of Fallot also had a persistent ductus. As she studied these patients in her clinic and followed several of them to the autopsy table, she began to appreciate the fact that children with both a persistent ductus and a tetralogy did reasonably well, but would begin to deteriorate if the ductus spontaneously closed later in childhood. Obviously, the ductus was serving to accomplish the opposite of what it did in the embryo: it allowed blood to pass from the high-pressure aorta into the low-pressure pulmonary artery beyond the obstruction. By shunting the circulation around the obstructed pulmonary outflow tract, it provided a bypass that markedly increased flow to the lungs. The logical solution for patients with tetralogy, then, was to surgically build a ductus. To Helen Taussig, the building of a ductus seemed a straightforward matter of plumbing—put a length of pipe in the right place, and thereby divert the blue blood around the narrowed pulmonary artery and into the lungs so

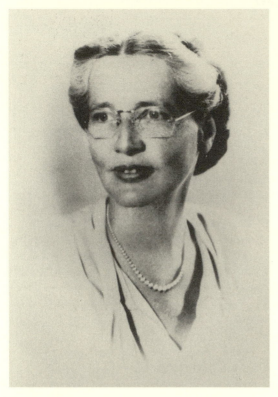

Helen Brooke Taussig (U.S. National Library of Medicine)

that it can be oxygenated. (Nuland 1988, 438)

In 1938 Taussig visited Maude Abbott at McGill University to learn all she could about heart defects. She met Alfred Blalock in 1941, and together they worked on perfecting an operation that many physicians of the time thought impossible. The Blalock-Taussig shunt successfully joined the subclavian artery to the pulmonary artery in a cyanotic child. Their accomplishment is one of the major milestones in medicine of the twentieth century. Their success in 1944 led to open-heart surgery.

Her book, *Congenital Malformations of the Heart*, published in 1947, was a major contribution to the field. "By means of this book the diagnosis of malformations of the heart is brought within the power of all physicians who are willing to devote time to its study and to practice its teachings" (Parks 1947, viii).

Another of Taussig's accomplishments was her work with Frances Kelsey, to ban thalidomide in the United States. Taussig confirmed Kelsey's fears, arising from her work at the FDA, and those of others by studying the situation in Germany, where already thousands of babies had been born with phocomelia—shorter bones in their legs and arms. Their mothers' taking of thalidomide while pregnant had caused the condition. Both Taussig and Kelsey testified before government officials, and the news spread that the disaster had been averted in the United States.

Shortly after this success, Taussig worked to institute tougher drug regulations.

I feel the situation should be brought to the immediate attention of the public in this country. It is also important to remember that in many instances the damage is done before the mother knows she is pregnant. Therefore, young women must learn to be cautious about new drugs. Until new laws have become effective, and indeed until research for the proper test on pregnant animals has been completed, physicians must bear in mind that sleeping tablets, tranquilizers, and other apparently innocent drugs may do terrible harm to the rapidly growing embryo and the unborn child. (Taussig 1962, 683)

Outspoken about abortion even in her early days, she felt the mother, not the government, should make the choice. She also spoke out about continually having to fight the antivivisectionists, a conflict both she and other scientists found frustrating. She was concerned as well that the United States did not have national health insurance that covered both adults and infants.

Many physicians who met or worked with her over the years remembered her fondly. One physician who referred a child to her later wrote, "I received a long, detailed letter from Dr. Taussig, but, although everything was made very clear, her letter was not just a technical report. That sweet lady wrote a very personal, homey message almost as if we were again face to face across a room. From time to time Teddy needed to return to Hopkins for checkups, and I always received another friendly, unpretentious letter. . . . Dr. Taussig will always be a heroine to me" (Carlisle 2001, 59). Taussig retired in 1963 but continued her work and stayed active in the field until she was killed in a car accident on May 21, 1986, in Kennett Square, Pennsylvania.

See also: Abbott, Maude Elizabeth Seymour; Kelsey, Frances Oldham

References: Carlisle, Richard C., "Helen Taussig—A Heroine," *Pharos of Alpha Omega Alpha–Honor Medical Society* 64, no. 1 (Winter 2001): 59; Grigg, William, "The Thalidomide Tragedy—25 Years Ago," *FDA Consumer* 21, no. 1 (February 1987): 14–17; Keene, Ann T., "Taussig, Helen Brooke," *American National Biography,* vol. 21, New York: Oxford University Press (1999); McNamara, Dan G., et al., "Historical Milestones: Helen Brooke Taussig: 1898–1986," *Journal of the American College of Cardiology* 10, no. 3 (September 1987): 662–671; Nuland, Sherwin B., *Doctors: The Biography of Medicine,* New York: Knopf (1988); Parks, Edward A., "Foreword," in Helen B. Taussig, *Congenital Malformations of the Heart;* Taussig, Helen B., *Congenital Malformations of the Heart,* New York: Commonwealth Fund (1947); Taussig, Helen B., "Dangerous Tranquility," *Science* 136, no. 3517 (25 May 1962): 683; Taussig, Helen B., "Little Choice and a Stimulating Environment," *Journal of the American Medical Women's Association* 36, no. 2 (February 1981): 43–44.

Thompson, Mary Harris
1829–1895

Mary Thompson was a physician and surgeon. She established a hospital and a medical college in Chicago so that women could gain both academic and practical experience in the field.

Born on April 15, 1829, she was the daughter of John Harris Thompson and Calista Corbin. She received her early educa-tion at Troy Conference Academy in West Poultney, Vermont, and Ft. Edward Collegiate Institute in New York. She had to teach in her teens in order to support her education. She was a gifted student and developed an early interest in physiology and anatomy, two subjects she was able to teach others.

In 1863 she received her medical degree from the New England Female Medical College, having spent one year at the New York Infirmary for Women and Children with the Blackwell sisters, where she gained some of her clinical experience. She then decided to try to establish a practice in Chicago.

She found employment with the Sanitary Commission, where she worked with women and children who had lost their husbands and fathers in the Civil War. She also helped many of the returning soldiers with their medical needs. It wasn't long before she decided to raise money for a hospital to tend to the overwhelming numbers of women and children seeking medical help. The Chicago Hospital for Women and Children opened in 1865. She became the surgeon and top physician.

Even though she had a medical degree, she applied to Rush Medical College for more training. The college denied her application until she enlisted the help of William Byford of Chicago Medical College. She graduated in 1870. More women were not able to follow due to numerous objections by male students and faculty. After graduation, she and Byford founded the Woman's Hospital Medical College in connection with her hospital.

She was a professor at the college and also maintained her position at the hospital, becoming one of the best-known women surgeons in the nation. She specialized in pelvic and abdominal surgery and also sought to improve current surgical instruments by inventing her own. Because of her competence, some males in the field who had doubts about a woman's capacity to practice medicine came to change their views. She published numerous articles on a variety of medical topics and used her influence to aid women in pursuing careers as physicians. She also opened a nurses-training program at her hospital in 1874. Thompson died of a cerebral hemorrhage on May 21, 1895, in Chicago.

References: Hast, Adele, "Thompson, Mary Harris," *American National Biography*, vol. 21, New York: Oxford University Press (1999).

Tilghman, Shirley Marie Caldwell
1946–

Shirley Tilghman greatly enhanced our knowledge of genes and their role in human development. She was a key designer of the Human Genome Project.

Born in Toronto, Ontario, in 1946, to Henry Caldwell and Shirley Carre Caldwell, Tilghman moved with her family very frequently and became interested in chemistry in high school in Winnipeg, Manitoba. She went on to study at Queen's University in Kingston, Ontario, receiving her degree in biochemistry in 1968. She decided to become a molecular biologist and earned a Ph.D. in biochemistry at Temple University in 1975.

She was a fellow at the National Institutes of Health and, with Philip Leder Tilghman, cloned the first mammalian gene. She worked later at the Fox Chase Cancer Center in Philadelphia, the University of Pennsylvania, and Princeton University. Currently she is director of the Institute for Genomic Analysis at Princeton.

Her research has focused on the genetic influence both parents have on the embryo. Her work with the Human Genome Project started before the project formally began in 1990. This project, which is vital to medical science, is a cooperative effort that aims to identify approximately 30,000 genes in the DNA of humans as well as discover the sequences of the billions of chemical bases that make up human DNA. Tilghman has two children with her former husband, Philip Tilghman.

References: Proffitt, Pamela, *Notable Women Scientists*, Detroit: Gale (1999).

Trout, Jennie Kidd
1841–1921

Jennie Trout was the first licensed female physician in Canada. She served many small towns in Ontario and established free dispensaries for the poor. She also founded the Women's Medical College at Queen's University in Kingston.

Born on April 21, 1841, in Kelso, Scotland, Trout emigrated with her family to Canada when she was a small child. They settled near Stratford, Ontario, on a farm. She was very bright, as demonstrated by her early education and successful efforts at teaching. She graduated from the Ontario Normal School in Toronto, which was one of the best at teacher preparation. She then taught for four years near Stratford, Ontario.

She married Edward Trout, a successful publisher, in 1865. She was ill much of her early life and was treated by electrotherapy. During her illness she determined to become a physician. No Canadian medical schools accepted women at that time, so she went to the Women's Medical College of Pennsylvania in Philadelphia and graduated in 1875. She returned to Canada and founded the Electro-Therapeutic Institute, a clinic that was well equipped to treat women with galvanic baths or electrical stimulation.

She then became interested in providing opportunities for women to pursue a medical education and in 1883 became the founder and trustee of the Kingston Women's Medical College. It merged with the Toronto Medical College in 1894 and was known as the Ontario Medical College for Women. She died on October 30, 1921, in Los Angeles.

References: Hacker, Carlotta, *The Indomitable Lady Doctors*, Toronto: Clarke, Irwin (1974); "Jennie Kidd Gowanlock Trout," http://www.rootsweb.com/~nwa/jennie.html; Rayson, Sandra, Robert A. Kyle, and Marc A. Shampo, "Dr. Jennie Kidd Trout— Pioneer Canadian Physician," *Mayo Clinic Proceedings* 68, no. 2 (February 1993): 189.

Turner-Warwick, Margaret
1924–

A British physician and immunologist, Margaret Turner-Warwick was the first woman president of the Royal College of Physicians.

Born on November 19, 1924, she received her early education in London. She then attended Oxford, earning her B.A. in 1946. She earned her medical degree at University College Hospital Medical School in London in 1956, and also earned a Ph.D. there in 1961.

Her early medical training involved posts at University College Hospital, Brompton Hospital, and the Elizabeth Garrett Anderson Hospital. She studied upper respiratory tract diseases, particularly tuberculosis and asthma. Her interests also expanded to immunology and thoracic medicine.

She became professor of medicine at the Cardiothoracic Institute in London in 1972, and wrote her textbook, *Immunology of the Lung*, which is still used by numerous medical schools today. From 1989 until 1992 she served as the first woman president of the Royal College of Physicians. In 1991 she was made a Dame Commander of the Order of the British Empire (DBE).

References: Haines, Catharine M. C., and Helen Stevens, *International Women in Science: A Biographical Dictionary to 1950*, Santa Barbara, CA: ABC-CLIO (2001); Turner-Warwick, Margaret, *Immunology of the Lung*, London: Edward Arnold (1978).

U

University of Bologna
1088?–

The first university in the world, the University of Bologna was founded about 1088. Although it became well-known mainly for law studies, prominent women professors in the sciences, including medicine, taught there. By the eighteenth century the Enlightenment had brought about more liberal views regarding women receiving higher education, as well as teaching. Beginning in 1772, Laura Bassi taught anatomy and physics at the University of Bologna.

See also: Bassi, Laura Maria Caterina
References: Rashdall, Hastings, *The Universities of Europe in the Middle Ages*, vol. 1: *Salerno, Bologna, Paris*, Oxford: Clarendon Press (1936).

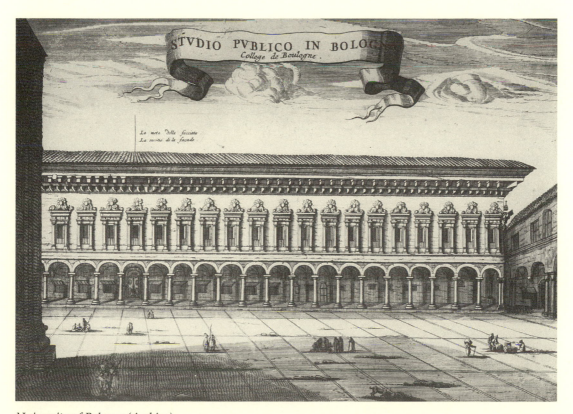

University of Bologna (Archive)

University of Salerno
fl. 900–1250

The medical school at the University of Salerno, in southern Italy, was the first medical school of medieval Europe. It flourished during the tenth through the beginning of the thirteenth centuries and was coeducational. It had as excellent a reputation for medicine as Bologna did for law and Paris for scholasticism. Frederick II, the Holy Roman Emperor, decreed in 1221 that the school at Salerno had to certify all physicians before they could practice legally.

References: Rashdall, Hastings, *The Universities of Europe in the Middle Ages*, vol. 1: *Salerno, Bologna, Paris*, Oxford: Clarendon Press (1936).

V

Van Hoosen, Bertha
1863–1952

Bertha Van Hoosen was a strong organizer of women in the medical field. She was an outstanding surgeon and founded the American Medical Women's Association in order to keep women abreast of current events, develop a voice for female physicians and enhance their image, and, most important, provide a supportive network for women physicians.

Born in Stony Creek, Michigan, on March 26, 1863, she was the daughter of a farmer, Joshua Van Hoosen, and a teacher, Sarah Ann Taylor. She attended school in Pontiac, Michigan, and then, despite her parents' misgivings and after teaching and nursing to earn the tuition, enrolled at the University of Michigan Medical School, from which she graduated in 1888. During her studies there she encountered much gender discrimination and fought for better clinical experience, as she wanted to become a surgeon. She gained more clinical experience after she went to the New England Hospital for Women and Children in Boston, and also had experience as an intern at the Women's Hospital of Detroit.

She opened her own practice in Chicago in 1892. In the early years, she found it very difficult to attract patients, but as her reputation grew, so did her practice. Her continued learning and teaching at various universities around Chicago culminated in her appointment in 1918 at Loyola University Medical School as a professor and head of obstetrics.

Believing that women had a right to bear children painlessly, she was a strong proponent of twilight sleep (the use of scopolamine-morphine) during childbirth, a controversial subject. Van Hoosen closely monitored patients using the drug and had a very good success rate in delivering healthy babies. She published a book on the use of scopolamine-morphine in 1915.

Responding to a growing need for a support system for women in the field, she founded the American Medical Women's Association in 1915. She was an excellent surgeon, looked up to by her students. Other women in the field best know her for her leadership qualities. She died in Romeo, Michigan, on June 7, 1952.

See also: American Women's Hospitals **References:** Lovejoy, Esther Pohl, *Women Doctors of the World*, New York: Macmillan (1957); McGovern, Constance M., "Van Hoosen, Bertha," *American National Biography*, vol. 22, New York: Oxford University Press (1999).

Vejjabul, Pierra Hoon
1909–

Pierra Vejjabul, a physician, worked to better the social standing of women in Thailand. Confronting many obstacles, she fought for the rights of all in her country, particularly children and the poor, to adequate living conditions and medical care.

Born in Lampang on November 27, 1909, Vejjabul was the daughter of Thongkich

Hoontrakul and Phon He, a third wife. Vejjabul witnessed some of the rivalry among her father's wives and was very much in support of monogamy at an early age.

A French doctor who helped her mother influenced her to go into medicine; she was also deeply affected by an unwed mother who committed suicide, dying in her arms. She decided to work on raising the status of women as well as advocating better relationships between children and mothers.

Her father was against her planned career, so she ran away to Saigon when she was only sixteen. Her father brought her back home. Later she ran away to Paris and went to the Sorbonne School of Medicine. She had to work and sell many of her personal belongings to make ends meet, but she managed to graduate in 1936 with a medical degree from the Sorbonne School of Medicine.

She went back to Thailand and worked for the government, combating venereal disease. She was strongly against prostitution and helped with blood tests for people from all walks of life to determine whether they had syphilis. She established some organizations to fight prostitution and worked to enact the law in 1960 that abolished it.

She also worked to aid the blind and assist poor mothers and children, taking numerous children into her own home until there was a place for them with a family. Premier Luang Pibul Songram dubbed her Vejjabul, or "complete doctor." She received much recognition and many awards for her work on educating the public about proper health care, including the Order of the White Elephant for meritorious service.

> In evaluating the pioneering humanitarian contributions that Dr. Pierra Vejjabul has made to the improvement of medical, sanitary, and moral standards in her country, journalists of the American press have called her the Jane Addams of Thailand and the Dr. Albert Schweitzer of Asia. A conventionally reared daughter of a well-to-do family, she defied tradition by becoming a doctor. Then as Dr. Pierra, the name by which her patients generally know her,

she boldly opposed unhygienic practices in child care, the custom of polygamy, legal prostitution, and some other customs of her people, in her determination to dignify women and to raise living conditions—especially among the underprivileged. ("Vejjabul" 1964, 455)

Currently Vejjabul lives in Thailand.

References: Lovejoy, Esther Pohl, *Women Doctors of the World*, New York: Macmillan (1957); "Vejjabul (Kunying) Pierra," *Current Biography Yearbook 1964*, New York: Wilson (1964).

Villa, Amelia Chopitea
1899?–1942

Amelia Villa was the first female physician in Bolivia. She graduated from the University of San Francisco Xavier in Sucre in 1926. She did some graduate work in Paris and also founded the Pabellon de Niños at the Oruro Hospital. The Bolivian government recognized her service.

References: Lovejoy, Esther Pohl, *Women Doctors of the World*, New York: Macmillan (1957).

Villa-Komaroff, Lydia
1947–

Lydia Villa-Komaroff was involved in the discovery that insulin could be produced from bacteria and has done extensive research to add to the knowledge of recombinant DNA. She is the third Mexican American who has earned a Ph.D. in a science field.

Born in Las Vegas, New Mexico, on August 7, 1947, she is the daughter of violinist and teacher John Vias Villa and Drucilla Jaramillo Villa, a social worker. She grew up with five siblings in a family where education was highly valued. She developed an early interest in science and pursued a college education.

She began her education at the University of Washington and then transferred to Goucher College along with her future husband, Anthony Komaroff. They married after Lydia graduated with a degree in biology in 1970. She went to work at the National Institutes of Health and became interested in molecular biology, pursuing further study at the Massachusetts Institute of Technology, where she obtained her Ph.D. in 1975.

Her work on recombinant DNA was useful in providing a technique to study genes within bacteria. This led to her work on cloning the insulin gene in rats, which eventually led to success in producing insulin for people from bacteria. Villa-Komaroff is currently vice-president for research at Northwestern University.

References: Proffitt, Pamela, *Notable Women Scientists*, Detroit: Gale (1999).

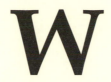

Wald, Florence Schorske
1917–

Florence Wald brought the hospice movement to the United States in 1974. She was inspired by her visit to St. Christopher's Hospice, which Cicely Saunders founded in Great Britain.

Wald was born in New York City on April 19, 1917, to Theodore Alexander Schorske and Gertrude Goldschmidt Schorske. She attended Mount Holyoke College and graduated in 1938. Wald received her master's in nursing from Yale University in 1941. She worked for the New York Visiting Nurses Association early in her career and also gained experience at Babies Hospital in New York City and Children's Hospital in Boston.

She spent six years in research at the Surgical Metabolism Unit of the New York College of Physicians and later taught psychiatric nursing at Rutgers State University. Following this work, she took a position at the Yale University School of Nursing as an assistant professor of psychiatric nursing. This is where she has spent most of her career and where she still works today. She was the dean of the School of Nursing for nine years.

In 1963, Cicely Saunders spoke at Yale, greatly impressing Wald. She felt Saunders was speaking to many of the issues she and her colleagues were confronting. She made a decision soon after to become involved in the hospice movement.

Wald was instrumental in the establishment of the first hospice in the United States, in Branford, Connecticut, and led the movement for better understanding of the issues facing those who were dying. She feels hospice is not for everyone, as some people want to fight to the end. Others who would have benefited have not always had the opportunity. "As more and more people—families of hospice patients and hospice volunteers—are exposed to this new model of how to approach end-of-life care, we are taking what was essentially a hidden scene, death, an unknown, and making it a reality. We are showing people that there are meaningful ways to cope with this very difficult situation" (Friedrich 1999, 1685).

Wald differs from Saunders on the question of physician-assisted suicide, feeling that there are times when this option should be available to patients; Saunders feels this approach is never justified. Wald has advocated and been supportive of better education for nurses and others involved with the care of the terminally ill. Her initial push for hospices in the United States has grown from the first hospice in Connecticut to over 2,500 nationwide. Wald lives in Westport, Connecticut, and is currently involved in hospice care in prisons. She married in 1959 and has two children.

See also: Saunders, Cicely Mary Strode
References: American Nurses Association, "The Hall of Fame Inductees, Florence S. Wald" (1996), http://www.nursingworld.org/hof/waldfs.htm; Friedrich, M. J., "Hospice Care in the United States: A Conversation with Florence S. Wald," *JAMA* 281, no. 18 (12 May 1999): 1683–1685; *Who's Who of*

American Women, 3d ed., Chicago: Marquis Who's Who (1963).

Wald, Lillian D.
1867–1940

Nurse, feminist, and health care reformer Lillian Wald advocated child-labor laws, brought to public consciousness the health care needs of the poor, and founded the famous Henry Street Settlement in New York City, one of the first settlement houses of its kind in a period of rapid industrialization in the United States. She founded the current concept of public health nursing.

Born in Cincinnati, Ohio, on March 10, 1867, she was the daughter of Max D. Wald and Minnie Schwarz Wald, both German immigrants. She grew up in an affluent German Jewish neighborhood in New York City. She became interested in nursing and graduated from the New York Hospital School of Nursing in 1889. She later attended the Women's Medical College of the New York Infirmary, founded by Elizabeth and Emily Blackwell, but did not become a physician. Instead she was asked by the Blackwells to begin training immigrants in New York in home nursing care.

She was appalled by the poverty in the streets of New York City and determined to do something about it. She and Mary Brewster started work with a little funding and found they were very welcome and needed.

> Gradually there came to our knowledge difficulties and conflicts not peculiar to any one set of people, but intensified in the case of our neighbors by poverty, unfamiliarity with laws and customs, the lack of privacy, and the frequent dependence of the elders upon the children. Workers in philanthropy, clergymen, orthodox rabbis, the unemployed, anxious parents, girls in distress, troublesome boys, came as individuals to see us, but no formal organization of our work was effected till we moved into the house on Henry Street, in 1895. (Wald 1915, 24)

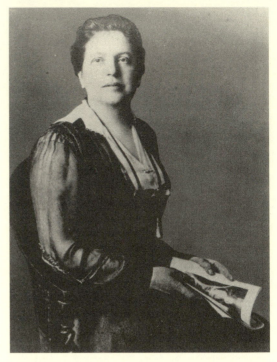

Lillian D. Wald (U.S. National Library of Medicine)

Over the years, Wald trained nurses at the Henry Street Settlement, cared for the sick and poor, listened to the illiterate, and worked to raise money as well as the consciousness of a nation. Her leadership led to the creation of the Visiting Nurses Services. Nurses in this organization cared for patients in their homes, saving the hospital beds for the critically ill. She also helped establish a school-nurses program to improve attendance at public schools. Children who attended school could be seen by a well-qualified nurse.

One of her biggest assets was her ability to raise funds from the affluent and from politicians. She wrote, gave lectures, and made the public better aware of the living and working conditions of the poor. Her work led to better child-labor laws and regulations on working conditions. Wald died in Westport, Connecticut, on September 1, 1940.

References: Daniels, Doris Groshen, *Always a Sister: The Feminism of Lillian D. Wald*, New York: Feminist Press at the City University of New York (1989); Daniels, Doris Groshen, "Wald, Lillian D.," *American National Biography*, vol. 22, New York: Oxford University Press (1999); Duffus, Robert Luther, *Lillian Wald, Neighbor and Crusader*, New York: Macmillan (1938); Wald, Lillian D., *The House on Henry Street*, New York: Henry Holt (1915).

Walker, Mary Broadfoot
1888–1974

Mary Walker was a Scottish pioneer in treating neurological disorders, particularly myasthenia gravis. She introduced physostigmine in treating this neuromuscular disorder in 1934. Only recently has this contribution been fully recognized.

Relatively unknown most of her life, Walker was born in Wigtown, Scotland, in 1888 and received her medical degree from the University of Edinburgh in 1913. She served the Royal Army Medical Corps in Malta and Salonika during World War I. She then worked at St. Alfege's Hospital in Greenwich for sixteen years. Later she served at several other hospitals, including St. Leonard's in Shoreditch, St. Francis's in Dulwich, and St. Benedict's in Tooting.

Her publication in 1934 of her discovery of the therapeutic effects of physostigmine on myasthenia gravis patients was a milestone in treatment of the disease. Her discovery generated some interest at the time, and medical practitioners asked to demonstrate her method a few times. However, for the most part, the medical community largely ignored her discovery during her lifetime. The Royal College of Physicians in London awarded her the Jean Hunter Prize in 1963 but did not elect her a fellow of the organization. Years after her death, many felt her shy personality and lack of a mentor or a laboratory for working on larger projects kept her amazing accomplishment in the dark. She died on September 13, 1974.

References: Kass-Simon, Gabriele, and Patricia Farnes, *Women of Science: Righting the Record*, Bloomington: Indiana University Press (1990); Keesey, John C., "Contemporary Opinions about Mary Walker: A Shy Pioneer of Therapeutic Neurology," *Neurology* 51, no. 5 (November 1998): 1433–1439; "Mary Broadfoot Walker," *Lancet* 2, no. 7893 (7 December 1974): 1401–1402; Schmidt, Jacob Edward, *Medical Discoveries: Who and When*, Springfield, IL: Thomas (1959).

Walker, Mary Edwards
1832–1919

Mary Walker was an early physician in the United States who fought many of society's standards for women, most notably the way they dressed, and proved a valuable physician and surgeon during the U.S. Civil War.

She was born in Oswego, New York, on November 26, 1832. Her father, Alvah Walker, was a farmer and physician. Her mother was Vesta Whitcomb Walker. She had four sisters and one brother who survived to adulthood. Her father was very supportive of some of the reform movements of the day, such as dress reform and women's rights.

Her early education covered the basics. Like her sisters, she attended Falley Seminary in Fulton and taught for a brief time. She decided to become a physician like her father and attended Syracuse Medical College, graduating in 1862. She married Albert E. Miller, also a physician, but the marriage ended in divorce. She practiced medicine in Columbus, Ohio, and Rome, New York.

During this period she was an avid crusader for dress reform. Reflecting her father's views, she disliked the restrictive clothing for women and objected to dresses altogether as bad for one's health and not conducive to proper hygiene. She chose to wear bloomers, pantaloons, or trousers, finding them more practical.

During the Civil War she volunteered when she was refused a commission. She worked in Washington, D.C., hospitals but wanted to go to the field and traveled extensively to see and tend to casualties. Eventually she became an assistant surgeon in the Union army, working near the front in many battles before being taken prisoner in Richmond, Virginia. She spent four months there as a captive of the Confederate army until she was released in a prisoner exchange.

When the war ended she was the first woman to receive a Congressional Medal of Honor for her heroism. She then traveled abroad and lectured on various subjects. When she returned home, she lectured and wrote about dress reform, marriage, the war, women's rights, health, and hygiene.

Walker was a colorful character with many interests who voiced her opinion whether asked or not. She aided in the progress of women in general and used her skills as a physician to save many a soldier during the Civil War.

Her Medal of Honor was rescinded in 1917 when Congress tried to change the requirements of the medal to make it more prestigious. Walker refused to return hers, wearing it daily until she died. President Carter reinstated her medal posthumously in 1977. Walker died in Oswego on February 21, 1919, just a little over a year before women gained the right to vote in the United States.

References: Chaff, S. L., "Walker, Mary Edwards," *Dictionary of American Medical Biography,* Westport, CT: Greenwood Press (1984); Snyder, Charles McCool, *Dr. Mary Walker: The Little Lady in Pants,* New York: Vantage Press (1962); Spiegel, Allen D., and Peter B. Suskind, "Mary Edwards Walker, M.D.: A Feminist Physician a Century ahead of Her Time," *Journal of Community Health* 21, no. 3 (June 1996): 211–235; Woodward, Helen Beal, *The Bold Women,* New York: Farrar, Straus and Young (1953).

Wars and Epidemics

Through the ages, the most optimal time for women to exercise their right to practice medicine seemed to be when countries waged war or were faced with overwhelming epidemics. When deaths were imminent and quickly occurring, even the most ardent antifemale medical professionals accepted whatever help was available. Florence Nightingale, Elizabeth Garrett Anderson, and Clara Barton are just a few women who were accepted as healers in times of great need. They then were able to use their experience to further their careers.

For centuries, women were seen as not capable of fruitful work.

> Roman men, as we have seen, were perceived as ambitious, energetic, resourceful, aggressive, and successful. In claiming their brides they demonstrate their manhood and give evidence of their ability to maintain a secure and prosperous household in the future. Women, on the other hand, were represented as weak, passive bearers of children whose active allegiance is evoked principally through their children, by appeal to the passions (*cupiditas* and *amor*), and by their own awareness of their helpless dependence on men. (Miles 1995, 215)

Women have been instrumental in coping with epidemics. In the seventeenth, eighteenth, and nineteenth centuries in the United States alone, there have been numerous regional outbreaks of influenza, typhoid fever, cholera, yellow fever, and measles. The yellow fever epidemic in 1852 affected the entire nation, with the most concentrated fatalities in the New Orleans area. In 1775 the influenza epidemic reached worldwide proportions and required women to travel long distances to care for the sick outside their own communities.

Women's vital work in times of crisis did not necessarily lead to a wholehearted belief in their competence as health care workers. Even as late as the twentieth century, many medical schools preferred male candidates. In Great Britain "the most comprehensible explanation of the medical schools' reaction against women students is in terms of simple 'backlash,' the reassertion of patriarchal prerogatives after the war, in the first instance, and in the context of competition for employment during the later 1920s" (Dyhouse 1998, 122).

Women's contributions in the medical field were only a small part of their war efforts. They also took the men's jobs while they served in the military. Yet whether in

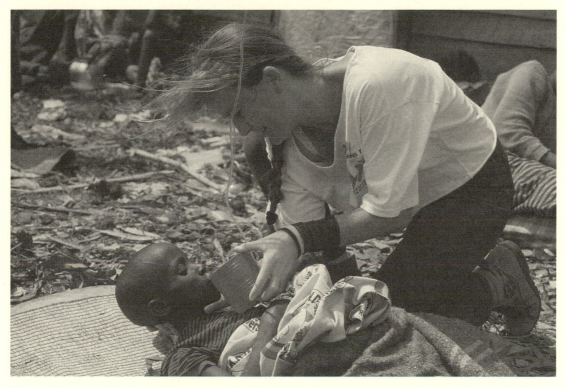

Women have served for centuries in wars and epidemics (Corbis)

the field tending to soldiers' wounds or at home doing the men's work, women still had very little power. They continued to be less valued both by society and under the law: "Employers in all nations paid women at standards well below wages for men with equivalent skills, denying them fringe benefits whenever possible" (Kolko 1994, 96).

In the medical field, women who had served on the battlefield often lost their status during peacetime. "During the First World War there really was nothing a woman doctor could not do in the war zone. They treated virtually every kind of wound and disease, they underwent the same hardships, privations and dangers as men, became prisoners of war, took part in devastating retreats, and worked under shells and bombs. None of this valuable experience advanced their career prospects. And it took the outbreak of another world war to gain medical women commissioned rank in the British army" (Leneman 1994, 177). In 1943 the U.S. Congress finally authorized the commissioning of women physicians as officers in the mili-

tary. During the Vietnam War and the Gulf War, women served in increasing numbers.

By World War II, professional bodies in Britain were more accepting of women physicians. The *Report of the Interdepartmental Committee on Medical Schools,* published in 1944, attests, "We believe that prudence and good sense dictate that the promise of developing into a good doctor shall be the overriding factor in the selection of students and that unsuitability for a medical career shall be the sole barrier to admission to a medical school" (Goodenough 1944, 97).

In the United States, women have continued to enter the medical profession in both the private and government sectors. From 1970 to 2000, the number of women physicians tripled in proportion to men (American Medical Association 2002, 316–317). Nursing continues to be a field dominated by women (Scanlon 2001, 21). Despite progress, however, some feel that women physicians will never gain equality with their male colleagues, particularly in the United States:

There is a "glass ceiling" on women physicians' upward mobility. They are kept from top-level positions, I will argue, through the subtle process of a kind of colleague boycott—not keeping them out entirely, but not including them in ways that allow them to replace the senior members of the medical community. This process is the "Salieri phenomenon"—a combination of faint praise and subtle denigration of their abilities to lead that delegitimates women physicians' bids to compete for positions of great authority. The reason men are so reluctant to allow women into the inner circles, I contend, is their fear that if too many women become leaders, the profession will "tip" and become women's work—and men will lose prestige, income and authority. (Lorber 1993, 63)

The fact that the male-dominated American Medical Association elected Nancy Dickey as its president in 1997 suggests that more women can achieve leadership roles with administrative power.

See also: Barriers to Success; Women of Color in Medicine

References: American Medical Association, "Physician Characteristics and Distribution in the United States, Chicago: Survey and Data Resources, American Medical Association (2002); Dyhouse, Carol, "Women Students and the London Medical Schools, 1914–39: The Anatomy of a Masculine Culture," *Gender and History* 10, no. 1 (1998): 110–132; Goodenough, William MacNamara, *Report of the Inter-Departmental Committee on Medical Schools*, London: His Majesty's Stationery Office (1944); Johnson, Samuel, *Letters of Samuel Johnson*, ed. George Birkbeck Hill, Oxford: Clarendon Press (1892); Kolko, Gabriel, *Century of War: Politics, Conflicts, and Society since 1914*, New York: New Press (1994); Leneman, Leah, "Medical Women at War, 1914–1918," *Medical History* 38, no. 2 (1994): 160–177; Livy, *The History of Rome*, vol. 1, London: George Bell (1906); Lorber, Judith, "Why Women Physicians Will Never Be True Equals in the American Medical Profession," in *Gender, Work, and Medicine: Women and the Medical Division of Labor*, edited by Elianna Riska and Katarina Wegar, London: Sage (1993); "Memories of War: How Vietnam-Era Nurses Are Coping Today," *USA Today* 121, no. 2574 (March 1993): 30–31; Miles, Gary B., *Livy: Reconstructing Early Rome*, Ithaca, NY: Cornell University Press (1995); Murray, Flora, *Women as Army Surgeons*, London: Hodder and Stoughton (1920); Scanlon, William S., "Nursing Workforce: Recruitment and Retention of Nurses and Nurse Aides Is a Growing Concern," Washington, DC: General Accounting Office (2001); Tannenbaum, R. J., "Earnestness, Temperance, Industry, the Definition and Uses of Professional Character among Nineteenth-Century American Physicians," *Journal of the History of Medicine and Allied Sciences* 49, no. 2 (April 1994): 251–283.

Wauneka, Annie Dodge
1910–1997

Annie Wauneka was a Navajo health care educator who taught her tribal members that proper hygiene and Western medicine were essential to ridding the community of tuberculosis. President John F. Kennedy awarded her the Presidential Medal of Freedom shortly before his assassination in 1963.

Born in the Navajo Nation near Sawmill, Arizona, on April 10, 1910, she was the daughter of Chief Henry Chee Dodge and his third wife, K'eehabah. She grew up with her father and tended the family flock. Her father was educated and had saved his money to provide well for his family. They lived in a Western-style home rather than the traditional hogan.

She received some education at a government boarding school in Fort Defiance, where she saw much sickness and disease. She helped care for some of her friends who were sick but saw many die. She later improved her spoken English at the Albuquerque Indian School.

When she was home she visited tribal

members with her father, a strong advocate of education and of helping the Navajo people, and began to realize the poverty of her tribe. She pursued further education with the U.S. Public Health Service.

In dealing with ailments in her tribe, she faced shortages of medical supplies, substandard living conditions, and age-old customs.

> Navajos classify diseases by cause rather than by symptom, maintaining that all trouble and illness are a result of a state of disharmony with the surrounding world, other people, and the supernatural environment. When all things in the universe are in tune, people have good health. But countless events can upset this harmony to cause sickness: a person can have a bad dream, break a taboo, or come into contact with such contaminating forces as spirits of the dead, non-Navajos, or Navajo witches. A whole range of animals, including snakes, bears, coyotes, and porcupines, can bring illness. Touching a tree struck by lightning or gathering and cooking with the wood from such a tree was thought to be a cause of tuberculosis. (Niethammar 2001, 87)

She married George Wauneka in 1929, and they reared six children. She was highly recognized for her good works during her lifetime.

"A humanitarian and advocate for better health, Dr. Annie, as she was known after she received an honorary doctorate degree from the Navajo Community College, has been credited with saving thousands of lives of tribal members when she almost single-handedly convinced Navajos to go to doctors to get treatment for tuberculosis" (Donovan 1997, A1). She died on November 10, 1997, from Alzheimer's disease.

References: Donovan, Bill, "Life Devoted to Health Care," *Navajo Times* 36, no. 44 (13 November 1997): A1; Niethammar, Carolyn J., *I'll Go and Do More: Annie Dodge Wauneka, Navajo Leader and Activist*, Lincoln: Univer-sity of Nebraska Press (2001); Suarez, Darlene Mary, "Annie Dodge Wauneka," in Frank Magill, ed., *Great Lives from History: American Women Series*, vol. 5, Pasadena, CA: Salem Press (1995).

Weizmann, Vera
1879–1966

Vera Weizmann was a physician and well-known as the first lady of Israel; her husband, Chaim Weizmann, became the country's first president in 1949. She worked to improve public health in Israel. Born in southern Russia in Rostov-on-Don as Vera Chatzman, she traveled to Geneva for a medical education. "The small group of young women to which Vira Chatzman belonged differed in a marked way from the general run of Jewish girl-students in the Swiss universities of that time. Their looks, their deportment, their outlook on life, set them apart. They were far more attractive than their contemporaries from the Pale of Settlement; they were less absorbed in Russian revolutionary politics; not that they were indifferent; but they paid more attention to their studies, and less to the public meetings and endless discussions which took up so much of the time of the average Russian student abroad" (Weizmann 1949, 95).

Like her husband, she was very active in Zionist causes and organizations. She also was instrumental in establishing health care and disease prevention programs in her country. Following her husband's death in 1952, she carried on the work he had started with the Weizmann Institute of Science in Rehovot, Israel.

She had two sons, Benjamin and Michael. Michael was killed in World War II. She died in September 1966.

References: Lovejoy, Esther Pohl, *Women Doctors of the World*, New York: Macmillan (1957); Weizmann, Chaim, *Trial and Error: The Autobiography of Chaim Weizmann*, New York: Harper (1949); "Weizmann, Vera" [obit], *New York Times* (25 September 1966): 85.

Western Reserve College
1826–

Founded in 1826 in Tallmadge, Ohio, this college was an early pioneer in educating women and African Americans, as well as white males, partly because Ohio was a major center of abolitionism. The school moved to Hudson, Ohio, a year after its founding.

Carroll Cutler, president of the college from 1870 to 1886, held the unconventional belief that women should have the same right as men to attend institutions of higher education, encouraging many women to enroll in the college in the late nineteenth century. Cutler had to continually defend his stance on women's rights to the faculty, and after he resigned in 1886, admittance of women ended for a brief time.

The name of the college changed to Western Reserve University in 1882. Both Emily Blackwell and Marie Zakrzewska obtained their medical degrees at Western Reserve University. In 1967, Western Reserve University merged with the neighboring Case School of Applied Science and became the current Case Western Reserve University.

References: Summerfield, Carol, and Mary Elizabeth Devine, eds., *International Dictionary of University Histories*, Chicago: Fitzroy Dearborn (1998).

Wetterhahn, Karen Elizabeth
1948–1997

Karen Wetterhahn was an established cancer researcher who also urged young women to enter the science field. She died prematurely from mercury poisoning, which brought international attention to the issue of laboratory safety.

Born in Plattsburgh, New York, on October 16, 1948, Wetterhahn was the daughter of Gustave George Wetterhahn and Mary Elizabeth Thibault Wetterhahn. She received an early education at St. Mary's High School in Champlain, New York, and then went on to study chemistry and mathematics at St. Lawrence University, graduating in 1970 at the top of her class.

She was a research fellow at Columbia University and earned a Ph.D. in 1975 in chemistry and both inorganic and physical biochemistry. She was a postdoctoral fellow at the National Institutes of Health for a year and then returned to Columbia to work at the Institute of Cancer Research. Soon thereafter she became the first female professor in chemistry at Dartmouth College.

She was a tireless researcher and writer, publishing more than eighty papers on cancer-causing chemicals and metals as well as how they interact with DNA. She also helped recruit female science students at Dartmouth in a program called the Women in Science Project (WISP), which served as a model for recruiting programs at several other colleges and universities.

After her tragic death from mercury poisoning on June 8, 1997, investigators discovered that the standard lab gloves she was wearing do not offer protection from dimethyl mercury. Her husband, Leon H. Webb, and a son and daughter survived her.

References: Proffitt, Pamela, *Notable Women Scientists*, Detroit: Gale (1999).

Whately, Mary Louisa
1824–1889

Mary Whately established a medical mission in Egypt after treating many people on her own. She was one of the first missionaries in Egypt.

Born August 31, 1824, at Halesworth in Suffolk, she was the daughter of Richard Whately, archbishop of Dublin, and Elizabeth Pope. She spent much of her early life in Dublin with frequent trips to England. She was deeply religious and early on became interested in the Irish Church's mission work abroad. She felt called to serve in Egypt, in the midst of the Islamic world.

In Cairo, she provided health care and worked to teach Muslims the Bible and convert them to Christianity. As a missionary in the field, she had to depend largely on her own resources. "No resident doctor was at this time near the scene of her work; and she herself administered constantly such remedies as she understood the use of, to the sick poor around her. Many a really serious case of eye disorder has been cured by her; many a wounded or otherwise injured hand or foot healed by her skilful hand" (Whately 1890, 61).

In 1879, Whately established a medical mission that served the needs of a poor community. To help with the patient load, she obtained the services of a Syrian medical missionary who had been trained at the American Medical College in Beirut. She died on March 9, 1889.

References: Cale, Patricia S., "A British Missionary in Egypt: Mary Louisa Whately," *Vitae Scholasticae* 3, no. 1 (1984): 131–143; Whately, Elizabeth Jane, *The Life and Work of Mary Louisa Whately*, London: Religious Tract Society (1890).

Widerstrom, Karolina
1856–1949

Karolina Widerstrom was the first woman doctor in Sweden. She paved the way for others by becoming a successful practicing gynecologist, social reformer, and writer.

Born in Sweden in 1856, Widerstrom became a physician in 1888. She was a teacher on sex and hygiene and wrote a book, *Hygiene for Women*, that was widely used for decades. Well ahead of her time, in 1897 she implemented sex education for girls' schools in Stockholm. She lectured on the needs of infants, the importance of training parents in childcare, and the detrimental effects of early parenthood.

Widerstrom was also concerned about the harm to society of the accepted profession of prostitution. Her success and good reputation were inspirational to future women physicians in Sweden. She died in 1949.

References: Andreen, Andrea, "Women Doctors in Sweden," *Journal of the American Medical Women's Association* 2, no. 2 (February 1947): 44; Lovejoy, Esther Pohl, *Women Doctors of the World*, New York: Macmillan (1957); Trost, Jan E., and Mai-Briht Bergstrom-Walan, "Sweden (Konungariket Sverige)," http://www.rki.de/GESUND/ ARCHIV/ IES/SWEDEN.HTM.

Williams, Anna Wessels
1863–1954

Anna Williams was a bacteriologist and pathologist who partnered with William Hallock Park to identify the bacillus *Corynebacterium diphtheriae*. This work led to the development of an antitoxin serum for the treatment of and immunization against diphtheria, which had caused the deaths of many children. Williams's research led to a greatly diminished occurrence of diphtheria around the world, and her findings are still useful to physicians today. Also important was her work in perfecting the diagnosis of rabies.

Born March 17, 1863, in Hackensack, New Jersey, she was the second of six children of William and Jane Williams. She received her early education at home from her parents before becoming a teacher at the New Jersey State Normal School in Trenton, New Jersey, in 1883. She taught for a few years and then decided to become a physician after her sister almost died from the delivery of a stillborn child. Her parents consented, and she entered the Women's Medical College, which had become a branch of the New York Infirmary for Women and Children.

After obtaining her medical degree, she stayed at the college in various teaching positions before furthering her education in Europe at several universities and hospitals. Her research on diphtheria began during an epidemic of the disease when she worked at a new diagnostic lab for the Health Department of the City of New York. She and Park worked with a mild tonsillar diphtheria to isolate a pure culture and develop an antitoxin to the disease.

Williams was also very good at writing for both the scientist and the layperson. She and Park coauthored the second, 1905, edition of the eleven-edition *Pathogenic Microorganisms Including Bacteria and Protozoa: A Practical Manual for Students, Physicians and Health Officers*. In 1929, she also collaborated with Park on *Who's Who among the Microbes,* a book for the nonprofessional.

Later, Williams worked on treatments for strep infections and pneumonia. She did research on scarlet fever and was the first person to fully understand that rabies began with a change in brain cells. This discovery led to diagnosis in the early stages of the disease. Williams was nationally recognized for her work. In 1907 she was appointed chair of the American Public Health Association's Committee on the Standard Methods for the Diagnosis of Rabies. Williams died on November 20, 1954.

References: Bailey, Martha J., *American Women in Science: A Biographical Dictionary,* Santa Barbara: ABC-CLIO (1994); Schafer, Elizabeth D., "Williams, Anna Wessels," in John A. Garraty and Mark C. Carnes, eds., *American National Biography,* vol. 23, New York: Oxford University Press (1999); Shearer, Benjamin F., and Barbara S. Shearer, *Notable Women in the Life Sciences: A Biographical Dictionary,* Westport, CT: Greenwood Press (1996).

Williams, Cicely Delphin
1893–1992

Cicely Williams was a British physician. She was the first to describe kwashiorkor, a disease of young children that can result in death.

Born on December 2, 1893, in Kew Park, Jamaica, she was the daughter of James Rowland Williams and Margaret E. C. Williams. Her father was the director of education in Jamaica. She received her early education at Bath High School for Girls, later attended Somerville College at Oxford, and then obtained her medical degree at Kings College.

She worked for the Colonial Medical Service from 1929 to 1948, serving on the African Gold Coast. It was here that she witnessed a large number of children suffering from kwashiorkor, a disease caused by a diet high in carbohydrates and low in protein. Older babies often suffered from this disease when the mother's breast milk was

not sufficient for both the newborn and the older child. Babies who lost their mothers or had mothers with health problems also suffered from the disease. These children were often passed around to female relatives who could take turns breast-feeding, but usually this practice did not provide enough milk to keep the child healthy.

The symptoms of kwashiorkor were slow to develop. "The baby might have been perfectly normal at birth, after four to twelve months of such a defective diet it would become highly irritable, lose weight, and have attacks of diarrhea. Its hands and feet would swell, and over a period of months its hair would gradually become pale and scanty, and its skin would turn a dull reddish color. If untreated at this stage, it would almost surely die of a progressive disease characterized by a terrible rash, an extensive sloughing of the skin, and an enlarged fatty liver" (Downs 1952, 443).

Williams wasn't able to perform any autopsies until she was in Accra in 1930. When children were about to die, the mothers would take them back to their tribal grounds. Some workers told Williams this practice was a matter of custom, but she listened to the mothers and discovered the real reason:

Apparently the bus companies charged more to transport a corpse and nothing for the live baby slung on its mother's back in a shawl. So Cicely offered to pay the extra fare if the mother would allow her to "do a small operation before the baby goes home." It was so simple, but no other European had thought of eavesdropping on the natives before. The nearest laboratory was two miles away and the body had to be taken immediately. . . . It was extremely difficult to define the certain cause of death because there would be so many contributory factors—inevitably worms, probably yaws, certainly evidence of improper diet—and frequently the child had died of pneumonia anyway. If the autopsy showed a lot of fat in the liver and oedema of the neck if not the whole of the gallbladder, she suspected a nutritional deficiency. (Craddock 1983, 63–64)

Williams began to treat the children with condensed milk, and their condition improved. She worked to educate many on recognition and prevention of the disease and on its treatment.

She taught at the American University in Beirut from 1959 to 1964 and in 1971 was a professor at Tulane University in the School of Public Health. She visited and lectured in many different countries on childhood diseases and health care for children and mothers. Williams died July 13, 1992.

References: Craddock, Sally, *Retired Except on Demand: The Life of Dr Cicely Williams*, Oxford: Green College (1983); Dally, Ann G., *Cicely: The Story of a Doctor,* London: Gollancz (1968); Downs, Elinor, "The Story of Kwashiorkor," *Journal of the American Medical Women's Association* 7, no. 12 (December 1952): 443–446; *Who's Who*, New York: St. Martin's Press (1992).

Women of Color in Medicine

Women of color faced a double hurdle in proving themselves intelligent and competent enough to pursue medical studies and practice as nurses and physicians. "If white women, black men, and poor whites, as many scholars argue, were outsiders in medicine, then black women, belonging as they did to two subordinate groups, surely inhabited the most distant perimeters of the professions" (Hine 1985, 107).

For many centuries, women themselves were well down in the class system, in many countries being traded as slaves. They often were illiterate. Until progress was made against gender discrimination, there was no hope of many cultures producing women educated for medicine.

Racism goes back to ancient times. The Hindu caste system was based on race; early cave drawings in Egypt represent racial differences. Many cultures show early signs of prejudice based on race, mainly because it is easiest to discriminate on the basis of color.

"From antiquity to approximately 1890, the Western world demonstrated an evolution of definite patterns in thoughts and actions toward those of other races" (Lauren 1996, 48). Colonizers have often discriminated against indigenous populations—"the Aborigines and Torres Strait Islanders in Australia, the Maori in New Zealand, the Uygur and the Hui in China, the Ainu in Japan, the Dayaks in Malaysia, the Papuans in Indonesia, the Andamans in India, the Saami in the Arctic regions of northern Europe, the Basarwa in Botswana, the Aka Pygmies of the Central African Republic, and the Ju/Wasi San in Namibia" (Lauren 1996, 313).

Race was an issue following both world wars, particularly after World War II, when nations were faced with the overwhelming evidence of Hitler's mass annihilations. Of interest during the two world wars was the perspective of some in minority groups that the white race might exhaust itself on war, providing other races with an opportunity to propel themselves to higher status. Mohammed Duse, editor of *African Times and Orient Review,* the first African-Asian journal, speculated that the nonwhite races of the world might benefit enormously from World War I: "We can only watch and pray. Unarmed, undisciplined, disunited, we cannot strike a blow, we can only await the event. But whatever that may be, all the combatants, the conquerors and the conquered alike, will be exhausted by the struggle, and will require years for their recovery, and during that time much may be done. Watch and wait! It may be that the non-European races will profit by European disaster" (Duse 1914, 450).

Racism continues to be a worldwide problem.

The first global attempt to speak for equality focused upon race. The first human rights provisions in the United Nations Charter were placed there because of race. The first international challenge to a country's claim of domestic jurisdiction and exclusive treatment of its own citizens centered upon race. The first binding treaty of human

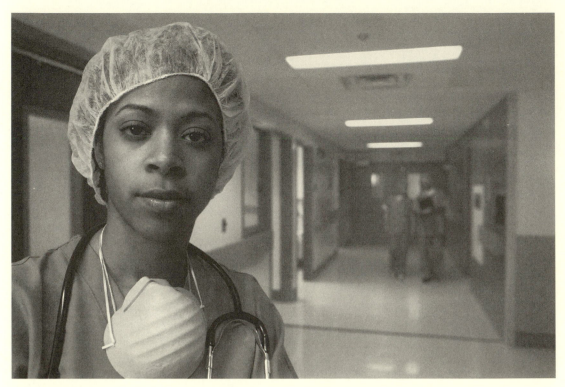

Women of color in medicine have to face both gender and racial discrimination (Corbis)

rights concentrated upon race. The international convention with the greatest number of signatories is that on race. Within the United Nations, more resolutions deal with race than with any other subject. And certainly one of the most long-standing and frustrating problems in the United Nations is that of race. (Lauren 1996, 4)

During World War I, black female nurses made some headway in Britain. After the war, they continued to fight for equal access to the profession. Having been refused by the Red Cross, all the armed forces, and other voluntary agencies, they finally achieved some success when in 1945 the U.S. Navy accepted nurses regardless of color.

During the end of World War II, Colonel Florence A. Blanchfield, the Army Nurse Corps superintendent, supported women of color in the ranks because more nurses were desperately needed. Like black servicemen, they had to work in segregated units in the beginning. One black soldier commented,

"Whenever we talked about the war and what the fighting was all about, someone would mention Hitler and his racist attitude toward blacks. We had no doubt about Hitler's prejudice because we had all heard the story about his snub of Jesse Owens during the 1936 Olympic Games. It never dawned on us that there was a real irony in the fact that the United States was trying to eradicate Nazi racism with a military formed along racist principles" (Conner 1985, 29).

Mary Mahoney opened a new profession for black women by graduating from the New England Hospital for Women and Children School of Nursing in Boston in 1879. In the early years of the National Association of Colored Graduate Nurses (NACGN), both Mahoney and Martha Franklin worked hard to organize black women. A major event was the dissolution of the NACGN in 1951 when the American Nurses Association (ANA) accepted blacks in the organization regardless of the policies of state units.

Most of the early black nurses could work in only a few hospitals. By the 1950s not much had changed, but the ANA worked to make the public aware of discrimination. Women of color have often found allies in white women who have struggled to gain credence and status in male-dominated societies and professions, and a combined force of both black and white nurses helped the cause of advancing black women nurses. In 1953, Marie Mink became an assistant professor in obstetric nursing at the University of Oklahoma. She was the first black woman to hold that position.

Black women physicians had the same problems as black nurses. Many women's medical schools lacked facilities for women to gain clinical experience, but white women could at least obtain a nursing position in order to observe doctors and surgeons. Most U.S. hospitals were segregated until the mid- to late twentieth century, and black hospitals were few in number. Hospitals with all-white staffs that allowed black women physicians to use their facilities were rare. As May Edward Chinn noted, "Even if a hospital was around the 'bend of the road' it was useless to us who were denied any privileges whatsoever of its facilities. We managed the best we could" (Warren 1999, 27).

Women of color in medicine still face barriers. A noticeable problem is the lack of role models for young girls of color. The contributions of blacks and other nonwhite groups, male or female, in medicine are often missing from history books. There is a "dearth of narratives or biographies of science-trained Blacks, particularly Black women" (Warren 1999, xiii).

Over the past few decades in the United States there has been emphasis on increasing the enrollments of students from underrepresented groups, but the effort has met with limited success. People of color are still underrepresented in the medical profession.

In North America, and specifically the United States, enrollment of black students in medical schools was only 2.2 percent in 1964, with the majority of them attending all-black schools: Howard University in Washington, D.C., and Meharry Medical College in Nashville, Tennessee (Nickens,

Ready, and Petersdorf 1994, 472). In the 1800s, some smaller liberal arts institutions had made an effort to educate blacks. The board of Oberlin College in 1835 "declared that 'the education of the people of color is a matter of great interest and should be encouraged and sustained in this institution'" (Duffy and Goldberg 1997, 137). Policies such as Oberlin College's remained the exception well into the twentieth century. "Prior to 1960, no selective college or university was making determined efforts to seek out and admit substantial numbers of African Americans" (Bowen and Bok 1998, 4). Even in the 1960s, civil rights awareness in education focused on men of color.

Numerous studies show that people of color perform as well as whites on licensing exams if they are given the same educational opportunities as whites. Many agree that the "pool size eventually can be increased by improving the socioeconomic well being for all African Americans" (Thomas 1999, 71). Thus the issue is social and political as well as educational.

In the medical profession, ethnic diversity is especially lacking in the specialties: "There is little doubt that women, African Americans, and Hispanics, have fewer opportunities to enter, or once in, to become contributing members of orthopaedic programs in the United States. The expressed reasons for this by faculty members sometimes sound reasonable, but on analysis all are spurious" (Mankin 1999, 85).

Hispanics and Native Americans as well as descendants of Oriental countries have had the same problems as blacks in addition to facing barriers specific to their ethnic groups. The women of these groups are also seen, many times, as inferior to their male counterparts as well as inferior to white females in the same occupation. Late in the nineteenth century and into the twentieth, many medical missionaries trained indigenous women to serve as nurses and physicians.

Women and even some men of color have taken advantage of the opportunity to serve minority populations. Many working-class neighborhood clinics have long waiting lines, and most white male physicians do not choose to work in underserved communities.

Most race research does not include females. Some have realized this oversight; for instance, in Great Britain, "a growing number of studies have begun to explore the interrelationship between racism and sexism, racial inequality and gender inequality and the position of African-Caribbean, Asian and other migrant women in British society. This has helped to overcome the gender blind approach of many studies of racial relations, though there are still many aspects of the position of black and ethnic minority women which have received little attention" (Solomos 1996, 13).

More research focused on women of color is needed to underscore empirical evidence that "abilities [are] separate and unrelated to gender, color, race, creed, language, religion, or country of origin. A scientist is a scientist, not an African American person who does science. A surgeon is a surgeon, not a woman from Honduras who speaks the language with an accent and also does hand surgery. Judge them only on what they are and are in fact, put on earth to do: care for patients, teach, and do research" (Mankin 1999, 86).

See also: Barriers to Success; Blanchfield, Florence Aby; Chinn, May Edward; Franklin, Martha Minerva; Mahoney, Mary Eliza; Wars and Epidemics

References: Bowen, William G., and Derek Bok, *The Shape of the River: Long-Term Consequences of Considering Race in College and University Admissions*, Princeton, NJ: Princeton University Press (1998); Conner, Douglas L., *A Black Physician's Story: Bringing Hope in Mississippi*, Jackson: University of Mississippi Press (1985); Duffy, Elizabeth A., and Idana Goldberg, *Crafting a Class: College Admissions and Financial Aid, 1955–1994*, Princeton, NJ: Princeton University Press (1997); Duse, Mohammed, "War!," *African Times and Orient Review* (4 August 1914): 449–450; Hine, Darlene Clark, "Co-Laborers in the Work of the Lord: Nineteenth Century Black Women Physicians," in Ruth J. Abrams, ed., *Send Us a Lady Physician: Women Doctors in America, 1835–1920*, New York: Norton (1985); Lauren, Paul Gordon, *Power and Prej-* udice: *The Politics and Diplomacy of Racial Discrimination*, Boulder, CO: Westview Press (1996); Mankin, Henry J., "Diversity in Orthopaedics," *Clinical Orthopaedics and Related Research: Issues of Minorities in Medicine and Orthopaedics* 363 (May 1999): 85–87; Nickens, Herbert W., Timothy P. Ready, and Robert G. Petersdorf, "Project 3000 by 2000: Racial and Ethnic Diversity in U.S. Medical Schools," *New England Journal of Medicine* 331, no. 7 (1994): 472–476; Solomos, John, *Racism and Society*, New York: St. Martin's Press (1996); Staupers, Mabel Keaton, *No Time for Prejudice: A Story of the Integration of Negroes in Nursing in the United States*, New York: Macmillan (1961); Thomas, Claudia L., "African Americans and Women in Orthopaedic Residency: The Johns Hopkins Experience," *Clinical Orthopaedics and Related Research: Issues of Minorities in Medicine and Orthopaedics* 363 (May 1999): 65–71; Warren, Wini, *Black Women Scientists in the United States*, Bloomington: Indiana University Press (1999); Watson, Wilbur H., *Against the Odds: Blacks in the Profession of Medicine in the United States*, New Brunswick, NJ: Transaction (1999).

Wong-Staal, Flossie
1946–

Flossie Wong-Staal codiscovered (with Robert Gallo) the human immunodeficiency virus (HIV) and was the first scientist to clone it. Known as one of the leading scientists in the fight against HIV/AIDS, Wong-Staal has remained at the forefront of knowledge on the deadly virus.

Born in Guangzhou, China, on August 27, 1946, she is the daughter of Sueh-fung Wang and his wife. She attended Catholic school and upon graduation decided on further study in the United States. She went to the University of California in Los Angeles (UCLA) and majored in molecular biology.

Upon graduation in 1968, she remained at UCLA and worked at the graduate level, earning a Ph.D. in 1972. She then went to Bethesda, Maryland, and worked for the National Cancer Institute, researching retroviruses with Robert Gallo. Her research group discovered the human T-cell leukemia virus (HTLV) and later two related retroviruses, one of which was HIV. Wong-Staal was the first scientist to clone HIV and to genetically map the virus. This step was critical to providing a blood test for the presence of HIV/AIDS.

In the following years, Wong-Staal wrote extensively to provide the scientific community with the necessary information for more research on the virus. In 1990 she became the director of the Center for AIDS Research at the University of California at San Diego. She believes in examining as many approaches as feasible, such as a vaccine and gene therapy. Not only does the virus reproduce very quickly but there are several strains, each of which may lend itself to a different treatment.

Wong-Staal married Steven Staal in 1971, and they had two daughters. They are now divorced, and she and her daughters live in San Diego, where she is currently codirector of the AIDS Research Institute at the University of California at San Diego.

References: Kelly, Patrick, "Wong-Staal, Flossie," *Current Biography* 62, no. 4 (April 2001): 87–90.

Wright, Jane Cooke
1919–

Jane Wright is a prominent cancer chemotherapy researcher whose work with various drugs and their effects on malignant tumors has provided great insight into cancer treatment. She has directed large hospital staffs as well as served as the dean of a medical college. Born in New York City on November 30, 1919, she is the daughter of Dr. Louis Tompkins Wright and Corinne Cooke Wright. Her family has a rich medical heritage with her father being one of the first black graduates of Harvard Medical School and a leader in the field of cancer chemotherapy; a grandfather was one of the first blacks to graduate from Meharry Medical College. Her father was also a civil rights leader.

After attending private schools in New

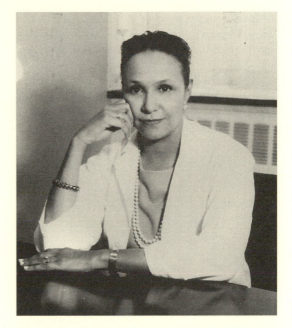

Jane Cooke Wright (U.S. National Library of Medicine)

York City, Wright entered Smith College in order to prepare for medical school. Upon graduation from Smith in 1942, she won a scholarship to New York Medical College. She obtained her M.D. and interned at Bellevue Hospital. She also worked at Harlem Hospital before getting married in 1947 to David D. Jones Jr., a Harvard Law School graduate.

She began working in internal medicine and was a school doctor in New York City until she took a position in 1949 at the Harlem Hospital Cancer Research Foundation as a clinician. It was here that she began studying the effects of drugs such as triethylene phosphoramide and triethylene melamine on malignant growths.

She moved on to become the director of cancer chemotherapy research at New York University Medical Center in 1955 and became an instructor in research surgery. She expanded her own clinical experience by doing surgical work at Bellevue and University Hospitals in New York City. By the 1960s, Wright believed, as did some other researchers, that cancer was caused by a virus. Her investigations based on this view included the drugs fluorouracil and steptonigrin. During this time she published quite extensively; she has an impressive bibliography documenting the chemotherapy research she was involved with.

She became the associate dean and professor of surgery at New York Medical College in 1967. Her duties broadened to heart disease and stroke as well as cancer. She has two daughters and lives in New York City.

References: "Wright, Jane C.," *Current Biography*, New York: H. W. Wilson (1968); Shearer, Benjamin F., and Barbara S. Shearer, *Notable Women in the Life Sciences*, Westport, CT: Greenwood Press (1996).

Yalow, Rosalyn Sussman
1921–

Rosalyn Yalow received the 1977 Nobel Prize for "the development of radioimmunoassay (RIA) of peptid hormones," a technique that she discovered in 1959 with her partner in research, Solomon Berson (Shearer and Shearer 1996, 409). The technique revolutionized endocrinology, and other fields soon found it indispensable.

She was born July 19, 1921, in New York City to Clara Zipper Sussman and Simon Sussman. Neither had much education, but they encouraged Rosalyn in her studies. She did very well in school and went to Hunter College in New York, which was free at the time; her family could not afford to pay for college.

She decided on a career in physics and graduated in 1941. She proceeded to the University of Illinois at Urbana-Champaign, earning a master's in 1942 and a Ph.D. in nuclear physics in 1945. She felt that nuclear physics was extremely exciting at the time and that it had medical applications.

She met Aaron Yalow, a fellow physicist graduate student, whom she married on June 6, 1943. They have two children, Benjamin and Elanna. Aaron was supportive of Rosalyn's career goals.

Yalow taught for a while upon earning her Ph.D. but then decided to work full-time at the Veterans' Administration Hospital in the Bronx, New York. There, she helped set up the hospital's radioisotope service and later teamed up with Berson, a physician, to work on insulin. During the

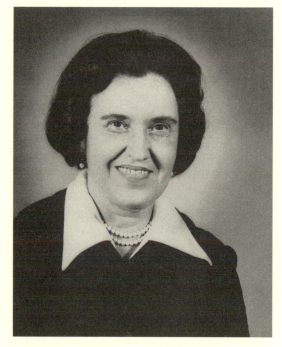

Rosalyn Sussman Yalow (U.S. National Library of Medicine)

1950s, they made great progress in using radioactively tagged insulin to determine how long insulin stayed in the diabetic's system. They deduced, correctly, that diabetics could build up antibodies to insulin. Before that time scientists didn't believe insulin molecules were large enough to incite an antibody. Their method of using radioactive substances then allowed them to test for many kinds of antibodies. Thus RIA was born.

"The introduction of radioimmunoassay . . . is probably the single most important advance in biological measurement of the past two decades. Together with related techniques it has revolutionised one major discipline—endocrinology—and has exerted a similar influence in other fields, notably haematology, pharmacology, and cancer detection" (Chard 1982, 1).

Yalow feels strongly that it is important for women to go into science or any other profession of their choosing as well as to become mothers. "Being a mother was an essential part of Rosalyn Yalow's plan for her life, and she insists that motherhood should fit into the lives of other women with careers in science" (Straus 1998, 186).

Some feel Berson deserved more credit for the development of RIA. Yalow has fully acknowledged his contribution during the years it took them to refine the process. Yalow's "work and methods advanced medical science in the areas of diagnosis, treatment, and prevention of disease. This was done by providing breakthroughs in the understanding of diabetes, in the diagnosis and treatment of many glandular disorders such as dwarfism and cretinism, and through providing a method to save countless people from acquiring liver disease from blood transfusions. She fought for what she wanted and for her beliefs" (Straus 1998, 257). Today Yalow is retired and lives in New York City.

References: Chard, T., *An Introduction to Radioimmunoassay and Related Techniques*, Amsterdam: Elsevier Biomedical Press (1982); McGrayne, Sharon Bertsch, *Nobel Prize Women in Science: Their Lives, Struggles, and Momentous Discoveries*, Secaucus, NJ: Carol (1998); Shearer, Benjamin, and Barbara S. Shearer, *Notable Women in the Life Sciences: A Biographical Dictionary*, Westport, CT: Greenwood Press (1996); Straus, Eugene, *Rosalyn Yalow, Nobel Laureate: Her Life and Work in Medicine: A Biographical Memoir*, New York: Plenum Trade (1998).

Yoshioka, Yayoi
1871–1959

Yaoi Yoshioka was an early Japanese female physician who struggled against oppression and social injustice to obtain a medical education. She founded the Tokyo Women's Medical College in 1899, which was finally recognized by the Japanese government in 1920.

She passed government examinations and became a gynecologist in 1893. With her husband, she established the Tokyo Women's Medical College, where she taught for fifty years. Yoshioka also established hospitals in Tokyo. She died of pneumonia in Tokyo on May 23, 1959, at the age of eighty-eight.

References: "Dr. Yayoi Yoshioka Dies," *New York Times* (24 May 1959): 88; Kawai, Yaeko, "Medical Women in Japan," *Journal of the American Medical Women's Association* 6, no. 9 (September 1951): 352–353; Lovejoy, Esther Pohl, *Women Doctors of the World*, New York: Macmillan (1957); "Yoshioka, Yayoi," *Kodansha Encyclopedia of Japan*, vol. 8, Tokyo: Kodansha (1983).

Z

Zakrzewska, Marie Elizabeth
1829–1902

Marie Zakrzewska was an early proponent of women becoming physicians and founded the New England Hospital for Women and Children after working with Elizabeth Blackwell and Emily Blackwell at the New York Infirmary for Women and Children and as a professor at the New England Female Medical College.

Born in Berlin, Germany, on September 6, 1829, Zakrzewska was the daughter of Ludwig Martin Zakrzewska and Caroline Fredericke Wilhelmina Urban. Her father worked in the military and later as a civil servant. They had very little money, and her mother worked as a midwife to help support the family. She had trained at the Royal Charity Hospital in Berlin.

Zakrzewska many times went with her mother on rounds and became interested in midwifery as a profession. She did well at the Royal Charity Hospital in Berlin and gained the position of head midwife in 1852. She stayed there less than a year before she left with her sister for New York City to become a physician.

After meeting Elizabeth Blackwell, she was inspired to go to Western Reserve College for a medical degree. She graduated in 1856, and the next year she helped the Blackwells establish the New York Infirmary for Women and Children. She worked as a resident physician for a few years, then moved on to become a professor of obstetrics in Boston at the New England Female Medical College, founded by

Samuel Gregory, because she wanted to further her education.

Gregory and she disagreed over the curriculum. She wanted to incorporate some laboratory practices into the students' work, such as dissection and the use of microscopes, but could not persuade him. She also wanted to establish more rigorous qualifications for diplomas. "But I found very little support, and I was told that it would be hard to disappoint some women who had perseveringly labored for a diploma. According to my ideas, which agree, I know, with the ideas of the profession generally, perseverance alone does not entitle persons to receive a diploma. Even should a disappointment prove to be a deathblow to the student, it is better that one should die rather than receive permission to kill many" (Zakrzewska 1924, 282). She felt compelled to leave the college and did so in 1862.

Upon her departure, she immediately went to work setting up the New England Hospital for Women and Children. She had helped the Blackwells set up the New York Infirmary because she could see female medical students' immediate need for clinical experience and the need for better health care for women and children. She saw the same need in Boston, and officially founded the hospital in 1862.

Zakrzewska had a very strong personality and worked hard to advance the status of women. She was an active suffragist and reformer. She was also very compassionate toward those she served. "At one time she was instrumental in having a lunch-room opened for poor working-girls, where for a few cents a nourishing and appetizing meal was provided" (NEHWC 1977, 19).

Zakrzewska effectively ran the New England Hospital for Women and Children until 1899. She was involved in all aspects of its operation. She continually urged women physicians to gain as much scientific knowledge as possible. She earned an excellent reputation as a physician, even among some of the male physicians of her day. She died in Boston on May 12, 1902.

See also: Blackwell, Elizabeth; New England Female Medical College; New England Hospital

References: New England Hospital for Women and Children (NEHWC), *Marie Elizabeth Zakrzewska: A Memoir*, Boston: New England Hospital for Women and Children (1902), reprinted in *History of Women Collection*, no. 5403, New Haven, CT: Research Publications (1977); Tuchman, Arleen Marcia, "Zakrzewska, Marie Elizabeth," *American National Biography*, vol. 24, New York: Oxford University Press (1999); Zakrzewska, Marie E., *A Woman's Quest: The Life of Marie E. Zakrzewska, M.D.*, ed. Agnes C. Vietor, New York: D. Appleton (1924).

Bibliography

Abrahams, Harold J. *The Extinct Medical Schools of Baltimore, Maryland.* Baltimore: Maryland Historical Society, 1969.

Ackerman, Jennifer. "Journey to the Center of the Egg." *New York Times,* sec. 6 (12 October 1997): 42.

Agris, Joseph. "Honoria Acosta Sison: Pioneer Gynecologist and Obstetrician." *Journal of Dermatologic Surgery and Oncology* 6:3 (March 1980): 178.

Alic, Margaret. *Hypatia's Heritage: A History of Women in Science from Antiquity to the Late Nineteenth Century.* London: Women's Press, 1986.

Allen, Nessy. "A Pioneer of Paediatric Gastroenterology: The Career of an Australian Woman Scientist." *Historical Records of Australian Science* 11:1 (June 1996): 35–50.

Alvord, Lori Arviso. "Navajo Surgeon Combines Approaches." *Health Progress* 80:1 (January–February 1999): 42.

Alvord, Lori Arviso, and Elizabeth Cohen Van Pelt. *The Scalpel and the Silver Bear.* New York: Bantam Books, 1999.

Ambrose, Paul. "Uniting Public Health and Medicine." *JAMA* 278:21 (3 December 1997): 1722.

American Medical Association. *Physician Characteristics and Distribution in the United States.* Chicago, IL: Survey and Data Resources, American Medical Association, 2002.

American Medical Missionary Society (AMMS). *A Great Field for Women.* Chicago: American Medical Missionary Society, 1880?. Reprinted in *History of Women,* reel 939, no. 8277. New Haven, CT: Research Publications, 1977.

American Men and Women of Science. 12th ed. New York: Bowker, 1972.

American Men and Women of Science. 20th ed. New York: Bowker, 1998.

American Nurses Association. "The Hall of Fame Inductees, Florence S. Wald." http://www.nursingworld.org/hof/waldfs.htm.

American Periodical Series, 1800–1850 [microfilm collection]. Ann Arbor: University of Michigan, 1946–1976.

Anderson, Charlotte M., and Valerie Burke, eds. *Paediatric Gastroenterology.* Oxford: Blackwell Scientific, 1975.

Andreen, Andrea. "Women Doctors in Sweden." *Journal of the American Medical Women's Association* 2:2 (February 1947): 44.

Andrews, Mary Raymond Shipman. *A Lost Commander: Florence Nightingale.* Garden City, NY: Doubleday, Doran, 1929.

Andrews, William L., Frances Smith Foster, and Trudier Harris, eds. *Oxford Companion to African American Literature.* New York: Oxford University Press, 1999.

"Anne Spoerry Tribute." *AMREF Current News.* http://www.amref.org/Spoerry.html.

Antler, Joyce. "Book Review: Toward a New Psychology of Women." *Social Policy* 18:3 (Winter 1988): 63–64.

"Apgar Scoring System." *Encyclopedia Britannica Online.* http://www.britannica.com/bcom/eb/article/4/0,5716,1694+1,00.html.

Apgar, Virginia. "A Proposal for a New Method of Evaluation of the Newborn Infant." *Current Researches in Anesthesia and Analgesia* 32 (July–August 1953): 260–267.

"Bachelor Mother." *Ebony* (September 1958): 92–96.

Bailey, Martha J. *American Women in Science: A Biographical Dictionary.* Santa Barbara: ABC-CLIO, 1994.

———. *American Women in Science, 1950 to the Present: A Biographical Dictionary.* Santa Barbara, CA: ABC-CLIO, 1998.

Baldwin, Richard S. *The Fungus Fighters.* Ithaca, NY: Cornell University Press, 1981.

Balfour, Lady Frances. *Dr. Elsie Inglis.* New York: George H. Doran, 1919.

Balfour, Margaret I., and Ruth Young. *The Work of Medical Women in India.* London: Oxford University Press, 1929.

Balmer, Randall, and John R. Fitzmier. *The Presbyterians.* Westport, CT: Greenwood Press, 1993.

Baly, Monica E. *Florence Nightingale and the Nursing Legacy.* London: Croom Helm, 1986.

Barbuto, Domenica M. *American Settlement Houses and Progressive Social Reform: An Encyclopedia of the American Settlement Movement.* Phoenix, AZ: Oryx Press, 1999.

Barker, Kristin. "Women Physicians and the Gendered System of Professions: An Analysis of the Sheppard-Towner Act of 1921." *Work and Occupations* 25:2 (May 1998): 229–255.

Barringer, Emily Dunning. *Bowery to Bellevue: The Story of New York's First Woman Ambulance Surgeon.* New York: W. W. Norton, 1950.

Barton, William E. *Life of Clara Barton, Founder of the American Red Cross.* Boston: Houghton Mifflin, 1922.

Bass, Elizabeth. "Esther Pohl Lovejoy, MD." *Journal of the American Medical Women's Association* 6:9 (September 1951): 354–355.

Benedict, Carol. *Bubonic Plague in Nineteenth-century China.* Palo Alto, CA: Stanford University Press, 1996.

Bickers, Robert A., and Rosemary Seton, eds. *Missionary Encounters: Sources and Issues.* Richmond, Surrey: Curzon Press, 1996.

Blackwell, Elizabeth. *Pioneer Work in Opening the Medical Profession to Women: Autobiographical Sketches.* New York: Source Book Press, 1970.

Bloch, Ernst. *The Principle of Hope.* Vol. 2. Cambridge, MA: MIT Press, 1986.

Bluemel, Elinor. *Florence Sabin: Colorado Woman of the Century.* Boulder, CO: University of Colorado Press, 1959.

Bowen, William G., and Derek Bok. *The Shape of the River: Long-Term Consequences of Considering Race in College and University Admissions.* Princeton, NJ: Princeton University Press, 1998.

Bowman, John S. *The Cambridge Dictionary of American Biography.* Cambridge, MA: Cambridge University Press, 1995.

Bren, Linda. "Frances Oldham Kelsey: FDA Medical Reviewer Leaves Her Mark on History." *FDA Consumer* 35:2 (March–April 2001): 24–29.

Brice-Finch, Jacqueline. "Seacole, Mary." *Oxford Companion to African American Literature.* New York: Oxford University Press, 1997.

Brownlee, Sibyl Ventress. *Out of the Abundance of the Heart: Sarah Ann Parker Remond's Quest for Freedom.* Ph.D. dissertation, University of Massachusetts, 1997.

Buck, Claire, ed. *Bloomsbury Guide to Women's Literature.* London: Bloomsbury, 1992.

Buckler, Georgina. *Anna Comnena: A Study.* London: Oxford University Press, 1929.

Bullough, Vern L., Olga Maranjian Church, and Alice Stein. *American Nursing: A Biographical Dictionary.* New York: Garland, 1988.

Burstein, Paul, and Marie Bricher. "Problem Definition and Public Policy: Congressional Committees Confront Work, Family, and Gender, 1945–1990." *Social Forces* 76:1 (September 1997): 135–168.

Burstyn, Linda. "Female Circumcision Comes to America." *Atlantic Monthly* 276:4 (October 1995): 28–35.

Burt, Olive Woolley. *Physician to the World: Esther Pohl Lovejoy.* New York: J. Messner, 1973.

Cadbury, William Warder, and Mary Hoxie Jones. *At the Point of a Lancet: One Hundred Years of the Canton Hospital, 1835–1935.* Shanghai: Kelly and Walsh, 1935.

Cale, Patricia S. "A British Missionary in Egypt: Mary Louisa Whately." *Vitae Scholasticae* 3:1 (1984): 131–143.

Calmes, Selma Harrison. "Virginia Apgar: A Woman Physician's Career in a Developing Specialty." *Journal of the American Medical Women's Association* 39:6 (November–December 1984): 184–188.

Calverley, Eleanor T. *My Arabian Days and Nights.* New York: Crowell, 1958.

Carlisle, Richard C. "Helen Taussig—A Heroine." *Pharos of Alpha Omega Alpha-Honor Medical Society* 64:1 (Winter 2001): 59.

Carnegie, Mary Elizabeth. *The Path We Tread: Blacks in Nursing Worldwide, 1854–1994.* New York: National League of Nursing Press, 1995.

Centers for Disease Control (CDC). "Achievements in Public Health, 1900–1999: Family Planning." *JAMA* 283:3 (19 January 2000): 326.

Ceskoslovensky Biograficky Slovnik. Prague: Academia, 1992.

Chard, T. *An Introduction to Radioimmunoassay and Related Techniques.* Amsterdam: Elsevier Biomedical Press, 1982.

Christy, Nicholas P. "Hattie E. Alexander, 1901–1968." *Journal of the College of Physicians and Surgeons of Columbia University* 17:2 (Spring 1997): http://cpmcnet.columbia.edu/news/journal/archives/jour_v17n2_0002.html.

Clarke, Edward H. *Sex in Education; or A Fair Chance for the Girls.* Boston: J. R. Osgood, 1873.

Cohen, Saul B. *The Columbia Gazetteer of the World.* New York: Columbia University Press, 1998.

Coles, Robert. *Anna Freud: The Dream of Psychoanalysis.* Reading, MA: Addison-Wesley, 1992.

Comfort, Nathaniel C. *The Tangled Field: Barbara McClintock's Search for the Patterns of Genetic Control.* Cambridge, MA: Harvard University Press, 2001.

Congdon-Martin, Elizabeth W. "Mary Washington Bacheler, M.D.: Enlisted for Life." *American Baptist Quarterly* 12:3 (1993): 271–282.

Conner, Douglas L. *A Black Physician's Story: Bringing Hope in Mississippi.* Jackson: University of Mississippi Press, 1985.

Contemporary Authors Online. Detroit: Gale, 1962– .

Contemporary Black Biography. Vol. 14. Detroit: Gale, 1997.

Cook, Sir Edward. *The Life of Florence Nightingale.* London: Macmillan, 1925.

Corner, George Washington. *A History of the Rockefeller Institute, 1901–1953: Origins and Growth.* New York: Rockefeller Institute Press, 1964.

Craddock, Sally. *Retired Except on Demand: The Life of Dr Cicely Williams.* Oxford: Green College, 1983.

Creese, Mary R. S. *Ladies in the Laboratory? American and British Women in Science, 1800–1900.* Lanham, MD: Scarecrow Press, 1998.

Crumpler, Rebecca. *A Book of Medical Discourses.* Boston: Cahsman, Keating, 1883.

Crystal, David. *The Cambridge Biographical Encyclopedia.* Cambridge: Cambridge University Press, 1998.

Cullis, W. C. "Scharlieb, Dame Mary Ann Dacomb." *Dictionary of National Biography, 1922–1930.* Oxford: Oxford University Press, 1937.

Curie, Eve. *Madame Curie: A Biography.* New York: Doubleday, 1937.

Current Biography Yearbook. New York: H. W. Wilson, 1993.

Dally, Ann G. *Cicely: The Story of a Doctor.* London: Gollancz, 1968.

"Dame Josephine Barnes." London *Times,* 29 December 1999, p. 19.

Damrosch, Douglas S. "Dorothy Hansine Andersen." *Journal of Pediatrics* 65:4 (October 1964): 477–479.

Daniels, Doris Groshen. *Always a Sister: The Feminism of Lillian D. Wald.* New York: Feminist Press at the City University of New York, 1989.

Darrow, Ruth Renter. "Icterus Gravis (Erythroblastosis) Neonatorum." *Archives of Pathology* 25 (1938): 378–417.

Davies, Mildred. "Valentina Dmitrieva." *Russian Women Writers.* Vol. 2. New York: Garland, 1999.

Davis, Althea T. *Early Black American Leaders in Nursing: Architects for Integration and Equality.* Boston: Jones and Bartlett, 1999.

"Dejerine, Augusta Klumpke." *The National Cyclopedia of American Biography,* vol. 31. New York: J. T. White, 1944.

Delaney, James J., Jr. "Roy Cleere and Florence Sabin." *Colorado Medicine* 80:2 (February 1983): 46–47.

Delmege, James Anthony. *Towards National Health; or, Health and Hygiene in England from Roman to Victorian Times.* New York: Macmillan, 1932.

De Vargas, Tegualda Ponce. "Women Doctors of Chile." *Journal of the American Medical Women's Association* 7:10 (October 1952): 389.

Diamond, Leila. "Charlotte Friend (1921–1987)." *Nature* 326:6115 (23 April 1987): 748.

Diamond, Leila, and Sandra R. Wolman. *Viral Oncogenesis and Cell Differentiation: The Contributions of Charlotte Friend.* New York: New York Academy of Sciences, 1989.

Dictionary of American Medical Biography. Westport, CT: Greenwood Press, 1984.

Dictionary of National Biography: 1941–1950. London: Oxford University Press, 1959.

Dictionary of National Biography: 1951–1960. London: Oxford University Press, 1971.

Dictionary of National Biography: 1981–1985. London: Oxford University Press, 1990.

Dictionary of National Biography: Missing Persons. Oxford: Oxford University Press, 1993.

Dictionary of New Zealand Biography, Vol. 4, *1921–1940.* Wellington: Bridget Williams Books and the Department of Internal Affairs, 1998.

Dictionary of Scientific Biography. New York: Scribner's, 1970–1980.

Dobell, A.R.C. "Maude Abbott." *Clinical Cardiology* 11:9 (September 1988): 658–659.

"Doctor Number One." *Holiday* 17:2 (February 1955): 92.

Donovan, Bill. "Life Devoted to Health Care." *Navajo Times* 36:44 (13 November 1997): A1.

Dossey, Barbara Montgomery. *Florence Nightingale: Mystic, Visionary, Healer.* Springhouse, PA: Springhouse Corp., 2000.

Downs, Elinor. "The Story of Kwashiorkor." *Journal of the American Medical Women's Association* 7:12 (December 1952): 443–446.

"Dr. Margaret D. Craighill, at 78, Former Dean

of Medical College." *New York Times* (26 July 1977): 32.

"Dr. Yayoi Yoshioka Dies." *New York Times* (24 May 1959): 88.

Drachman, Virginia G. *Hospital with a Heart: Women Doctors and the Paradox of Separatism at the New England Hospital, 1862–1969*. Ithaca, NY: Cornell University Press, 1984.

Drake, Fred W. *Ruth V. Hemenway, MD: A Memoir of Revolutionary China, 1924–1941*. Amherst: University of Massachusetts Press, 1977.

Dries, Angelyn. "Dengel, Anna." *Biographical Dictionary of Christian Missions*. New York: Macmillan, 1998.

Du Boulay, Shirley. *Cicely Saunders, Founder of the Modern Hospice Movement*. New York: Amaryllis Press, 1984.

Duffin, Jacalyn. "The Death of Sarah Lovell and the Constrained Feminism of Emily Stowe." *Canadian Medical Association Journal* 146:6 (15 March 1992): 881–888.

———. "Apgar, Virginia." *American National Biography*, 1999.

Duffus, Robert Luther. *Lillian Wald, Neighbor and Crusader*. New York: Macmillan, 1938.

Duffy, Elizabeth A., and Idana Goldberg. *Crafting a Class: College Admissions and Financial Aid, 1955–1994*. Princeton, NJ: Princeton University Press, 1997.

Dunn, Thelma Brumfield. *The Unseen Fight against Cancer: Experimental Cancer Research— Its Importance to Human Cancer*. Charlottesville, VA: Batt Bates, 1975.

Duse, Mohammed. "War!" *African Times and Orient Review* (4 August 1914): 449–450.

Elders, M. Joycelyn, and David Chanoff. *Joycelyn Elders, M.D.: From Sharecropper's Daughter to Surgeon General of the United States of America*. New York: Morrow, 1996.

Elion, Gertrude B. "The Purine Path to Chemotherapy." In Tore Frangsmyr and Jan Lindsten, eds., *Physiology or Medicine: 1981–1990*. River Edge, NJ: World Scientific, 1993.

Elliott, S. D. "Obituary: Rebecca Craighill Lancefield, 1895–1981." *Journal of General Microbiology* 126:1 (September 1981): 1–4.

Encyclopedia Britannica. Chicago: Encyclopedia Britannica, 1997.

Encyclopedia of World Biography. Detroit: Gale Research, 1999.

Engel, Barbara Alpern. *Mothers and Daughters: Women of the Intelligentsia in Nineteenth Century Russia*. Cambridge: Cambridge University Press, 1983.

Epstein, Eric Joseph, and Philip Rosen.

Dictionary of the Holocaust: Biography, Geography, and Terminology. Westport, CT: Greenwood Press, 1997.

"Expert on Cell Surfaces to Deliver Lucy W. Pickett Lecture November 20." *College Street Journal* (Mount Holyoke College), http://138.110.28.9/offices/comm/csj/111700/pickett.shtml.

Fahimi, Miriam. "Homa Shaibany, M.B.B.S.: First Woman Surgeon of Iran." *Journal of the American Medical Women's Association* 7:7 (July 1952): 272–273.

Fairbanks, Virgil F. "In Memoriam: Winifred M. Ashby, 1879–1975." *Blood* 46:6 (December 1975): 977–978.

Fedoroff, Nina, and David Botstein, eds. *The Dynamic Genome: Barbara McClintock's Ideas in the Century of Genetics*. Cold Spring Harbor, NY: Cold Spring Harbor Laboratory Press, 1992.

Finkelstein, David. "A Woman Hater and Women Healers: John Blackwood, Charles Reade, and the Victorian Women's Medical Movement." *Victorian Periodicals Review* 28:4 (Winter 1995): 330–352.

Flanagan, Sabina. *Hildegard of Bingen, 1098–1179: A Visionary Life*. London: Routledge, 1998.

Fleming, Leslie A. *Women's Work for Women: Missionaries and Social Change in Asia*. Boulder, CO: Westview Press, 1989.

Flexner, Abraham. *Medical Education in the United States and Canada: A Report to the Carnegie Foundation for the Advancement of Teaching*. New York: Carnegie Foundation for the Advancement of Teaching, 1910.

Folkers, Karl. "Gladys Anderson Emerson (1903–1984): A Biographical Sketch." *Journal of Nutrition* 115:7 (July 1985): 837–841.

Ford, Bonnie. "Lydia Folger Fowler." In *Great Lives from History, American Women Series*. Vol. 2. Pasadena, CA: Salem Press, 1995.

Foster, Pauline Poole. *Ann Preston, M.D. (1813–1872): A Biography—The Struggle to Obtain Training and Acceptance for Women Physicians in Mid-Nineteenth Century America*. Pittsburgh: University Press of Pennsylvania, 1984.

Fountain, Henry. "Mary Ellen Jones, 73, Crucial Researcher on DNA." *New York Times* (7 September 1996): 13.

Franklin, James Henry. *Ministers of Mercy*. New York: Missionary Education Movement of the United States and Canada, 1919.

Friedrich, M. J. "Hospice Care in the United States: A Conversation with Florence S. Wald." *JAMA* 281:18 (12 May 1999): 1683–1685.

"From the Centers for Disease Control and Prevention: Achievements in Public Health, 1900–1999—Family Planning." *JAMA* 283:3 (19 January 2000): 326–327, 331.

Fryer, Mary Beacock. *Emily Stowe: Doctor and Suffragist.* Toronto: Hannah Institute, Dundurn Press, 1990.

Fullton, Mary H. *"Inasmuch": Extracts from Letters, Journals, Papers, etc.* West Medford, MA: Central Committee on the United Study of Foreign Missions, 1915.

Gabor, Andrea. "Married, with Househusband." *Working Woman* 20:11 (November 1995): 46–50.

Garraty, John A., and Mark C. Carnes, eds. *American National Biography.* New York: Oxford University Press, 1999.

Gartner, Carol B. "Fussell's Folly: Academic Standards and the Case of Mary Putnam Jacobi." *Academic Medicine* 71:5 (May 1996): 470–477.

———. "Jacobi, Mary Corinna Putnam." *American National Biography.* New York: Oxford University Press, 1999.

Gelbart, Nina Rattner. "The Monarchy's Midwife Who Left No Memoirs." *French Historical Studies* 19:4 (Fall 1996): 997–1023.

———. *The King's Midwife: A History and Mystery of Madame du Coudray.* Berkeley: University of California Press, 1998.

Gerritsen Women's History [microfilm collection]. Sanford, NC: Microfilming Corporation of America, 1975– .

Gill, Derek L. T. *Quest: The Life of Elisabeth Kubler-Ross.* New York: Harper & Row, 1980.

Gladwin, Mary E. *The Red Cross and Jane Arminda Delano.* Philadelphia: W. B. Saunders, 1931.

Glazer, Penina Migdal, and Miriam Slater. *Unequal Colleagues: The Entrance of Women into the Professions, 1890–1940.* New Brunswick, NJ: Rutgers University Press, 1987.

Glusker, Jenny P. "Dorothy Crowfoot Hodgkin." *Protein Science* 3:12 (December 1994): 2465–2469.

Gordon, Doris Jolly. *Doctor Down Under.* London: Faber and Faber, 1958.

Green, Monica H. *The Trotula: A Medieval Compendium of Women's Medicine.* Philadelphia: University Press of Pennsylvania, 2001.

Greene, Gayle. *The Woman Who Knew Too Much: Alice Stewart and the Secrets of Radiation.* Ann Arbor: University of Michigan Press, 1999.

Grigg, William. "The Thalidomide Tradedy—25 Years Ago." *FDA Consumer* 21:1 (February 1987): 14–17.

Grinstein, Louise S., Carol A. Biermann, and Rose K. Rose, eds. *Women in the Biological Sciences: A Biobibliographic Sourcebook.* Westport, CT: Greenwood Press, 1997.

Grinstein, Louise S., Rose K. Rose, and Miriam H. Rafailovich. *Women in Chemistry and Physics: A Biobibliographic Sourcebook.* Westport, CT: Greenwood Press, 1993.

Grosskurth, Phyllis. *Melanie Klein: Her World and Her Work.* New York: Knopf, 1986.

Guillain, Georges, and Pierre Mathieu. *La Salpêtrière.* Paris, France: Masson, 1925.

Gundersen, Herdis. "Medical Women in Norway." *Journal of the American Medical Women's Association* 6:7 (July 1951): 281.

Gutman, Israel. *The Encyclopedia of the Holocaust.* New York: Macmillan, 1990.

Hacker, Carlotta. *The Indomitable Lady Doctors.* Toronto: Clarke, Irwin, 1974.

Haden-Guest, Leslie. *Votes for Women and the Public Health.* London: Women's Freedom League, 1912.

Haines, Catharine M. C., and Helen Stevens. *International Women in Science: A Biographical Dictionary to 1950.* Santa Barbara, CA: ABC-CLIO, 2001.

Hannam, June. "Rosalind Paget: The Midwife, the Women's Movement and Reform before 1914." In *Midwives, Society, and Childbirth: Debates and Controversies in the Modern Period.* Edited by Hilary Marland and Anne Marie Rafferty. London: Routledge, 1997.

Harvey, Abner McGehee. "A New School of Anatomy: The Story of Franklin P. Mall, Florence R. Sabin, and John B. MacCallum." *Johns Hopkins Medical Journal* 136:2 (February 1975): 83–94.

Hays, Elinor Rice. *Those Extraordinary Blackwells: The Story of a Journey to a Better World.* New York: Harcourt, Brace & World, 1967.

"Helen Dyer, 103, Cancer Researcher." *Washington Times* (22 September 1998): C6.

Hellstedt, Leone McGregor. *Women Physicians of the World: Autobiographies of Medical Pioneers.* Washington, DC: Hemisphere, 1978.

Heureaux, Mercedes A. "Oldest University in America." *Journal of the American Medical Women's Association* 10:7 (July 1955): 249.

Hiestand, Wanda C. "Think Different: Inventions and Innovations by Nurses, 1850 to 1950." *American Journal of Nursing* 100:10 (October 2000): 72.

Hine, Darlene Clark. "Co-Laborers in the Work of the Lord: Nineteenth-Century Black Women Physicians." In *Send Us a Lady Physician: Women Doctors in America,*

1835–1920. Edited by Ruth J. Abrams. New York: W. W. Norton, 1985.

———. *Black Women in America: An Historical Encyclopedia.* Brooklyn, NY: Carlson, 1993.

———, ed. *Facts on File Encyclopedia of Black Women in America.* Vol. 11. New York: Facts on File, 1997.

History of Women [microfilm collection]. New Haven, CT: Research Publications, 1975– .

Hong, Fan. *Footbinding, Feminism, and Freedom: The Liberation of Women's Bodies in Modern China.* London: F. Cass, 1997.

Hoobler, Icie Gertrude Macy. *Boundless Horizons: Portrait of a Pioneer Woman Scientist.* Smithtown, NY: Exposition Press, 1982.

Horney, Karen. *The Unknown Karen Horney: Essays on Gender, Culture, and Psychoanalysis.* New Haven: Yale University Press, 2000.

Hughes, Muriel Joy. *Women Healers in Medieval Life and Literature.* New York: King's Crown Press, 1943.

Hume, Edward Hicks. *Doctors Courageous.* New York: Harper, 1950.

Hume, Ruth Fox. *Great Women of Medicine.* New York: Random House, 1964.

Hunt, Caroline Louisa. *The Life of Ellen H. Richards.* Boston: Whitcomb & Barrows, 1912.

Hurd-Mead, Kate Campbell. *A History of Women in Medicine from the Earliest Times to the Beginning of the Nineteenth Century.* Haddam, CT: Haddam Press, 1938.

International Who's Who of Women. London: Europa, 1997.

Jacobs, Aletta. *Memories: My Life as an International Leader in Health, Suffrage, and Peace.* New York: Feminist Press, 1996.

James, L. Stanley. "Fond Memories of Virginia Apgar." *Pediatrics* 55:1 (1975): 1–4.

Jeffery, Mary Pauline. *Dr. Ida: India—The Life Story of Ida S. Scudder.* New York: Fleming H. Revell, 1938.

"Jennie Kidd Gowanlock Trout." http://www.rootsweb.com/~nwa/jennie.html.

Jensen, Rita Henley. "Mimi Ramsey." *Ms.* 6:4 (January 1996): 50–52.

Johnson, Samuel. *The Letters of Samuel Johnson, with Mrs. Thrale's Genuine Letters to Him.* Oxford: Clarendon Press, 1952.

Jordan, Louis Garnett. *Up the Ladder in Foreign Missions.* Nashville, TN: National Baptist Publishing Board, 1903.

Jurdak, Hania. "The Late Adma Abu Shdeed: AUB's First Woman Doctor." *AUB Bulletin* 35:2 (March 1993): 12–13.

Kagan, Helenah. *Reshit darki bi-Yerushalayim.* Tel Aviv: Vitso, Histadrut 'olamit le-nashim Tsiyoniyot; Tel-Yitshak: ha-midrashah ha-Liberalit 'a. s. Dr. Y. Forder, 1980.

Kass-Simon, G., and Patricia Farnes. *Women of Science: Righting the Record.* Bloomington: Indiana University Press, 1990.

Kaufman, Martin, Stuart Galishoff, and Todd L. Savitt, eds. *Dictionary of American Medical Biography.* Westport, CT: Greenwood Press, 1984.

Kawai, Yaeko. "Medical Women in Japan." *Journal of the American Medical Women's Association* 6:9 (September 1951): 352–353.

Kay, Virginia. "Stewart, Alice." *Current Biography* 61:7 (July 2000): 70–76.

Keesey, John C. "Contemporary Opinions about Mary Walker: A Shy Pioneer of Therapeutic Neurology." *Neurology* 51:5 (November 1998): 1433–1439.

Keller, Evelyn Fox. *A Feeling for the Organism: The Life and Work of Barbara McClintock.* San Francisco: W. H. Freeman, 1983.

Kelly, Catriona. *An Anthology of Russian Women's Writing, 1777–1992.* Oxford: Oxford University Press, 1994.

Kelly, Howard Atwood, and Walter L. Burrage. *Dictionary of American Medical Biography: Lives of Eminent Physicians of the United States and Canada, from the Earliest Times.* New York: D. Appleton, 1928.

Kelly, Patrick. "Wong-Staal, Flossie." *Current Biography* 62:4 (April 2001): 87–90.

Kendall, Florence P. "Sister Elizabeth Kenny Revisited." *Archives of Physical Medicine and Rehabilitation* 79:4 (April 1998): 361–365.

Kenny, Elizabeth. *And They Shall Walk.* New York: Dodd, Mead, 1943.

Kenyon, Josephine Hemenway. *Healthy Babies Are Happy Babies: A Complete Handbook for Modern Mothers.* Boston: Little, Brown, 1934.

"Kenyon, Josephine Hemenway." [Obit.] *JAMA* 192:1 (5 April 1965): 75.

Kessler, James H. *Distinguished African American Scientists of the 20th Century.* Phoenix, AZ: Oryx Press, 1996.

Kester-Shelton, Pamela, ed. *Feminist Writers.* Detroit: St. James Press, 1996.

Koch, Harriett Rose Berger. *Militant Angel.* New York: Macmillan, 1951.

Kodansha Encyclopedia of Japan. Vol. 6. Tokyo: Kodansha, 1983.

Krajewska, Teodora Kosmowska. *Pamietnik.* Krakow: Krajowa Agencja Wydawnicza, 1989.

Kroll, J. Simon, and Robert Booy. "*Haemophilus influenzae*: Capsule Vaccine and Capsulation Genetics." *Molecular Medicine Today* 2:4 (April 1996): 160–165.

Kubler-Ross, Elisabeth. *On Death and Dying.* New York: Macmillan, 1969.

———. *The Wheel of Life: A Memoir of Living and Dying.* New York: Scribner's, 1997.

Kyle, Robert A., and Marc A. Shampo. "Honoria Acosta-Sison." *JAMA* 246:11 (11 September 1981): 1191.

Lacy, Cherilyn. "Science or Savoir-Faire? Domestic Hygiene and Medicine in Girls' Public Education during the Early Third French Republic, 1882–1914." *Proceedings of the Annual Meeting of the Western Society for French History* 24 (1997): 25–37.

Lal, Maneesha. "The Politics of Gender and Medicine in Colonial India: The Countess of Dufferin's Fund, 1885–1888." *Bulletin of the History of Medicine* 68:1 (Spring 1994): 29–66.

Lambert, Bruce. "Dr. Florence B. Seibert, Inventor of Standard TB Test, Dies at 93." *New York Times* (31 August 1991): 12.

Lanker, Brian. *I Dream a World: Portraits of Black Women Who Changed the World.* New York: Stewart, Tabori, and Chang, 1989.

Lauren, Paul Gordon. *Power and Prejudice: The Politics and Diplomacy of Racial Discrimination.* Boulder, CO: Westview Press, 1996.

Laurie, Rev. Thomas. *Women and the Gospel in Persia.* New York: Fleming H. Revell, 1887.

Lazarus, Hilda. "Message from India." *Journal of the American Medical Women's Association* 3:6 (June 1948): 250.

Lecompte, Nancy. "The Last of the Androscoggins: Molly Ockett, Abenaki Healing Woman." http://www.avcnet.org/ne-do-ba/bio_moly.html.

Ledley, Robert S. "Dayhoff, Margaret Oakley." *American National Biography.* Vol. 2. New York: Oxford University Press, 1999.

Leneman, Leah. *In the Service of Life: The Story of Elsie Inglis and the Scottish Women's Hospitals.* Edinburgh: Mercat Press, 1994.

———. "Medical Women at War, 1914–1918." *Medical History* 38:2 (1994): 160–177.

Levi-Montalcini, Rita. *In Praise of Imperfections: My Life and Work.* New York: Basic Books, 1988.

Limentani, Adam. *Between Freud and Klein: The Psychoanalytic Quest for Knowledge and Truth.* London: Free Association Books, 1989.

"Lina and the Brain." *Time* 49:9 (3 March 1947): 45–46.

Linenthal, Arthur J. *First a Dream: The History of Boston's Jewish Hospitals, 1896 to 1928.* Boston: Beth Israel Hospital/Francis A. Countway Library of Medicine, 1990.

Livy. *The History of Rome.* Vol. 1. London: George Bell, 1906.

Lloyd, Thomas. "Rh-Factor Incompatibility: A Primer for Prevention." *Journal of Nurse-Midwifery* 32, no. 5 (September–October 1987): 297–307.

Logan, Rayford W., and Michael R. Winston. *Dictionary of American Negro Biography.* New York: W. W. Norton, 1982.

Lorber, Judith. "Why Women Physicians Will Never Be True Equals in the American Medical Profession." In *Gender, Work, and Medicine: Women and the Medical Division of Labour.* Edited by Elianne Riska and Katarina Wegar. London: Sage, 1993.

Lovejoy, Esther Pohl. *Women Physicians and Surgeons: National and International Organizations.* Livingston, NY: Livingston Press, 1939.

———. *Women Doctors of the World.* New York: Macmillan, 1957.

Lucas, Marion Brunson. *A History of Blacks in Kentucky.* Vol. 1. Frankfort: Kentucky Historical Society, 1992.

Mabie, Catharine L. *Our Work on the Congo: A Book for Mission Study Classes and for General Information.* Philadelphia: American Baptist Publication Society, 1917.

———. *Congo Cameos.* Philadelphia: Judson Press, 1952.

MacDermot, Hugh Ernest. *Maude Abbott: A Memoir.* Toronto: Macmillan, 1941.

Magill, Frank, ed. *Great Lives from History, American Women Series.* Pasadena, CA: Salem Press, 1995.

Mangan, Katherine S. "First Female President: Texas A&M Professor Prepares to Lead AMA." *Chronicle of Higher Education* 44 (10 October 1997): A10.

———. "Enlisting the Spirit in Medical Treatment." *Chronicle of Higher Education* 45:42 (25 June 1999): A12.

Mankin, Henry J. "Diversity in Orthopaedics." *Clinical Orthopaedics and Related Research: Issues of Minorities in Medicine and Orthopaedics* 362 (May 1999): 85–87.

Manley, Albert E. *A Legacy Continues: The Manley Years at Spelman College, 1953–1976.* Lanham, MD: University Press of America, 1995.

Manton, Jo. *Elizabeth Garrett Anderson.* New York: Dutton, 1965.

Marshall, Helen E. *Mary Adelaide Nutting: Pioneer of Modern Nursing.* Baltimore, MD: Johns Hopkins University Press, 1972.

"Mary Broadfoot Walker." *Lancet* 2:7893 (7 December 1974): 1401–1402.

McCarty, Maclyn. "Rebecca Craighill Lancefield." *Biographical Memoirs.* Vol. 57.

New York: National Academy of Sciences, 1987.

McGee, Anita Newcomb. *The Nurse Corps of the Army.* Carlisle, PA: Association of Military Surgeons, 1902. Reprinted in *History of Women Collection,* no. 10001. New Haven, CT: Research Publications, 1977.

McGrayne, Sharon Bertsch. *Nobel Prize Women in Science: Their Lives, Struggles, and Momentous Discoveries.* Secaucus, NJ: Carol, 1998.

McIntosh, Rustin. "Hattie Alexander." *Pediatrics* 42:3 (September 1968): 544.

McKown, Robin. *She Lived for Science: Irene Joliot-Curie.* New York: J. Messner, 1961.

McLaren, Eva Shaw. *A History of the Scottish Women's Hospitals.* London: Hodder & Stoughton, 1919.

McMaster, Philip D., and Michael Heidelberger. "Florence Rena Sabin." *Biographical Memoirs.* Vol. 34. New York: National Academy of Sciences, 1960.

McMurray, Emily J. *Notable Twentieth-Century Scientists.* Detroit: Gale, 1995.

McNamara, Dan G., J. A. Manning, M. A. Engle, R. Whittemore, C. A. Neill, and C. Ferencz. "Historical Milestones: Helen Brooke Taussig, 1898–1986." *Journal of the American College of Cardiology* 10:3 (September 1987): 662–671.

"Medical Women's International Association." *London Times* (15 July 1924): 17f.

"Memories of War: How Vietnam-Era Nurses Are Coping Today." *USA Today* 121:2574 (March 1993): 30–31.

Miller, Helen S. *Mary Eliza Mahoney, 1845–1926: America's First Black Professional Nurse.* Atlanta, GA: Wright, 1986.

Miller, Jean Baker. *Toward a New Psychology of Women.* Boston: Beacon Press, 1976.

Miller, Jean Baker, and Irene Pierce Stiver. *The Healing Connection: How Women Form Relationships in Therapy and in Life.* Boston: Beacon Press, 1997.

Mintz, Morton. "'Heroine' of FDA Keeps Bad Drug off of Market." *Washington Post* (15 July 1962): A1.

Morais, Herbert M. *The History of the Negro in Medicine.* 3d ed. New York: Publishers Co., 1969.

Morani A. D. "Reflections." *Clinics in Plastic Surgery* 10:4 (October 1983): 669–670.

Morantz-Sanchez, Regina Markell. *Sympathy and Science: Women Physicians in American Medicine.* New York: Oxford University Press, 1985.

———. *Conduct Unbecoming a Woman: Medicine on Trial in Turn-of-the-Century Brooklyn.* New York: Oxford University Press, 1999.

More, Ellen Singer. *Restoring the Balance: Women Physicians and the Profession of Medicine, 1850–1995.* Cambridge, MA: Harvard University Press, 1999.

Muir, Hazel. *Larousse Dictionary of Scientists.* Edinburgh: Larousse, 1994.

Murray, Flora. *Women as Army Surgeons: Being the History of the Women's Hospital Corps in Paris, Wimereux, and Endell Street, September 1914–October 1919.* London: Hodder & Stoughton, 1920.

Murray, Jocelyn. "Brown, Edith Mary." *Biographical Dictionary of Christian Missions.* New York: Macmillan, 1998.

National Encyclopedia of American Biography. Vol. 57. Clifton, NJ: James T. White, 1977.

Navratil, Michal. *Almanach Ceskych Lekaru.* Prague: Náklaem Spisovatelov m, 1913.

Necas, Ctibor. "Prvni Uredni Lekarka V Bosnen." *Casopis Matice Moravske* (Czechoslovakia) 102:3–4 (1983): 245–257.

———. "Dr. Med. Teodora Krajewska, Lekarka Urzedowa W Dol. Tuzle I Sarajewie." *Archiwum Historii i Filozofii Medycyny* (Poland) 50:1 (1987): 75–98.

New Catholic Encyclopedia. New York: McGraw-Hill, 1967.

New England Hospital for Women and Children (NEHWC). *Marie Elizabeth Zakrzewska: A Memoir.* Boston: New England Hospital for Women and Children, 1902. Reprinted in *History of Women,* no. 5403. New Haven, CT: Research Publications, 1977.

Niethammar, Carolyn J. *"I'll Go and Do More": Annie Dodge Wauneka, Navajo Leader and Activist.* Lincoln: University of Nebraska Press, 2001.

Nightingale, Florence. *Notes on Nursing: What It Is, and What It Is Not.* New York: D. Appleton, 1860. Reprinted in *History of Women,* reel 343, no. 2366. New Haven, CT: Research Publications, 1975.

"NIH Lectures." http://www1.od.nih.gov/oir/sourcebook/ir-communictns/lecture-info.htm#Pitt.

Notable American Women 1607–1950. Cambridge, MA: Belknap Press, 1971.

Notable Black American Scientists. Detroit: Gale, 1998.

Notable Twentieth-Century Scientists. Detroit: Gale, 1995.

Notable Twentieth-Century Scientists Supplement. Detroit: Gale, 1998.

Nuland, Sherwin B. *Doctors: The Biography of Medicine.* New York: Knopf, 1988.

Nusslein-Volhard, Christiane, and Jorn Kratzschmar, eds. *Of Fish, Fly, Worm, and*

Man: Lessons from Developmental Biology for Human Gene Function and Disease. Berlin: Springer, 2000.

Ogilvie, Marilyn, and Joy Harvey, eds. *The Biographical Dictionary of Women in Science: Pioneering Lives from Ancient Times to the Mid-20th Century.* New York: Routledge, 2000.

Ohles, Frederik, Shirley M. Ohles, and John G. Ramsay. *The Biographical Dictionary of Modern American Educators.* Westport, CT: Greenwood Press, 1997.

Olkkonen, Tuomo. "Suomen Ensimmainen Naistohtori." *Opusculum* 5:3 (1985): 122–128.

Organ, Claude H., and Margaret M. Kosiba. *Century of Black Surgeons: The U.S.A. Experience.* Norman, OK: Transcript Press, 1987.

Osborn, June Elaine. "AIDS and the Politics of Compassion." *Hospitals* 66:18 (20 September 1992): 64.

———. "Infections." *Journal of Urban Health* 75:2 (June 1998): 251–257.

"Outstanding Uruguayan Women." http://www.correo.com.uy/filatelia/frames/MujeresDestacadas_ingles.htm.

Pagel, Walter. "Hildegard of Bingen." *Dictionary of Scientific Biography.* Vol. 6. New York: Scribner's, 1970–1980.

Paris, Bernard J. *Karen Horney: A Psychoanalyst's Search for Self-Understanding.* New Haven, CT: Yale University Press, 1994.

Park, William Hallock, and Anna W. Williams. *Who's Who among the Microbes.* New York: Century, 1929.

Parks, Edward A. "Foreword." In Helen B. Taussig, *Congenital Malformations of the Heart.* New York: Commonwealth Fund, 1947.

Parrish, Rebecca. *Orient Seas and Lands Afar.* New York: Fleming H. Revell, 1936.

Parry, Melanie, ed. *Chambers Biographical Dictionary.* Edinburgh: Chambers, 1997.

Peitzman, Steven J. *A New and Untried Course: Women's Medical College and Medical College of Pennsylvania, 1850–1998.* New Brunswick, NJ: Rutgers University Press, 2000.

"Petermann, Mary, Ph.D." [Obit.] *New York Times* (16 December 1975): 42.

Pflaum, Rosalynd. *Grand Obsession: Madame Curie and Her World.* New York: Doubleday, 1989.

———. *Marie Curie and Her Daughter Irene.* Minneapolis, MN: Lerner Publications, 1993.

Pliny, the Younger. *Letters.* Vol. 1. London: W. Heinemann, 1915.

Preston, Ann. "The Status of Women-Physicians." *Medical and Surgical Reporter* 16:18 (4 May 1867). Reprinted in *American Periodical Series 1800–1850,* new series.

Pringle, Rosemary. *Sex and Medicine: Gender, Power, and Authority in the Medical Profession.* Cambridge: Cambridge University Press, 1998.

"Prof. Lina Stern, Physiologist, 89." *New York Times* (9 March 1968): 29.

Proffitt, Pamela, ed. *Notable Women Scientists.* Detroit: Gale, 1999.

"Profile: Alma Dea Morani, MD." *Journal of the American Medical Women's Association* 38:5 (September–October 1983): 137.

Pruitt, Ida. *A Daughter of Han.* New Haven, CT: Yale University Press, 1945.

Putnam, Ruth. *Life and Letters of Mary Putnam Jacobi.* New York: G. P. Putnam's Sons, 1925.

Quinn, Susan. *A Mind of Her Own: The Life of Karen Horney.* New York: Summit Books, 1987.

———. *Marie Curie: A Life.* New York: Simon & Schuster, 1995.

Raju, T. N. "The Nobel Chronicles." *Lancet* 356:9223 (1 July 2000): 81.

Rashdall, Hastings. *The Universities of Europe in the Middle Ages,* vol. 1: *Salerno, Bologna, Paris.* Oxford: Clarendon Press, 1936.

Rayson, Sandra, Robert A. Kyle, and Marc A. Shampo. "Dr. Jennie Kidd Trout—Pioneer Canadian Physician." *Mayo Clinic Proceedings* 68:2 (February 1993): 189.

Rich, Mari. "Canady, Alexa." *Current Biography* 61:8 (August 2000): 11–15.

Richards, Linda. *Reminiscences of Linda Richards, America's First Trained Nurse.* Boston: Whitcomb & Barrows, 1915.

Riska, Elianne. "Women's Careers in Medicine: Developments in the United States and Finland." *Scandinavian Studies* 61 (Spring/Summer 1989): 185–198.

Roland, Charles G. "Maude Abbott, MD, 'Madonna of the Heart.'" *Medical and Pediatric Oncology* 35:1 (July 2000): 64–65.

Rose, Kenneth W. *A Survey of Source at the Rockefeller Archive Center for the Study of Twentieth Century Africa.* North Tarrytown, NY: Rockefeller Archive Center, 1996.

Ross, Ishbel. *Child of Destiny: The Life Story of the First Woman Doctor.* New York: Harper, 1949.

Rossiter, Margaret W. *Women Scientists in America: Struggles and Strategies to 1940.* Baltimore, MD: Johns Hopkins University Press, 1982.

Rozett, Robert, and Shmuel Spector. *Encyclopedia of the Holocaust.* New York: Facts on File, 2000.

Rubinstein, Murray A. *The Origins of the Anglo-American Missionary Enterprise in China,*

1807–1840. Lanham, MD: Scarecrow Press, 1996.

Salber, Eva Juliet. "Payment for Health Care in the United States: A Personal Statement." *Journal of Public Health Policy* 4:2 (June 1983): 202–206.

———. *The Mind Is Not the Heart: Recollections of a Woman Physician.* Durham, NC: Duke University Press, 1989.

Sammons, Vivian Ovelton. *Blacks in Science and Medicine.* New York: Hemisphere, 1990.

Sapriza, Graciela. "Clivajes de la Memoría: Para una Biografía de Paulina Luisi." *Uruguayos Notables.* Montevideo: Fundación BankBoston, 1999.

Saunders, Cicely. "A Personal Therapeutic Journey." *British Medical Journal* 313:7072 (21–28 December 1996): 1599–1601.

Sayre, Anne. *Rosalind Franklin and DNA.* New York: W. W. Norton, 1975.

Scharlieb, Mary Ann Dacomb Bird. *Reminiscences.* London: Williams and Norgate, 1924. Reproduced in the Gerritsen Collection of Women's History, no. 2518.2. Sanford, NC: Microfilming Corporation of America, 1980.

Schiebinger, Londa. *The Mind Has No Sex? Women in the Origins of Modern Science.* Cambridge, MA: Harvard University Press, 1989.

Schmidt, Jacob Edward. *Medical Discoveries: Who and When.* Springfield, IL: Thomas, 1959.

Schneider, Keith. "Scientist Who Managed to 'Shock the World' on Atomic Workers' Health." *New York Times* (3 May 1990): A20.

"Scientist." *Ebony* 15:10 (August 1960): 44.

Seacole, Mary. *Wonderful Adventures of Mrs. Seacole in Many Lands.* New York: Oxford University Press, ca. 1857. Reprinted 1988.

Segal, Hanna. *Melanie Klein.* New York: Viking Press, 1980.

Seibert, Florence Barbara. *Pebbles on the Hill of a Scientist.* St. Petersburg, FL: St. Petersburg Printing, 1968.

Seppanen, Anni. "Medical Women in Finland." *Journal of the American Medical Women's Association* 5 (1950): 291.

Shampo, Marc A., and Robert A. Kyle. "Barbara McClintock—Nobel Laureate Geneticist." *Mayo Clinic Proceedings* 70:5 (May 1995): 448.

Shearer, Benjamin F., and Barbara S. Shearer. *Notable Women in the Life Sciences: A Biographical Dictionary.* Westport, CT: Greenwood Press, 1996.

———. *Notable Women in the Physical Sciences: A Biographical Dictionary.* Westport, CT: Greenwood Press, 1997.

Sheehy, Noel, Antony J. Chapman, and Wendy A. Conroy. *Biographical Dictionary of Psychology.* London: Routledge, 1997.

Sherratt, Tim. "No Standing Back: Dame Jean MacNamara." *Australasian Science* 13:4 (Summer 1993): 64.

Sherrow, Victoria. *Women and the Military: An Encyclopedia.* Santa Barbara, CA: ABC-CLIO, 1996.

Siim, Birte. *Gender and Citizenship: Politics and Agency in France, Britain, and Denmark.* New York: Cambridge University Press, 2000.

Sivulka, Juliann. "From Domestic to Municipal Housekeeper: The Influence of the Sanitary Reform Movement on Changing Women's Roles in America, 1860–1920." *Journal of American Culture* 22:4 (Winter 1999): 1–7.

Smillie, Wilson George. *Public Health: Its Promise for the Future; A Chronicle of the Development of Public Health in the United States, 1607–1914.* New York: Macmillan, 1955.

Smith, Warren Hunting. *Hobart and William Smith: The History of Two Colleges.* Geneva, NY: Hobart and William Smith Colleges, 1972.

Snodgrass, Mary Ellen. *Historical Encyclopedia of Nursing.* Santa Barbara, CA: ABC-CLIO, 1999.

Snyder, Charles McCool. *Dr. Mary Walker: The Little Lady in Pants.* New York: Vantage Press, 1962.

Solomos, John. *Racism and Society.* New York: St. Martin's Press, 1996.

Spain, Daphne. *How Women Saved the City.* Minneapolis: University of Minnesota Press, 2001.

Spiegel, Allen D., and Peter B. Suskind. "Mary Edwards Walker, M.D.: A Feminist Physician a Century ahead of Her Time." *Journal of Community Health* 21:3 (June 1996): 211–235.

Spoerry, Anne. *They Call Me Mama Daktari.* Norval, ON: Moulin, 1996.

Stapleton, Stephanie. "Former NIH Chief to Lead Red Cross." *American Medical News* 42, no. 29 (2 August 1999): 24.

Staupers, Mabel Keaton. *No Time for Prejudice: A Story of the Integration of Negroes in Nursing in the United States.* New York: Macmillan, 1961.

Straus, Eugene. *Rosalyn Yalow, Nobel Laureate: Her Life and Work in Medicine; A Biographical Memoir.* New York: Plenum, 1998.

Summerfield, Carol, and Mary Elizabeth Devine, eds. *International Dictionary of University Histories.* Chicago: Fitzroy Dearborn, 1998.

Swain, Clara A. *A Glimpse of India: Being a Collection of Extracts from the Letters of Dr. Clara A. Swain, First Medical Missionary to India of the Woman's Foreign Missionary Society* of the Methodist Episcopal Church in America. New York: J. Pott, 1909. Reprinted in *History of Women,* no. 6170. New Haven, CT: Research Publications, 1977.

Taussig, Helen B. "Dangerous Tranquility." *Science* 136:3517 (25 May 1962): 683.

———. "Little Choice and a Stimulating Environment." *Journal of the American Medical Women's Association* 36:2 (February 1981): 43–44.

Taylor, Richard R., William S. Mullins, and Roger J. Parks. *Medical Training in World War II. United States. Surgeon-General's Office.* Washington, DC: Office of the Surgeon General, Department of the Army, 1974.

Terry, John Mark, Ebbie Smith, and Justice Anderson. *Missiology: An Introduction to the Foundations, History, and Strategies of World Missions.* Nashville, TN: Broadman and Holman, 1998.

Thomas, Claudia L. "African Americans and Women in Orthopaedic Residency: The Johns Hopkins Experience." *Clinical Orthopaedics and Related Research: Issues of Minorities in Medicine and Orthopaedics* 362 (May 1999): 65–71.

Thomas, David Hurst, Betty Ballantine, and Ian Ballantine. *The Native Americans: An Illustrated History.* Atlanta, GA: Turner, 1993.

Tobey, James Alner. *Riders of the Plagues: The Story of the Conquest of Disease.* New York: Scribner's, 1930.

Tong, Benson. *Susan La Flesche Picotte, M.D.: Omaha Indian Leader and Reformer.* Norman: University of Oklahoma Press, 1999.

Tooley, Sarah A. *The Life of Florence Nightingale.* London: Cassell, 1914.

"Tracing Nightingale's Steps." *Nursing* 31:1 (January 2001): 44–48.

Traut, Thomas. "Biographical Memoirs: Mary Ellen Jones." http://www.nap.edu/ readingroom/books/biomems/mjones.html.

Trost, Jan E., and Mai-Briht Bergstrom-Walan. "Sweden (Konungariket Sverige)." http:// www.rki.de/gesund/archiv/ies/sweden. htm.

Tucker, Sara W. "Opportunities for Women: The Development of Professional Women's Medicine at Canton, China, 1879–1901." *Women's Studies International Forum* 13:4 (1990): 357–368.

Tufts, Henry. *The Autobiography of a Criminal.* New York: Duffield, 1930.

Turner, Allan. "Healthy, Irrepressible Perspective: AMA's First Female President Breaks through Perceived 'Old Boys' Network." *Houston Chronicle* (29 June 1997): 1.

Turner-Warwick, Margaret. *Immunology of the Lung.* London: Edward Arnold, 1978.

Van der Does, Louise Q., and Rita J. Simon. *Renaissance Women in Science.* Lanham, MD: University Press of America, 1999.

Vare, Ethlie Ann, and Greg Ptacek. *Mothers of Invention: From the Bra to the Bomb—Forgotten Women and Their Unforgettable Ideas.* New York: Morrow, 1988.

Waddington, Ivan. *The Medical Profession in the Industrial Revolution.* Dublin: Gill and Macmillan, 1984.

Wade-Gayles, Gloria. "Britton, Mary E." *Black Women in America: An Historical Encyclopedia.* Vol. 1. Brooklyn, NY: Carlson, 1993.

Waite, Frederick Clayton. *History of the New England Female Medical College.* Boston, MA: Boston University School of Medicine, 1950.

Wald, Lillian D. *The House on Henry Street.* New York: Henry Holt, 1915.

Walton, John, Paul B. Beeson, and Ronald Bodley Scott, eds. *The Oxford Companion to Medicine.* Oxford: Oxford University Press, 1986.

Wang, Ping. *Aching for Beauty: Footbinding in China.* Minneapolis: University of Minnesota Press, 2000.

Ward, Kevin, and Brian Stanley. *The Church Mission Society and World Christianity, 1799–1999.* Grand Rapids, MI: Eerdmans, 2000.

Warren, Wini. *Black Women Scientists in the United States.* Bloomington: Indiana University Press, 1999.

Watson, Wilbur H. *Against the Odds: Blacks in the Profession of Medicine in the United States.* New Brunswick, NJ: Transaction, 1999.

Weizmann, Chaim. *Trial and Error: The Autobiography of Chaim Weizmann.* New York: Harper, 1949.

"Weizmann, Vera." [Obit.] *New York Times* (25 September 1966): 85.

Welch, Amy S. "Learning from Women." *Women & Therapy* 17:3–4 (1995): 335–346.

Welch, Rosanne. *Women in Aviation and Space.* Santa Barbara, CA: ABC-CLIO, 1998.

Wells, Susan. *Out of the Dead House: Nineteenth-Century Women Physicians and the Writing of Medicine.* Madison: University of Wisconsin Press, 2000.

Whately, Elizabeth Jane. *The Life and Work of Mary Louisa Whately.* London: Religious Tract Society, 1890.

White, Kerr L., and Julia E. Connelly, eds. *The Medical School's Mission and the Population's Health—Medical Education in Canada, the United Kingdom, the United States, and*

Australia. New York: Springer-Verlag, 1992.

Who Was Who, 1941–1950. London: A & C Black, 1951.

Who Was Who among English and European Authors, 1931–1949. Detroit: Gale, 1978.

Who Was Who in America with World Notables, Vol. 6, *1974–1976.* Chicago: Marquis Who's Who, 1976.

Who's Who. New York: St. Martin's Press, 1992.

Who's Who in Australia. Melbourne: Information Australia, 1998.

Who's Who in Lebanon 1988–1989. Beirut: Publitec, 1988.

Who's Who of American Women. 3d ed. Chicago: Marquis Who's Who, 1963.

Who's Who of American Women. 5th ed. Chicago: Marquis Who's Who, 1968.

Who's Who of American Women. 17th ed. Chicago: Marquis Who's Who, 1991.

Who's Who of American Women. 22d ed. New Providence, NJ: Marquis Who's Who, 2000.

Williams, Ralph Chester. *The United States Public Health Service, 1798–1950.* Washington, DC: Commissioned Officers Association of the U.S. Public Health Service, 1951.

Winslow, Charles-Edward Amory. "The Untilled Fields of Public Health." *Science* 51 (1920): 23.

———. *The Evolution and Significance of the Modern Public Health Campaign.* New Haven, CT: Yale University Press, 1923.

Wintrobe, Maxwell M. *Blood, Pure and Eloquent: A Story of Discovery, of People, and of Ideas.* New York: McGraw-Hill, 1980.

Woodham-Smith, Cecil. *Florence Nightingale, 1820–1910.* London: Constable, 1950.

Woodward, Helen Beal. *The Bold Women.* New York: Farrar, Straus & Young, 1953.

Wool, Ira G. "Ribosomes." *Encyclopedia of Human Biology.* 2d ed. Vol. 7. San Diego: Academic Press, 1997.

"Wright, Jane C." *Current Biography.* New York: H. W. Wilson, 1968.

Wyly, M. Virginia. "Apgar, Virginia." *Dictionary of American Biography, Supplement 9, 1971–1975.* New York: Scribner's, 1994.

Yedidia, Michael J., and Janet Bickel. "Why Aren't There More Women Leaders in Academic Medicine? The Views of Clinical Department Chairs." *Academic Medicine* 76:5 (May 2001): 453–465.

Young, Helen Praeger. "From Soldier to Doctor: A Chinese Woman's Story of the Long March." *Science and Society* 59:4 (Winter 1995–1996): 531–547.

Zakrzewska, Marie E. *A Woman's Quest: The Life of Marie E. Zakrzewska, M.D.* New York: D. Appleton, 1924.

Zwar, Desmond. *The Dame: The Life and Times of Dame Jean Macnamara, Medical Pioneer.* South Melbourne: Macmillan, 1984.

Index

About the Author

Laura Lynn Windsor is a health sciences reference librarian at Ohio University. She has been a reference librarian at public and academic libraries for more than fifteen years. She is a member of the American Library Association and the Medical Library Association.